Acute Leukemias

Edited by Pier Paolo Piccaluga

Published in London, United Kingdom

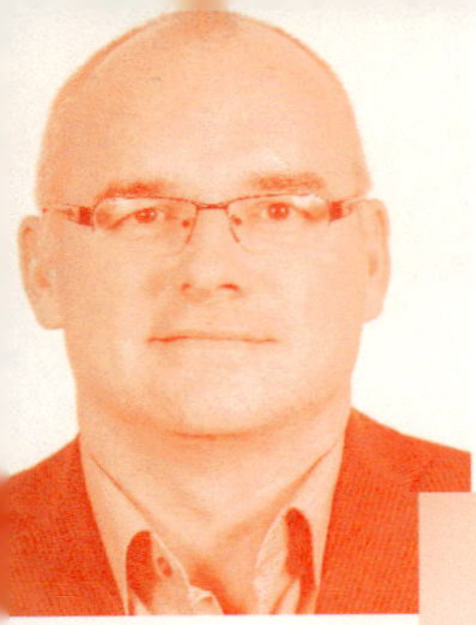
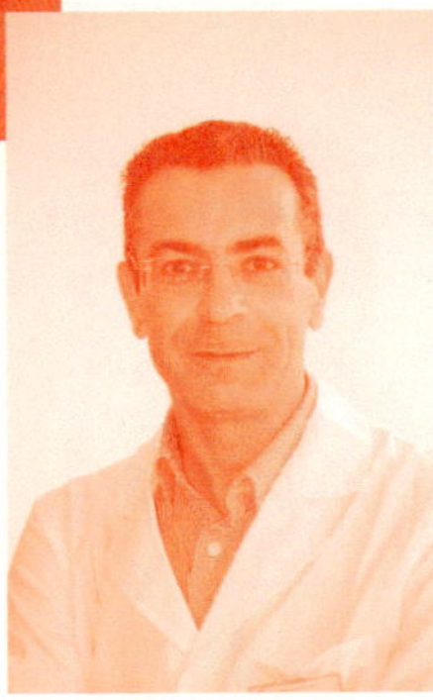
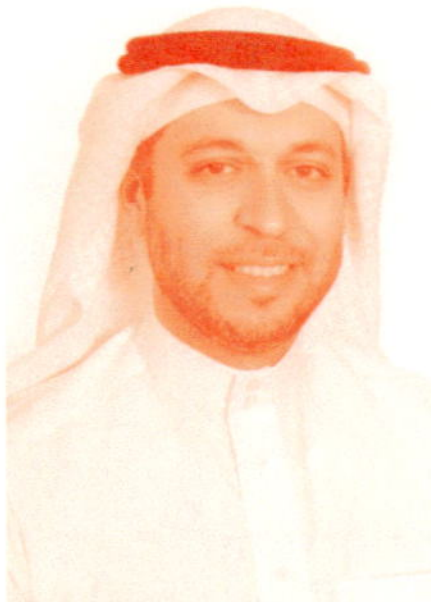
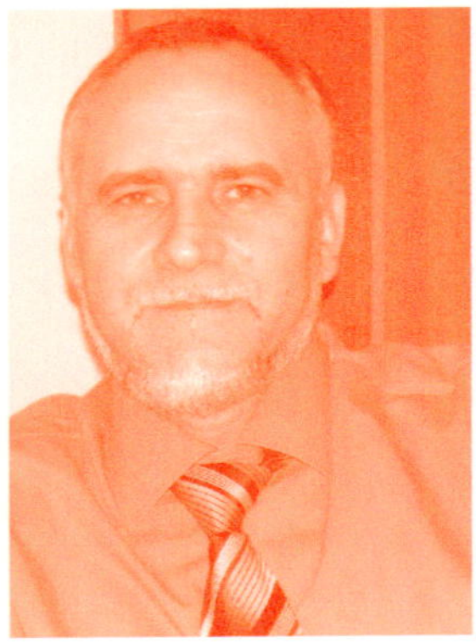
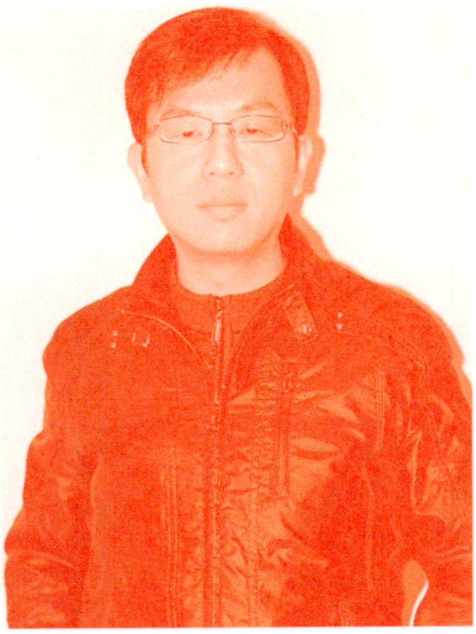
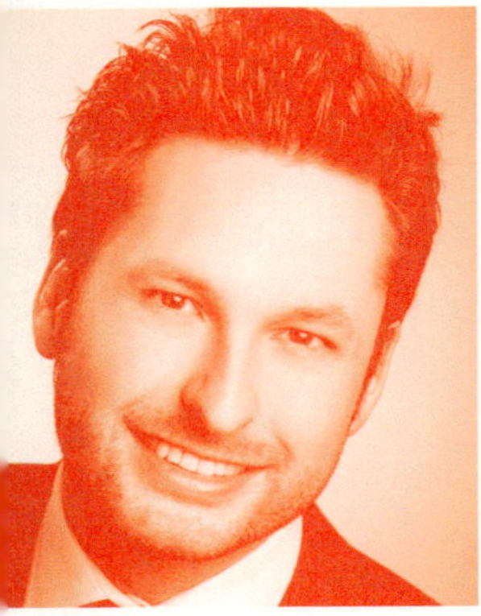
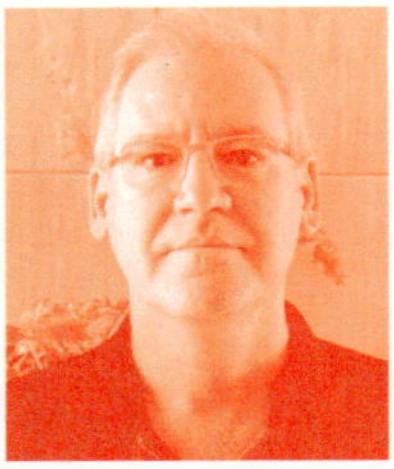

IntechOpen

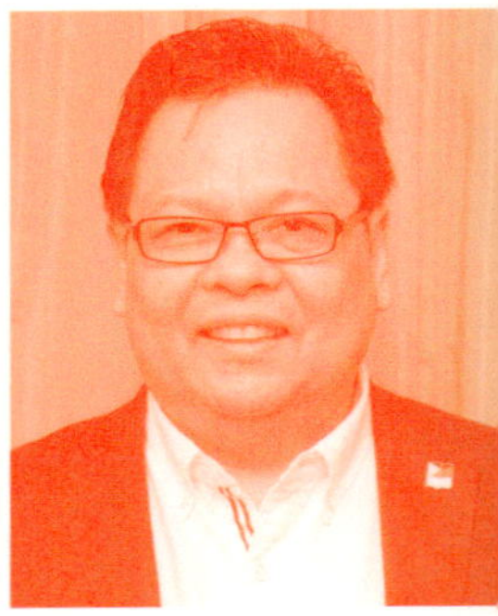
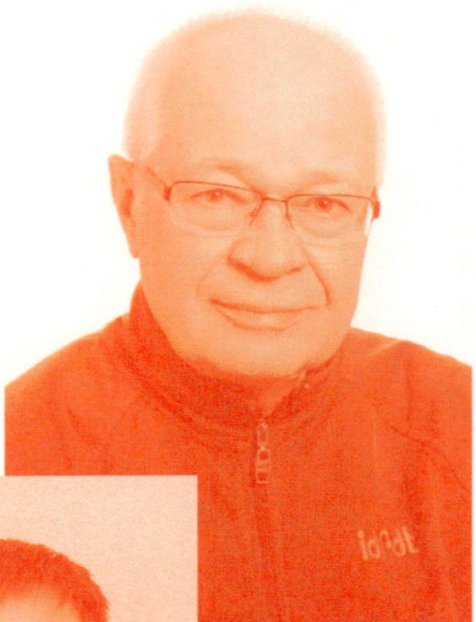
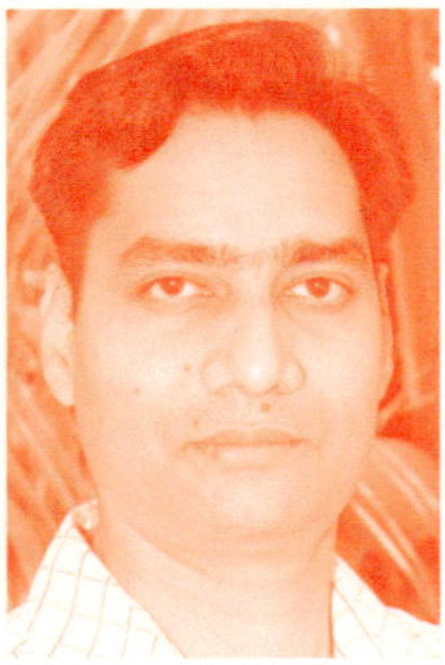
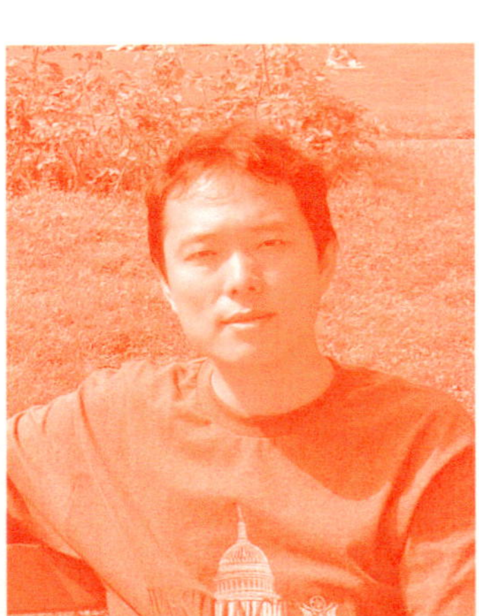
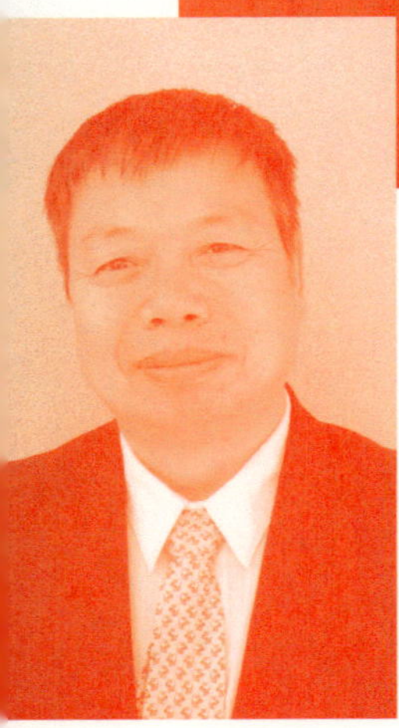
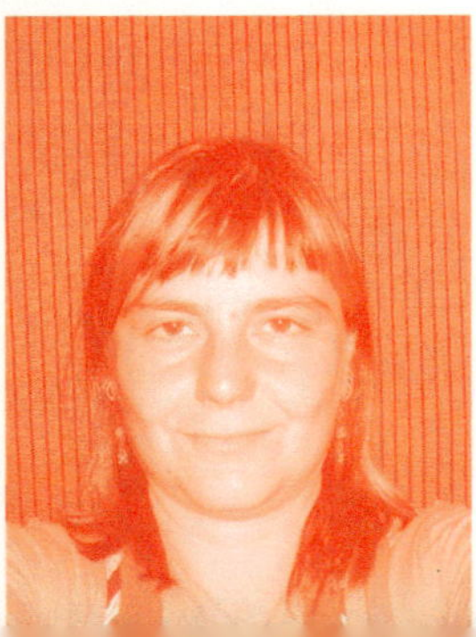

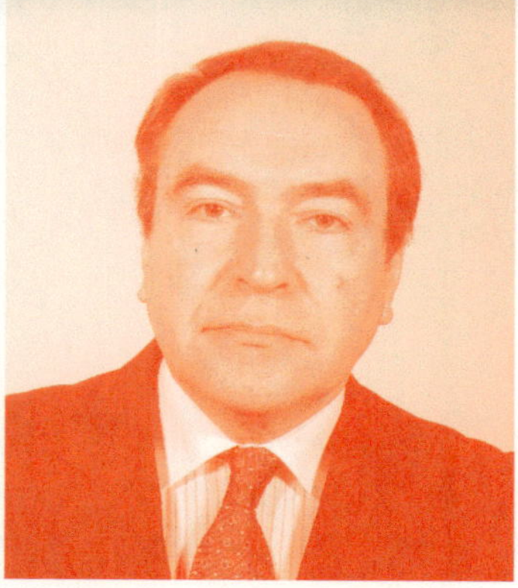
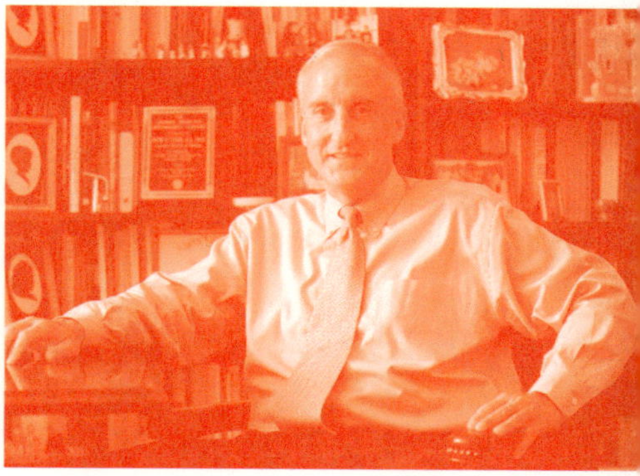
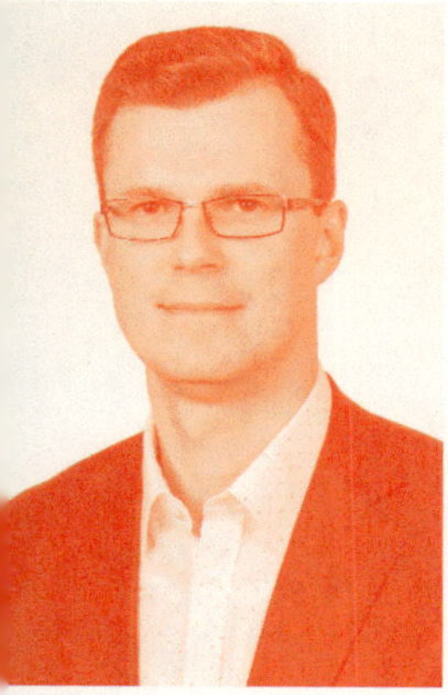
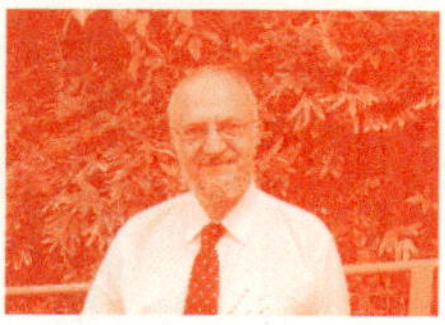
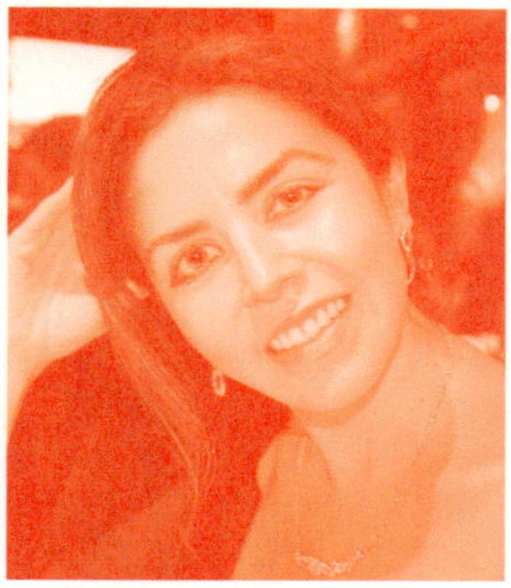

Supporting open minds since 2005

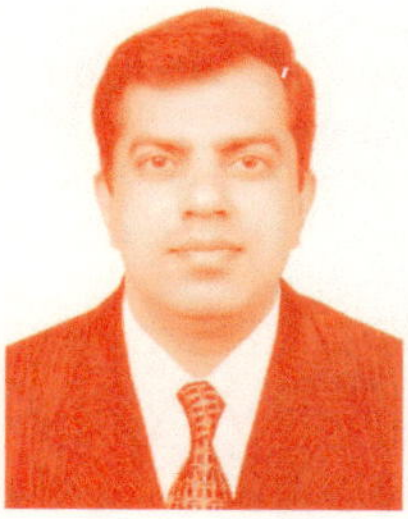
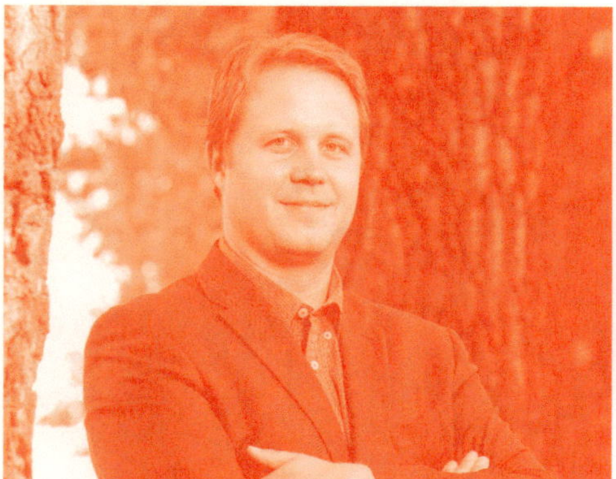
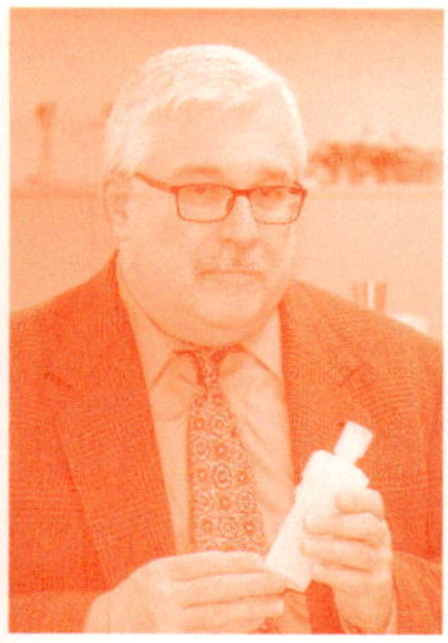
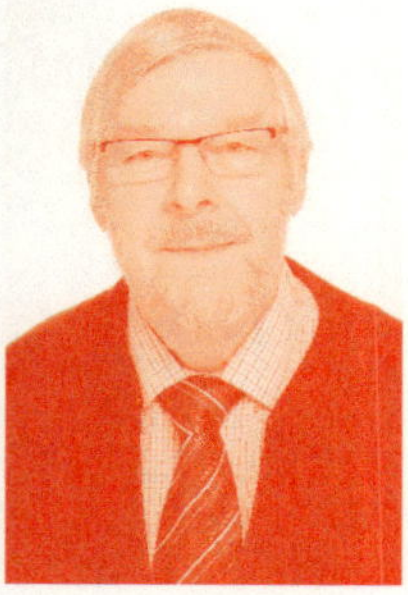
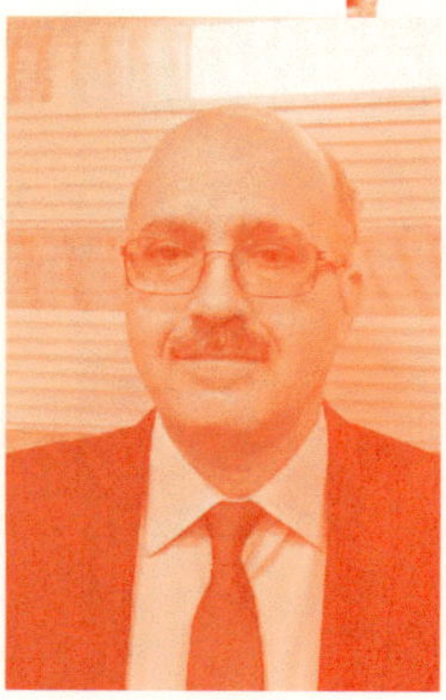
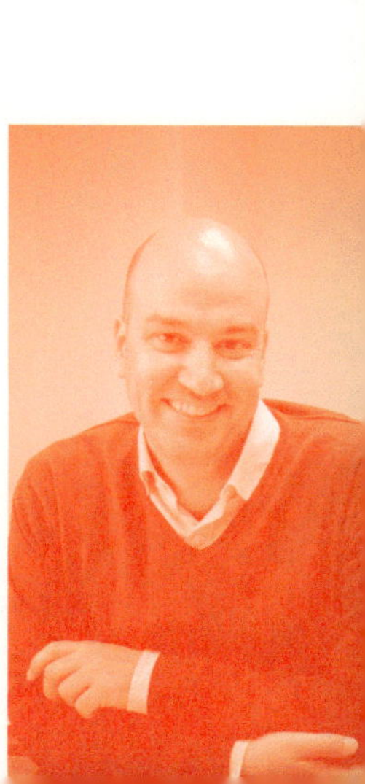
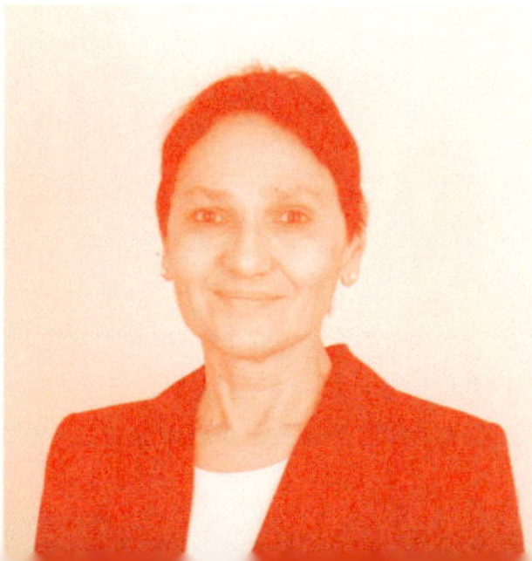

Acute Leukemias
http://dx.doi.org/10.5772/intechopen.87292
Edited by Pier Paolo Piccaluga

Contributors
Ashraf Abdullah Saad, Debora Capelli, Francesco Saraceni, Diego Menotti, Alessandro Fiorentini, Attilio Olivieri, Omer Jamy, Sravanti Rangaraju, Vasko Graklanov, Martha Alvarado-Ibarra, José Antonio De la Peña Celaya, Luara Luz Arana-Luna, Eleazar Hernández-Ruiz, José Luis Alvarez Vera, María Eugenia Espitia Ríos, Juan Manuel Pérez Zúñiga, Giuseppe Milone, Annalisa Condorelli, Salvatore Leotta, Giovanni Schininà, Alessandra Cupri, Roberta Sciortino, Guray Saydam, Fahri Sahin, Fatma Keklik Karadag, Arturo Solis Herrera, Ruth-Isabel Solís-Arias, Luis Fernando Torres- Solis, Jenny Y. Wang, Jonason Yang, Nunki Hassan, Sheng Xiang Franklin Chen, Jayvee Datuin, Irina Panovska-Stavridis, Gerwin Huls, Jacobien Hilberink, Elena Arriazu, Javier Marco, Irene Peris, Carmen Vicente, Paulina Podszywalow-Bartnicka, Magdalena Wolczyk, Katarzyna Piwocka, Guadalupe Garcia-Alcocer, Edgardo Becerra, Alex Tonks, Andrew Robinson, Richard Darley, Pier Paolo Piccaluga

First published in London, United Kingdom, 2021 by IntechOpen
IntechOpen is the global imprint of INTECHOPEN LIMITED, registered in England and Wales, registration number: 11086078, 5 Princes Gate Court, London, SW7 2QJ, United Kingdom
Printed in Croatia

British Library Cataloguing-in-Publication Data
A catalogue record for this book is available from the British Library

Additional hard and PDF copies can be obtained from orders@intechopen.com

Acute Leukemias
Edited by Pier Paolo Piccaluga
p. cm.
Print ISBN 978-1-83881-168-6
Online ISBN 978-1-83881-169-3
eBook (PDF) ISBN 978-1-83881-173-0

For EU product safety concerns:
IN TECH d.o.o., Prolaz Marije Krucifikse Kozulić 3, 51000 Rijeka, Croatia, info@intechopen.com or visit our website at intechopen.com.

Meet the editor

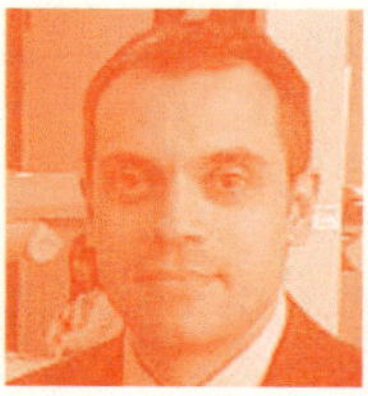

Pier Paolo Piccaluga, Prof., MD, Ph.D., is currently Associate Professor of Pathology at the Department of Experimental, Diagnostic and Specialty Medicine, Bologna University School of Medicine—Institute of Hematology and Medical Oncology, and has been responsible for many years for the Molecular Pathology Laboratory. In 2018, he was appointed for teaching at the Queen Mary University of London and Jomo Kenyatta University of Agriculture and Technology, Nairobi, Kenya. He is the author of several international publications in journals such as Nature Medicine, Journal of Clinical Investigation, Journal of Experimental Medicine, Journal of Clinical Oncology, Blood, Lancet Oncology, and Lancet Infectious Diseases. Dr. Piccaluga is ranked a Top Italian Scientist (TIS) by VIA-Academy.

Contents

Preface

Acute leukemia, which can be either myeloid or lymphocytic, is currently the thirteenth cause of morbidity and the tenth cause of mortality among cancers worldwide (**Figure 1**). Despite differences in epidemiology among the various subtypes (e.g., myeloid leukemia is more common in older adults, whereas lymphocytic leukemia is more common in children), the overall incidence of leukemia is continuously, though slowly, increasing.

In the last two decades, tremendous efforts have been made to understand the pathophysiology and especially the molecular pathogenesis of acute leukemias. Massive parallel sequencing has allowed for the identification of multiple mutations as well as hypotheses about a hierarchy in the sequence of genetic events. This has led to a more refined classification, progressively moving from a morphology-based classification (FAB classification, 1974) to a largely molecular based one (WHO classification, 2017).

This book presents a brief overview of the history of leukemia diagnosis and treatment. It also examines the biology and diagnosis of acute leukemia through a series of chapters dealing with molecular events as well as stem cell biology. As such, the book largely focuses on conventional therapy of acute myeloid leukemia (AML) and acute lymphocytic leukemia (ALL) based on age subgroups. Highlighted are new low-toxicity approaches for adolescents.

Despite signs of progress in chemotherapy, stem cell transplantation remains a major tool to achieve cure in acute leukemia patients. Thus, the book presents different treatment strategies as well as diagnostic methods for monitoring minimal residual disease after transplant.

Finally, the book summarizes targeted therapies, including those already approved for first- and second-line treatments as well as the molecular mechanisms determining drug sensitivity or resistance.

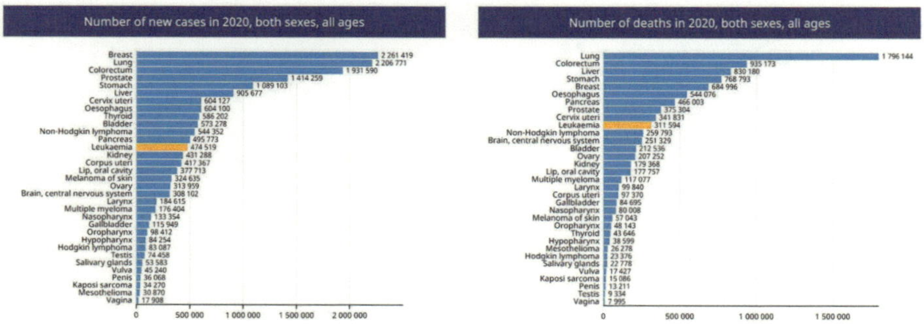

Figure 1.
Cancer incidence and mortality statistics worldwide and by region.

This book is intended for all health professionals, particularly those involved in the diagnosis and treatment of oncological diseases, as well as medical students and fellows.

I am grateful to IntechOpen for the opportunity to edit this volume. I would like to thank Ms. Dajana Pemac, Ms. Ana Simic, and Ms. Sara Gojevic-Zrnic for their help and support, as well as all the contributors who dedicated their time and effort.

Pier Paolo Piccaluga, MD, PhD
Professor,
Institute of Hematology and Medical Oncology,
Department of Experimental, Diagnostic and Specialty Medicine,
Bologna University School of Medicine,
Bologna, Italy

Section 1

Introduction

Chapter 1

Introductory Chapter: A Brief History of Acute Leukemias Treatment

Pier Paolo Piccaluga

1. The early history

The first case of leukemia had been probably described by Velpeau in 1827 [1]. Literally, he described his patient as '*A florist and seller of lemonade who had abandoned himself to the abuse of spirituous liquor and of women, without, however, becoming syphilitic*' [1, 2] that presented with abdomen distention, fatigue, fever, and side effects of urinary stones. At physical examination, severe hepatosplenomegaly was described, while the blood appeared "like gruel" [1, 2]. The patients actually died as soon as hospitalized [1, 2]. Despite probably depicting an acute leukemia (AL) case, a formal diagnosis was not made. Indeed, the first description of AL was dated in 1845, when two young pathologists, the German Rudolf Virchow and the British John Bennett, described it at the same time. Virchow suggested to name it "*leukämie*" (ie leukemia), a disease originating in the tissue producing blood cells; conversely, Bennett described it as "*leukocypenia*", being a type of pyemia, a suppuration of the blood [2]. The real nature of leukemia was then recognized in about 20 years, confirming Virchows theory (**Table 1**). Since then, attempts to cure it were made with scares success. At that time, the most widely used approach radiation, arsenic, and mesothorium (thorium-X).

Year	Development
1600 BC	First written description of cancer in ancient Egypt
1670*	Examination of the blood with the compound microscope
1827	First clinical description of leukemia by *Alfred-Armand-Luois-Marie Velpeau*
1847	Term "leukemia" coined by *Rudolph Virchow*
1872	*Franz-Ern-Christian Neumann* suggested that leukemia is a disease of the bone marrow
1877	*Paul Ehrlich* introduced histochemical staining
1913	Distinction of acute and chronic, lymphoid and myeloid leukemias
1914	*Theodor Boveri* proposed that leukemia arises from a single cell through chromosomal changes
1974	FAB classification of leukemias based on cytology
2008	WHO classification of leukemia including molecular subtypes

Table 1.
Evolution in leukemia diagnosis.

In 1930, Dr. Gloor from the Naegeli's clinic in Zurich [3], described "*the case of an American businessman*" whose white blood cell count reached 100x10^9/L, with fever and anemia, a classical presentation of AL [2, 3]. He received radiation, arsenic, and mesothorium, and blood transfusion, achieving complete remission. Curiously (and possibly dramatically), when Dr. Gloor tried to publish this first successfully treated AL case, he lost his job and was outcasted in a small clinic in a peripheral canton, only a "fool or a knave" [2] possibly believing to cure AL. The patient, Eugene Metzger, died fifty years later, at the age of 102, in New York. Noteworthy, arsenic is nowadays a pillar of acute promyelocytic leukemia treatment, as established by Francesco Lo Coco and Colleagues [4]. A grapping hypothesis suggests that the curative effect might be due to the blood transfusion, acting as the first stem cell transplant, rather than on anti-leukemic agents only.

2. The advent of chemotherapy

In 1948, based on the evidence that AL children receiving folic acid did worsen, Dr. Farber proposed the first rational treatment for AL [2, 5]. He correctly guessed

Year	Development
1865	*Heinrich Lissauer* administered potassium arsenite to a woman with chronic myelogenous leukemia
1895	Radiation therapy was administered with transient benefit
1930	*Walther Gloor* cured the first leukemic patient with arsenic trioxide, irradiation, mesothorium and transfusion
1943	Isolation of folic acid
1948	Nitrogen mustard for Hodgkin disease; Antifols: aminopterin then amethopterin (methotrexate) for acute lymphoblastic leukemia
1951	Adrenocorticotropic hormone then prednisone for acute lymphoblastic leukemia
1953	Mercaptopurine, methotrexate licensed by the FDA
1955	Prednisone licensed by FDA
1958	Dexamethasone licensed by FDA
1958	Cyclophosphamide licensed by FDA
1963	Vincristine licensed by FDA
1969	Cytarabine licensed by FDA
1978	Native L-asparaginase licensed by FDA
1979	Daunorubicin licensed by FDA
1983	Etoposide licensed by FDA
1987	Mitoxantrone licensed by FDA
1994	Pegylated L-asparaginase licensed by FDA
1995	All-trans-retinoic acid approved for acute promyelocytic leukemia
2000	Arsenic trioxide licensed for acute promyelocytic leukemia by FDA
2001	Imatinib licensed for chronic myelogenous leukemia by FDA*

**During XXI century, several novel targeted agents were then approved.*

Table 2.
Development of anti-leukemia treatments (adapted from Paul S. Gaynon, Toska J. Zomorodian, and Donald Pinkel. History of leukemia: Historical perspectives. In childhood Leukemias: Third edition, by Ching-hon Pui, Ed. Cambridge university press 978–0–521–19661–1).

Date	Development
1873	Blood transfusion first applied to leukemic patients (*Callender*)
1901	First description of human blood groups (*Landsteiner*)
1937	First hospital blood bank
1954	Introduction of platelet transfusion
1957	First successful syngeneic bone marrow transplantation
1968	First successful sibling donor bone marrow transplant (immunodeficiency)
1972	First successful matched sibling donor marrow transplantation (aplastic anemia)
1974	Anthony Nolan Bone Marrow Donor Registry (UK)
1977	Evidence of survivals >1 for 18/110 patients with advanced leukemia transplanted from matched donors
1979	Report of Success >50% for matched sibling donor marrow transplantation for acute myeloid leukemia in first remission
1986	National Marrow Donor Registry Program (USA)
1983	First successful haploidentical T-cell depleted bone marrow transplant
1989	First successful transplant using umbilical cord blood
1997	First reduced-intensity bone marrow transplantation
2002	First generation CAR-T cells
2017	The FDA approves CD19-directed CAR T cells for the treatment of relapsed, refractory acute lymphoblastic leukemia in children and young adults.

Table 3.
Evolution of transfusion services and stem cell transplantation.

that blocking folic acid metabolism could on the contrary avoid leukemic cells growth. Based on that, he wrote "we may now with some justice hope that aminopterin, or some as yet unsynthesized substance related to it, will afford a substantial basis for real hope in this now hopeless disease" [5].

Despite Farber intuition, the prognosis of AL patients remained very poor throughout the 1950s and the 1960s. When Boggs, Wintrobe, and Cartwright examined the overall outcome of AL patients treated with 6- mercaptopurine (6-MP) and methotrexate, they were discouraged, and concluded that, "*the possibility of spontaneous remission must be entertained whenever a patient with acute leukemia becomes apparently well yet, so far as known, practically all such patients subsequently died in relapse. Of the extremely rare case in which the patient did not die, it may be said that the original diagnosis was incorrect*" [2, 6].

Conversely, in the pediatric setting, progressive and impressive improvements were seen starting in the 1960s, especially due to the big efforts of Don Pinkel and Colleagues at St. Jude Institute [7, 8]. Particularly, they systematically changed and improved their chemotherapy regimens, documenting a terrific improvement in a few decades in the prognosis of children affected by AL, an almost invariably fatal disease till then [7, 8].

By contrast, the prognosis remained dismal in adults. However, largely following pediatric studies, the treatment of lymphoid (ALL) and non-lymphoid (myeloid, AML) leukemias became progressively distinct. Eventually, in 1973, the combination of daunorubicin and cytarabine, administered according to the 3 + 7 scheme was documented to be effective in acute myeloid leukemia [9], while post-induction intensification was further developed for ALL (see a schematic timeline of anti-leukemia treatments development in **Table 2**).

In the 1950s, pre-clinical experiments led to the evidences that bone marrow engraftment after sub-lethal irradiation was associated to leukemia disappearance in mice [10]. This prompted further clinical research in humans and in 1957 Donald Thomas described the first intravenous infusion of bone marrow in humans [11]. In the following decades, tremendous progresses were made and successful bone marrow transplantations were recorded in acute leukemia patients, wither with relapsed/refractory disease and in complete remission [12–14]. By time, bone marrow transplantation evolved to stem cell transplantation, with different sources being available such as marrow, peripheral blood, and umbilical cord blood. At the same time, donation was not limited to siblings but extended to voluntary matched donors, the first registry being funded in UK in 1974, and even only partially compatible ones, in the so called haploidentical transplant (**Table 3**).

Overall, however, the success of anti-leukemic treatments was achieved not only by developing new drugs and schemes (**Table 2**) [15] but also by dramatically improving supportive cares (**Table 3**) [15], especially as far as blood and derivates transfusion as well as anti-microbe drugs were concerned. Particularly, after the first blood transfusion in a leukemic patient in 1873, the most significant advancement was represented by blood groups description in 1901 by Landsteiner et al. Eventually, in 1937 the first hospital blood bank was established and blood products such as platelets were successfully administered in 1954 [15].

3. From chemotherapy to targeted drugs

The most recent advances, spanned across the last 3 decades, can be largely attributed to a terrific improvement in technology and a definitely better knowledge of leukemia biology (**Table 4**) [15]. Specifically, after the first recognition of recurrent genomic imbalances in the 1970s, patients' risk of recurrence, and therefore the most appropriate treatment (more or less intensified), were defined by cytogenetic analyses [16–17]. Subsequently, quantitative polymerase chain reaction (PCR) based techniques allowed an accurate and reliable quantitation of the residual

Year	Development
1670*	Examination of the blood with the compound microscope
1877	*Paul Ehrlich* introduced histochemical staining
1934	Flow cytometry
1960*	Metaphase cytogenetics; *Peter Nowell* and *David Hungerford* describe the Philadelphia chromosome
1975	Production of monoclonal antibodies
1978	Thiopurine methyltransferase polymorphisms related to response and toxicity
1980	Fluorescent in situ hybridization
1985	Polymerase chain reaction
1996	Gene expression arrays
1998	Minimal residual disease by the polymerase chain reaction
2001	Classification of AML risk based on cytogenetic features
2008	First whole genome sequencing in AML
2016	Genomic Classification and Prognosis in Acute Myeloid Leukemia
2017	Integration of Next-Generation Sequencing to Treat Acute Lymphoblastic Leukemia

**Approximately.*

Table 4.
Evolution of technologies that re-defined leukemia diagnosis and prognostication.

disease, this becoming a major factor in determining the choice of treatment (more or less intensified chemotherapy, stem cell transplantation, and targeted drugs) especially in ALL [18]. Finally, next generation sequencing, the first AML genome studied in 2008 [19], quickly led to a refined molecular classification of both AML and ALL [20–21], unveiling new therapeutic targets and hopefully nearing the new era of personalized medicine. Indeed, in the current century, a series of amazing new drugs have been licensed for acute leukemia treatment, including tyrosine kinase inhibitors, BCL2 inhibitors, IDH2 inhibitors, demethylating agents, and monoclonal antibodies including the novel bispecific T-cell engagers (**Table 3**). On the other hand, the latest frontier of cellular therapy relies on the chimeric antigen receptor T-cell therapies (CAR-T), firstly demonstrated to be effective in younger ALL patients [22].

We may certainly expect that further improvements in our understanding of leukemogenesis will lead to later significant success in curing these still terrible diseases.

Author details

Pier Paolo Piccaluga
Department of Experimental, Diagnostic and Specialty Medicine, Institute of Hematology and Medical Oncology, Bologna University School of Medicine, Bologna, Italy

*Address all correspondence to: pierpaolo.piccaluga@unibo.it

References

[1] Gunz FW. Leukemia in the past. In: Henderson ES, Lister TA (eds). Leukemia. WB Saunders Company: Philadelphia, 1990, pp 3-11.

[2] Beutler E. The treatment of acute leukemia: past, present, and future. Leukemia (2001) 15, 658-661

[3] Gloor W. Ein fall von geheilter Myeloblasten leukamie. Munch Med Wochenschr 1930; 77: 1096-1098

[4] Lo Coco F, Avvisati G, Vignetti M, et al. Retinoic Acid and Arsenic Trioxide for Acute Promyelocytic LeukemiaN Engl J Med 2013; 369:111-121

[5] Farber S, Diamond LK, Mercer RD, Sylvester RF Jr, Wolff JA. Temporary remissions in acute leukemia in children produced by folic acid antagonist, 4-aminopteroyl-glutamic acid (aminopterin). New Engl J Med 1948; 238: 787-793

[6] Boggs DR, Wintrobe MM, Cartwright GE. The acute leukemia. Analysis of 322 cases and review of the literature. Medicine (Baltimore) 1962; 41: 163-225.

[7] Pui CH. Childhood leukemias. New Engl J Med 1995; 332: 1618-1630.

[8] Pui CH, Evans WE. Treatment of acute lymphoblastic leukemia. N Engl J Med 354: 166-178

[9] Yates JW, Wallace HR, Ellison RR, Holland JF: Cytosine arabinoside (NSC-63878) and daunorubicin (NSC-83142) therapy in acute nonlymphocytic leukemia. Cancer Chemother Rep 57:485, 1973.

[10] Barnes, D.W.H., Corp, M.J., Loutit, J.F. & Neal, F.E. (1956) Treatment of murine leukaemia with X-rays and homologous bone marrow. British Medical Journal, ii, 626-627.

[11] Thomas, E.D., Lochte, H.L., Jr, Lu, W.C. & Ferrebee, J.W. (1957). Intravenous infusion of bone marrow in patients receiving radiation and chemotherapy. New England Journal of Medicine, 257, 491-496

[12] Thomas, E.D., Buckner, C.D., Banaji, M., et al (1977) One hundred patients with acute leukemia treated by chemotherapy, total body irradiation, and allogeneic marrow transplantation. Blood, 49, 511-533

[13] Thomas, E.D., Buckner, C.D., Clift, R.A., et al (1979) Marrow transplantation for acute non-lymphoblastic leukemia in first remission. New England Journal of Medicine, 301, 597-599

[14] Thomas, E.D., Sanders, J.E., Flournoy, N., et al (1979) Marrow transplantation for patients with acute lymphoblastic leukemia in remission. Blood, 54, 468-476

[15] Paul S. Gaynon, Toska J. Zomorodian, and Donald Pinkel. History of leukemia: historical perspectives. In Childhood Leukemias: Third Edition, by Ching-Hon Pui, Ed. Cambridge University Press 978-0-521-19661-1.

[16] C.D. Bloomfield, L.M. Secker-Walker, A.I. Goldman, et al. Six-year follow-up of the clinical significance of karyotype in acute lymphoblastic leukemia, Cancer Genetics and Cytogenetics, Volume 40, Issue 2, 1989, Pages 171-185.

[17] Visani, G., Bernasconi, P., Boni, M. et al. The prognostic value of cytogenetics is reinforced by the kind of induction/consolidation therapy in influencing the outcome of acute myeloid leukemia – analysis of 848 patients. Leukemia 15, 903-909 (2001).

[18] Cavé H, van der Werff ten Bosch J, Suciu S, et al. Clinical significance of minimal residual disease in childhood acute lymphoblastic leukemia. European Organization for Research and Treatment of Cancer--Childhood Leukemia Cooperative Group. N Engl J Med. 1998 Aug 27;339(9):591-8.

[19] Ley TJ, Mardis ER, Ding L, et al. DNA sequencing of a cytogenetically normal acute myeloid leukaemia genome. Nature. 2008 Nov 6;456(7218):66-72.

[20] Papaemmanuil E, Gerstung M, Bullinger L, et al. Genomic Classification and Prognosis in Acute Myeloid Leukemia. N Engl J Med. 2016 Jun 9;374(23):2209-2221.

[21] Inaba H, Azzato EM, Mullighan CG. Integration of Next-Generation Sequencing to Treat Acute Lymphoblastic Leukemia with Targetable Lesions: The St. Jude Children's Research Hospital Approach. Front Pediatr. 2017 Dec 4; 5:258.

[22] Pehlivan KC, Duncan BB, Lee DW. CAR-T Cell Therapy for Acute Lymphoblastic Leukemia: Transforming the Treatment of Relapsed and Refractory Disease. Curr Hematol Malig Rep. 2018 Oct;13(5):396-406.

Section 2

Biology and Diagnosis of Acute Leukemias

Chapter 2

Juvenile Myelomonocytic Leukemia (JMML): A Mimicker of *KMT2A*-Rearranged Acute Myeloid Leukemia (AML)

Ashraf Abdullah Saad

Abstract

Juvenile myelomonocytic leukemia (JMML) is the most confusing mimicker of *KMT2A*-rearranged acute myeloid leukemia (AML). Clinical presentation, age of susceptibility (infancy or early childhood) and abnormal monocytosis are common clinical features. To complicate matters, JMML morphologically resemble acute myelomonocytic leukemia (AML M4) and distinction must be made based on accurate blast and promonocyte counts. As treatment significantly varies, AML/JMML overlap can lead to catastrophic consequences that can be avoided by timely management. Therefore, meticulous knowledge of JMML is essential to treat patients with hematologic malignancies. The pathognomic feature of JMML is increased infiltration of the peripheral blood, bone marrow, and viscera by abnormal myelomonocytic cells. Molecular diagnostics has generated substantial dividends in dissecting the genetic basis of JMML. We can now molecularly confirm the diagnosis of JMML in approximately over 90% of patients who harbor driver mutations in *KRAS, NRAS, PTPN11, NF1*, or *CBL* genes. The presence of monosomy 7 is a classic feature of JMML that can support the diagnosis in many cases. On the other hand, cytogenetics and Fluorescence in situ hybridization analysis (FISH) are indispensable to differentiate *KMT2A*-rearranged AML from JMML. In particular, AML with t(9;11) is associated with monocytic features that can be easily mistaken for JMML.

Keywords: JMML, *KMT2A*, DNA hypermethylation, p-STAT5, azacitidine

1. Introduction

JMML is a rare aggressive clonal hematopoietic neoplasm of infancy and early childhood that combines excessive proliferation of the granulocytic and monocytic lineages with dysplasia making JMML analogous to chronic myelomonocytic leukemia (CMML). Therefore, the current WHO classification of myeloid neoplasms and acute leukemia envisages JMML as an overlap myeloproliferative/myelodysplastic neoplasm. The diagnosis of JMML is mainly based on the clinical presentation in combination with morphology of the peripheral blood smears and the molecular analysis of leukemic cells. The peripheral blood and bone marrow of

JMML diagnostic criteria
I. Clinical and hematologic features (all 4 features mandatory):
• PB monocyte count ≥1 x 10^9/L.
• Blast percentage in PB and BM <20%.
• Splenomegaly.
• Absence of Philadelphia chromosome (*BCR/ABL1* rearrangement).
II. Genetic studies (1 finding sufficient):
• Somatic mutation in *PTPN11* or *KRAS* or *NRAS* (Germ line mutations -indicating Noonan syndrome- need to be excluded).
• Clinical diagnosis of NF1 or *NF1* mutation.
• Germ line *CBL* mutation and loss of heterozygosity of CBL.
III. For patients without genetic features, besides the clinical and hematologic features listed under I, the following criteria must be fulfilled:
• Monosomy 7 or any other chromosomal abnormality or at least 2 of the following criteria:
• Hemoglobin F increased for age.
• Myeloid or erythroid precursors on peripheral blood smear.
• GM-CSF hypersensitivity in colony assay.
• Hyperphosphorylation of STAT5.
[1]*Arber DA, Orazi A, Hasserjian R, et al. The 2016 revision to the World Health Organization classification of myeloid neoplasms and acute leukemia.* Blood. *2016;127(20):2391–2405. doi:10.1182/blood-2016-03-643,544*

Table 1.
The diagnostic criteria for juvenile myelomonocytic leukemia[1].

children with JMML may display features of both myeloproliferative and myelodysplastic disorders (ie, immature and dysplastic forms), as well as cytopenias due to marrow infiltration and/or splenomegaly. Splenomegaly, lymphadenopathy, and skin rashes are common clinical features but the clinical picture of JMML can be somewhat non-specific. JMML is frequently confused with viral infections, immunodeficiency syndromes, myelodysplastic syndromes, myeloproliferative neoplasms or other forms of leukemia [1]. Moreover, JMML has diverse molecular subtypes with contrasting features and varied clinical outcomes. The broad overlap in clinical and laboratory features in combination with the heterogeneity of JMML itself made the diagnosis of JMML a hurdle to most hematologists. Consequently, the diagnosis of JMML almost always relies on the diagnostic criteria (**Table 1**). The chief backbone of the diagnostic criteria is the associated molecular and/or cytogenetic abnormalities. In particular, the genomic landscape of JMML had revolutionized our understanding of leukemogenesis of this greatly equivocal disease. JMML is a predominantly fatal disease but the clinical course can be highly variable. At both extremes of the disease, a third of patients follow a relatively indolent course while approximately 15% of cases develop AML, the so called 'blast crisis' [2].

2. Clinical features

- Patients present with splenomegaly, fever, thrombocytopenia, monocytosis, and elevated HbF.

- Leukocytosis is common in JMML, but a presenting white blood count <10 x 10^9/L is occasionally noted.

- Anemia is generally not a leading symptom and rarely requires red blood cell (RBC) transfusion.
- Most patients present with evidence of infection or constitutional symptoms that may mimic viral infections.
- Polyclonal hypergammaglobulinemia and presence of autoantibodies.
- The hallmark of the disease is the overproduction of myelomonocytic cells (monocytic and granulocytic cells) that infiltrate skin and vital organs (spleen, liver, and lungs) leading to various clinical manifestations as follows [3]:

1. Lungs: dry cough, tachynoea and interstitial infiltrates on chest X-ray are signs of pulmonary infiltration.
2. Skin: Cafe-au-lait spots might be indicative of an underlying germline conditions such as Neurofibromatosis type 1 (NF1) or Noonan syndrome-like disorder. Neurofibromas occur in patients with NF1. About 25% of patients have pleomorphic skin rashes in the forms of:
   - Eczematous eruptions (cradle cap).
   - Indurated raised lesions with central clearing.
   - Sweet syndrome.
3. Gut infiltration may predispose patients to diarrhea—sometimes with bloody features—and gastrointestinal infections.
4. Lymph nodes: About half of all patients have lymphadenopathy. Leukemic infiltrates may give rise to markedly enlarged tonsils.
5. There is generally marked splenomegaly/hepatosplenomegaly:
   - Hepatomegaly is generally less prominent than splenomegaly.
   - Approximately 7–10% of JMML patients will not have splenomegaly at diagnosis but virtually all patients will develop splenomegaly within weeks to months of initial presentation (spleen size rapidly increases with time).

3. Pathologic features

3.1 Peripheral blood

The peripheral blood (**Figure 1**) is the most important specimen for diagnosis [4]. It typically shows leukocytosis and thrombocytopenia. The vast majority of JMML patients have thrombocytopenia with the exception of children with NF1- mutated JMML, who show platelet counts within the normal range in most cases. The median reported white blood cell counts are 25–30 x 10^9/L. The leukocytosis consists mainly of neutrophils, with some immature cells (e.g. promyelocytes and myelocytes)

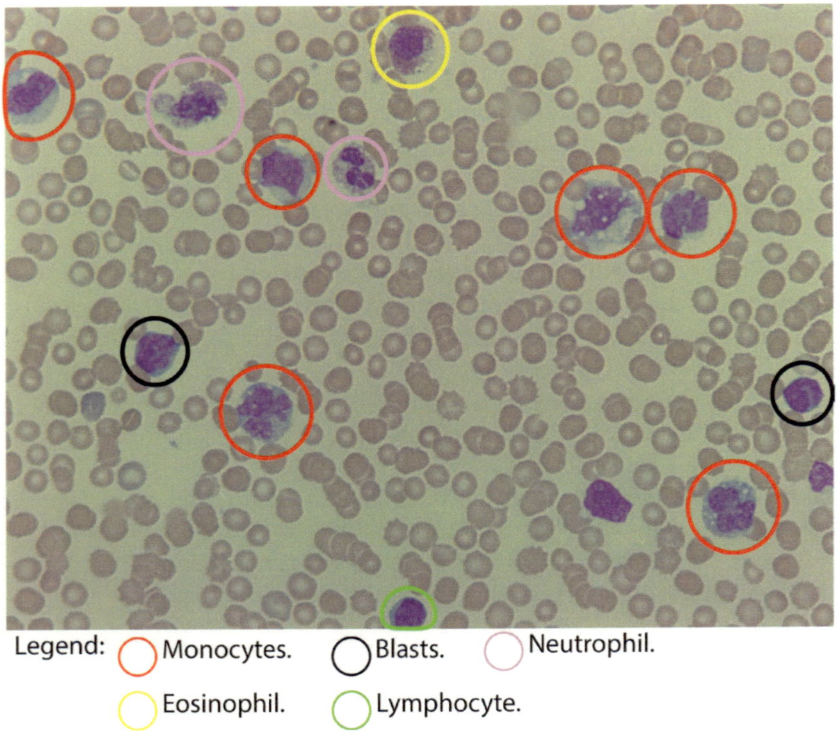

Figure 1.
Peripheral blood of a 13 months old boy with PTPN11-mutated JMML. Photomicrograph shows leukocytosis with neutrophilia and monocytosis. There is left shift, toxic granulation and vacuolation. Occasional primitive cells (~ 2%) are present. No nucleated RBCs are seen.

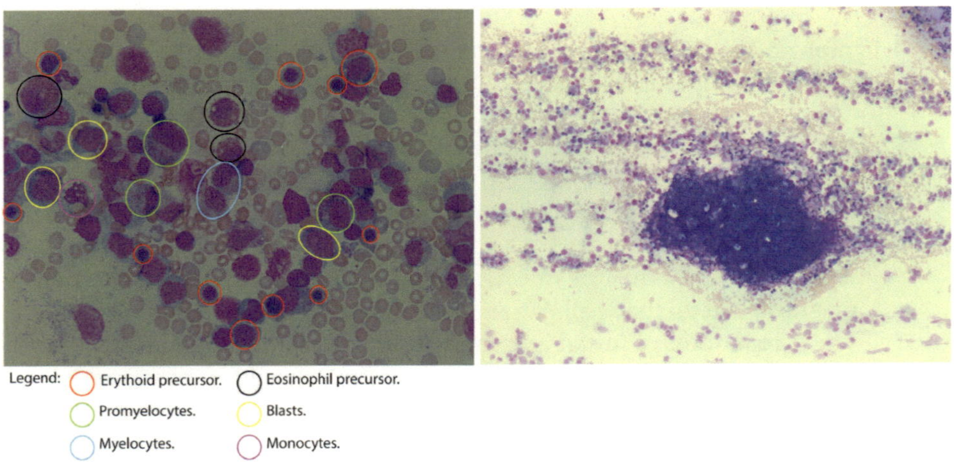

Figure 2.
Bone marrow aspirate demonstrates a hypercellular marrow (100 – Age = %normal cellularity) with left shift and increased myeloid and monocyte lineages. Blast count is about 4%. There is occasional evidence of hemophagocytosis and mild erythroid dysplastic features.

and monocytes. Although most cases show a striking monocytosis, often with dysplastic forms, the absolute monocyte count can be <1 x 10^9/L. Blasts (including promonocytes) usually account for <5% of the white blood cells, and always <20%. Eosinophilia and basophilia are observed in a minority of cases. Nucleated red blood cells are often seen. Red blood cell changes include macrocytosis (particularly in patients with monosomy 7), but normocytic red blood cells are more common.

3.2 Bone marrow

Bone marrow (**Figure 2**) findings are consistent with the diagnosis of JMML but are not per se diagnostic. However, bone marrow aspiration is necessary to exclude AML M4. The most consistent finding in bone marrow specimens is the reduced number or absence of megakaryocytes in about two third of cases. The bone marrow aspirate and biopsy are hypercellular with granulocytic proliferation, although in some patients erythroid precursors may predominate. Monocytes in the bone marrow are often less prominent than in the peripheral blood, generally accounting for 5–10% of the bone marrow cells. The marrow blasts (including promonocytes) can be moderately elevated, but does not reach the level seen in acute leukemia (account for <20% of the bone marrow cells). Auer rods are never present. Dysplasia is usually minimal; however, dysgranulopoiesis (including pseudo-Pelger-Huet neutrophils and hypogranularity) may be noted in some cases, and erythroid precursors may be enlarged. No specific immunophenotypic abnormalities have been reported in JMML.

4. Differential diagnosis

4.1 *KMT2A*-rearranged AML masquerading as JMML

Unlike in AML, the bone marrow in patients with JMML demonstrates no blockage of differentiation of myeloid elements. Rather, as is seen in chronic myeloid leukemia (CML), the bone marrow in JMML displays myeloid hyperplasia with increased production of monocytic cells along the full spectrum of differentiation, including blast forms, promonocytes, monocytes, and macrophages. The marrow blast count may be slightly elevated but in classic JMML it does not reach the counts seen in AML. Nevertheless, differentiating JMML from AML is nearly impossible on clinical grounds alone as significant hepatosplenomegaly and respiratory failure can occur in both. Moreover, blood counts and hematologic features may mimic AML. This especially holds true for infants with the lysine methyltransferase 2A (*KMT2A*) rearrangements who occasionally present with hepatosplenomegaly and low blast count resembling JMML [5]. A puzzling interface between *KMT2A*-rearranged AML and JMML therefore exists. Recent reports have validated the close mimicry between *KMT2A*-rearranged AML and JMML [6]. Unless unveiled by cytogenetics, JMML can conceal the clinical diagnosis of *KMT2A*-rearranged AML. Age of susceptibility (infancy or early childhood) and abnormal monocytosis have blurred the line between these distinct entities. Specifically, JMML may mimic AML with t(9;11). t(9;11) is the most frequent molecular subtype involving the *KMT2A* gene (*KMT2A-MLLT3*) in AML. t(9;11)-positive AML/JMML overlap was well-characterized in the medical literature [7]. Both conditions have increased immature monocytes and blasts. I reported a 14-month-old girl with t(9;11)-positive AML who died as she received JMML-directed therapy. The clinical picture, peripheral smear and the suboptimal blast count of only 10% had stealthily impersonated JMML [8].

Chromosomal rearrangements involving the *KMT2A* gene do not exist in the genomic landscape of JMML. KMT2A gene rearrangements are common genetic mutations in pediatric AML with an incidence of 15–25% (50–60% in children younger than two years). However, both KMT2A-rearranged AML and JMML share common morphologic features. *KMT2A*-rearranged AML is usually AML M4 or M5, and both are characterized by increased numbers of monoblasts or abnormal monocytes. JMML morphologically resemble AML M4 and distinction must be made based on accurate blast and promonocyte counts.

Differentiating AML from JMML is vital for survival. Chemotherapy regimens for JMML are mainly cytoreductive as a bridge to hematopoietic stem cell transplantation (HSCT) rather than curative as for AML. Therefore, any delay in establishing the correct diagnosis and/or administration of wrong treatment can be lethal. Molecular diagnosis has become the mainstay to distinguish between AML and JMML. Cytogenetics and FISH should be immediately performed to detect *KMT2A* gene rearrangements in every suspicious case.

4.2 JMML masquerading as RALD

JMML is closely related to RAS-associated autoimmune leukoproliferative disorder (RALD) [9]. RALD is a non-malignant, non-infectious leukoproliferative disease that resembles the autoimmune lymphoproliferative syndrome (ALPS) caused by mutations affecting the FAS/FASL pathway.

Similar to patients with ALPS, RALD patients present with lymphadenopathy, massive splenomegaly, increased circulating B cells, hypergammaglobulinemia, and autoimmunity. However, RALD was separated from ALPS as:

1. In contrast to ALPS, biomarkers such as $CD4^-/CD8^-$ double negative T-cell receptor αβ ($TCR\alpha\beta^+$) T cells and serum vitamin B12 levels are not always increased.

2. Germline or somatic mutations in *FAS, FASL, or CASP10* are absent in RALD.

RALD is a RAS-associated somatic disorder characterized by myelomonocytic and lymphoid hyperplasia that shares identical somatic *KRAS* or *NRAS* mutations found in up to 25% of JMML patients. It is thought that RAS activation itself can alter selection patterns of autoreactive B cells and antibody production leading to autoimmune manifestations. Overlap features of both JMML and RALD include:

1. Cytopenias, lymphadenopathy, and splenomegaly.

2. Persistent absolute or relative monocytosis is a cardinal feature of RALD.

3. Bone marrow and peripheral blood smear findings overlap with those of JMML in children or CMML in older patients.

4. Morphologic features compatible with dysplasia, such as hyposegmented pelgeroid neutrophils, can also be seen in RALD further obscuring the distinction between RALD and JMML.

5. Autoimmunity can be noted in up to 25% of children with JMML, whereas hypergammaglobulinemia is present in more than 50% of cases.

6. Nearly all patients with RALD meet the revised diagnostic criteria for JMML.

Distinguishing RALD from JMML can be impossible on clinical grounds alone. However, this distinction has an important prognostic value as RALD is characterized by an indolent clinical course whereas JMML can be fatal if left untreated. The most definitive diagnostic distinction between RALD and JMML occurs in the setting of a cytogenetic abnormality (eg, monosomy 7), which excludes RALD and favors a malignant process. However, normal bone marrow cytogenetics has been reported in around 65% of JMML patients.

JMML/RALD overlap can lead to inappropriate treatment decisions. In some patients, RALD was misdiagnosed as JMML and vice versa. It is the author's experience that a patient with KRAS-mutated JMML was misdiagnosed as RALD for many weeks until he developed full -blown JMML. It is noteworthy that RALD can occur as the initial presentation and transform to JMML several years later. Indeed, JMML/RALD represents a continuum of two different phenotypes of the same disorder. Although both RALD and JMML share common RAS mutations, the transition from RALD to JMML is caused by additional genetic or epigenetic events. Therefore, patients with RALD should be very closely monitored for acquisition of additional dysplastic, molecular, or clonal karyotypic abnormalties that may herald malignant transformation [10].

4.3 JMML masquerading as myeloproliferative neoplasms (MPNs)

JMML can mimic myeloproliferative malignancies with receptor tyrosine kinase translocations. Identification of these cases is crucial, because patients may benefit from receptor tyrosine kinase–targeted inhibitors.

4.4 Nonmalignant disorders mimicking JMML

- Viral infections such as human herpes virus-6 (HHV-6), parvovirus, or cytomegalovirus (CMV). Occasionally, patients with JMML may present with these viral infections in addition to their underlying hematologic malignancy. Differentiation between CMV-related disease and JMML in infants excreting CMV is sometimes difficult, because clinical and laboratory findings of CMV infection can overlap with those of JMML.

- Leukocyte adhesion deficiency variants.

- Wiskott Aldrich syndrome: need to be considered in male infants.

- Infantile malignant osteopetrosis (IMO): can mimic all clinical and hematological features of JMML.

- Hemophagoytic lymphohistiocytosis (HLH).

- Autoimmune diseases, including rheumatoid arthritis and systemic lupus erythematosus.

5. Genomics

5.1 The central role of the RAS signaling pathway

JMML is an oncogenic RAS mutant cancer where approximately 90% of patients carry either somatic or germline gain of function mutations in *PTPN11, KRAS, NRAS, CBL, or NF1* genes that lead to constitutive activation of the RAS signaling pathway (**Figure 3**). The RAS signaling pathway is a component of multi-step signal transduction pathway that controls the cellular proliferation, differentiation,

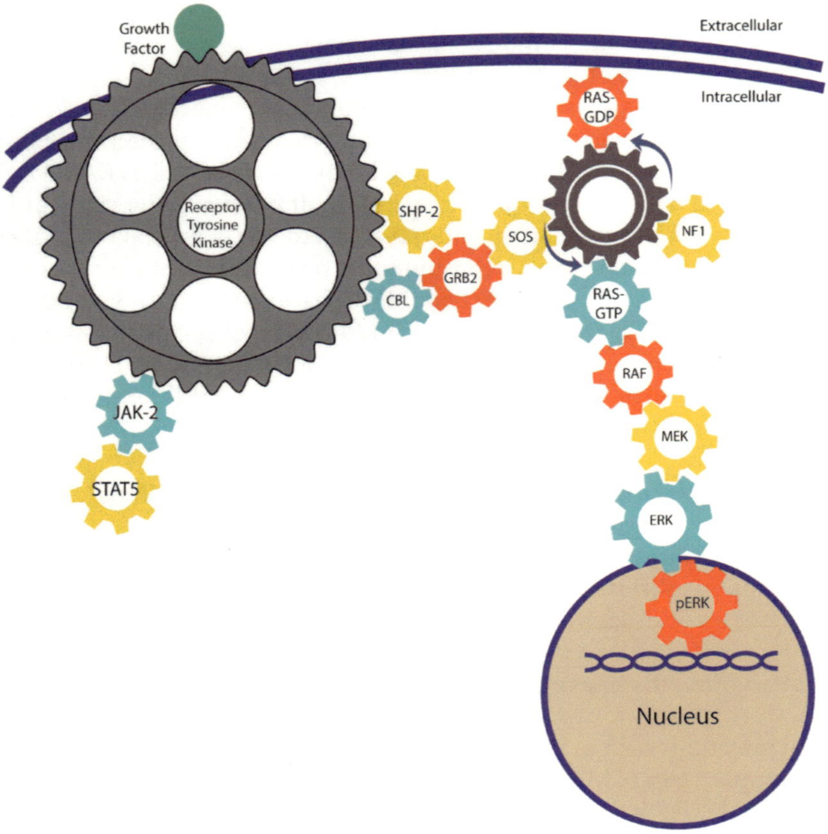

Figure 3.
Illustrative representation of the RAS signaling pathway portraying the transmission of extracellular signals in a gear train to the nucleus. Upon stimulation, a docking site for GRB2 is created which binds to GEF (SOS). The GRB2-SOS interaction converts RAS-GDP to RAS-GTP. The RAS-GTP initiates a cascade of phosphorylations on RAF, MEK and, lastly, ERK. The phospho-ERK then translocates into the nucleus. A counteracting force by GAP (neurofibromin) accelerates the conversion of RAS-GTP to RAS-GDP to restrain the activation of the RAS signaling pathway. Mutations of RAS pathway prevent the conversion of RAS-GTP to RAS-GDP to induce the constitutive activation of the RAS signaling pathway, the characteristic feature of JMML.

and survival. It relays extracellular stimuli such as growth factors to the nucleus where the response to those stimuli is executed by an induced transcriptional program [11].

The RAS family include the proto-oncogenes *HRAS, NRAS and KRAS* which represent a subset of a superfamily of small membrane-localized GTPases. Like other small GTPases, RAS proteins function as molecular switches that cycle between an inactive guanosine diphosphate (GDP)-bound and an active guanosine triphosphate (GTP)-bound conformations. RAS is activated when the receptor tyrosine kinases (RTKs, a large superfamily of receptors for a wide array of growth factors) are activated by growth factor binding leading to RTK autophosphorylation and the creation of docking sites for adaptor molecules like growth factor receptor-bound protein 2 (GRB2). The amount of GTP-RAS generated is regulated by two opposing regulatory mechanisms [12]:

a. Guanine nucleotide exchange factors (GEFs) are necessary for the conversion of GDP-RAS into GTP-RAS. The Son of Sevenless (SOS) is the GEF for the RAS signaling pathway. SOS is recruited by the adaptor protein GRB2 in response to RTK activation. The binding of SOS to GBR2 localizes it to the plasma membrane, where it can activate the membrane bound RAS. Gain of function of the Src-homology tyrosine phosphatase 2 (SHP-2) results in activation of the GEFs and in this way to a continuous activation of RAS. SHP-2 is the encoded gene product of *PTPN11*, the most commonly mutated gene in JMML.

b. GTPase activating proteins (GAPs), like neurofibromin act antagonistically to inactivate RAS by increasing their intrinsic rate of GTP hydrolysis to the inactive form (RAS-GDP) leading to the termination of the RAS signaling. Neurofibromin is the encoded gene product of the tumor suppressor gene *NF1,* the gene implicated in Neurofibromatosis type 1.

Cancer-associated RAS mutations typically alter amino acids G12, G13 or Q61. These mutant RAS proteins display impaired GTPase activity which renders them resistant to GTPase activating proteins (GAPs). Mutant RAS proteins are therefore locked in the signal-transmitting GTP- bound form (the cytosolic ratio of GTP is much higher than GDP at 10:1). The active GTP-RAS in turn activates the RAF kinase, resulting in a downstream proliferative effect.

The *CBL* gene (11q23.3) is a proto-oncogene that encodes three distinct homologs which represent the mammalian CBL family of proteins. Members of the CBL protein family (Cbl/c-Cbl, Cbl-b, and Cbl-c/Cbl-3) are E3 ubiquitin ligases that functions as a negative regulator of many signal transduction pathways by promoting degradation by ubiquitination of activated RTKs (and nonreceptor tyrosine kinases). Studies in animal models and genetic analyses in human cancer have firmly established that CBL proteins function as tumor suppressors. The mutant CBL (lacking E3 ligase activity)- dependent oncogenesis is driven by loss of ubiquitination-dependent degradation of activated RTKs resulting in a synergistic increase in signaling. Mutant CBL proteins may indeed promote oncogenesis in JMML via the RAS signaling pathway. In addition, CBL is an adaptor protein that positively regulates signal transduction. Approximately 150 proteins are associated with or are regulated by CBL proteins. Among these proteins is the adaptor GRB2 that binds to CBL. The CBL-GRB2 interaction modulates the interaction between GRB2 and SOS and hence it is also possible that CBL-GRB2 interactions lead to activation of the RAS pathway.

5.2 GM-CSF–dependent hypersensitivity

Granulocyte-macrophage colony-stimulating factor (GM-CSF) and the related cytokines interleukin 3 (IL-3) and interleukin 5 (IL-5) regulate hematopoietic cell survival, proliferation, differentiation, migration, and perform effector functions such as phagocytosis or reactive oxygen species release. Unlike other cytokine receptors, GM-CSF receptor (GMR) has a significant nonredundant role in macrophage-mediated acute and chronic inflammation, pulmonary homeostasis, allergic diseases, and myeloid haematologic malignancies [13]. GMR is found in myeloid cells and some non-hematopoietic cells, but it is not expressed by lymphoid cells such as T cells. GMR is composed of a ligand-specific α chain (GMR α) and a β common (βc) signaling subunit, which is shared with the IL-3 and IL-5 receptors. Both of which are members of the cytokine receptor family. The binding of GM-CSF to the ligand specific GMRα promotes the formation of a higher-order signaling complex that leads to the activation of non-receptor tyrosine kinases JAK2 and Src family kinases (c-Src and Lyn), which subsequently phosphorylate GMRβc to create docking sites for adapters and signal relay molecules (such as SHP-2) initiating downstream signaling. GM-CSF, IL-3, and IL-5 activate at least three downstream pathways: the JAK/STAT pathway, the RAS signaling pathway, and PI

3-kinase activation pathway. These pathways should not be viewed as being mutually exclusive and may have substantial overlap [14].

RAS signaling pathway mutations might potentiate JAK/STAT signaling by stabilizing or directly activating the GM-CSF receptor or its associated signaling molecules. In particular, the dysregulated SHP-2 (a non-receptor protein tyrosine phosphatase) by JMML-associated mutations is normally essential for efficient STAT5 activation in myeloid cells that are stimulated with IL-3 (SHP-2 is recruited to phosphorylated tyrosine residues on the activated β subunit of the GMR). Elevated levels of RAS-GTP might also increase the degree and/or duration of JAK2 kinase activity. The disturbed GMR signaling in JMML leads to an aberrant response to GM-CSF which can be tested by 2 laboratory assays:

5.2.1 CFU-GM assay (the traditional methylcellulose assay)

The selective hypersensitivity of myeloid progenitor cells of JMML to the GM-CSF in hematopoietic colony formation assays (CFAs) results in spontaneous growth of colony-forming units -granulocyte/macrophage (CFU-GM) in the absence of exogenous growth factors. JMML cells are cultured in semisolid methylcellulose media producing excess number of monocyte–macrophage colonies in the absence of added exogenous growth factors. This spontaneous proliferation of JMML myeloid progenitor cells is primarily due to the striking hypersensitivity of progenitors to GM-CSF in vitro.

This phenomenon, and hallmark of the disease, was first described in 1991. The CFU-GM assay has 2 main pitfalls. The assay is not standardized across diagnostic laboratories and although sensitive it is rather a non-specific assay. Viral infections such as HHV-6 and CMV have also been reported to cause GM-CSF hypersensitivity. Although the hypersensitive pattern of CFU-GM colony growth in methylcellulose is neither necessary nor sufficient to establish a diagnosis of JMML, it used as a minor diagnostic criterion for those 10 percent of JMML patients who do not have identifiable molecular abnormalities affecting the RAS signaling pathway.

5.2.2 p-STAT5 phospho-specific flowcytometry assay

Low-dose GM-CSF can induce hyperphosphorylation of STAT5 in either $CD33^+$/$CD34^+$ (myeloid precursor cells) or $CD33^+$/$CD34^-$/$CD14^+$/$CD38^{low}$ population (represents the more mature monocytic cells) in patients with JMML. In contrast to $CD34^+$/$CD33^+$ cells, neither $CD34^-$/$CD33^+$ (mature myeloid cells) nor $CD34^+$/$CD33^-$ (non-myeloid precursors), demonstrated any STAT5 hyperphosphorylation in response to GM-CSF. These results indicate that the peculiar STAT5 hyperphosphorylation signature specifically resides in the myeloid compartment of hematopoietic progenitor cells [15].

After binding of GM-CSF to its receptor, Janus-kinase-2 (JAK-2) is recruited to the cytoplasmic domain of the β chain, and activation of JAK-2 occurs, which subsequently induces STAT-5 phosphorylation. This signaling pathway induces migration of STAT-5 dimers to the nucleus and promotes the transcription of various genes such as pim-1 and CIS to induce cell differentiation. This cytokine-specific response is exclusively present in JMML patients compared with healthy controls or other pediatric MPNs, indicating that it is critical for disease pathogenesis. The aberrant response of phospho-STAT5 (p-STAT5) to sub-saturating doses of GM-CSF is demonstrated by phospho-specific flow-cytometry assay. This assay is superior to the traditional CFU-GM assay in the following aspects [16]:

1. As compared to CFU-GM assay, p-STAT5 profiling is a rapid diagnostic tool for JMML. CFU-GM assay takes up to several weeks of culture as it requires monocyte depletion.

2. p-STAT5 profiling could discriminate JMML from diseases mimicking JMML, such as CMV infection and transient myeloproliferative disorder in Noonan syndrome (NS/MPD) that also exhibit GM-CSF hypersensitivity by in vitro colony assay but not by phospho-specific flowcytometry.

Interestingly, CMML (the adult equivalent of JMML) also displays GM-CSF-dependent hypersensitivity. Primary CMML samples demonstrate GM-CSF–dependent hypersensitivity by hematopoietic CFAs and phospho-STAT5 (pSTAT5) flowcytometry compared with healthy donors. Among CMML patients, the pSTAT5 hypersensitive response positively correlated with high-risk disease, peripheral leukocytes, monocytes, and signaling associated mutations.

The p-STAT5 response to low doses of GM-CSF was also detectable in AML M4/M5. JMML, CMML, and M4/M5 AML are related entities in which hyperactive RAS and aberrant JAK2/STAT5 signaling are early or initiating events. As such, M4/M5 AML might be distinct from other subtypes of AML, in which aberrant transcription factor fusions such as PML-RARA and AML1-ETO likely represent primary leukemogenic events. This has important therapeutic implications, as M4/M5 AML might be highly dependent on RAS and JAK2/STAT5 signaling, and therefore sensitive to inhibitors of these pathways. Because GM-CSF signaling is critical for monocyte differentiation and survival, targeting GM-CSF in the therapeutics of JMML in vitro and AML in vivo has been reported, with varying degrees of success [17].

The absence of the p-STAT5 phospho-flow signature in conditions that are phenotypically similar to JMML highlights the importance of the signaling disruptions that we observe specifically in JMML. The flow cytometric p-STAT5 profiling is a reliable, sensitive and specific diagnostic tool for identifying patients with JMML that was added in the 2016 revision to the World Health Organization classification of myeloid neoplasms and acute leukemia as a minor diagnostic criterion for those 10 percent of JMML patients who do not have identifiable molecular abnormalities affecting the RAS signaling pathway.

In fact, hyperphosphorylation of STAT5 does not only add to the genetic mapping of JMML but it has significant therapeutic implications. Kotecha et al. demonstrated that p-STAT5 phospho-flow signature may identify children with NRAS and PTPN11 mutations who will have a benign clinical course and can be observed closely without aggressive treatment. p-STAT5 phospho-flow signature was also absent in infants with NS/MPD which indicates that phospho-flow cytometry provides a more specific readout of the rewired signaling networks found in JMML. Remarkably, p-STAT5 signaling response can indicate disease status as the p-STAT5 responsive population was shown to disappear in remission and reappear during relapse. Differences in GM-CSF-stimulated phospho-STAT5 levels might be utilized to identify targeted agents with potential efficacy as well as to follow response to treatment, relapse, or transformation to AML [18].

5.3 JMML interlacing with RASopathies

As opposed to the somatic mutations found in cancer, germline mutations of genes that encode components or regulators of the RAS signal transduction pathway result in clinically defined group of human genetic syndromes collectively termed as “RASopathies” or “neuro- cardio-facio cutaneous syndromes (NCFCS) [19]. The RASopathies are one of the largest known groups of malformation syndromes with an incidence of around 1 in 1000 individuals. They exhibit numerous overlapping phenotypic features such as neurodevelopmental dysmorphic features, an increased risk of autoimmunity and predisposition to cancer and abnormal myelopoiesis in infancy. The RAS signal transduction pathway plays an essential role in regulating the cell cycle and cellular growth, differentiation, and senescence, all of which are critical to normal development. Therefore, it is not surprising that RAS signal transduction pathway dysregulation has detrimental effects on both embryonic and later stages of development. RASopathies include:

1. Noonan syndrome: PTPN11, KRAS, SOS1, RAF1, NRAS.

2. Costello: HRAS.

3. Cardiofacio-cutaneous syndromes (KRAS, BRAF, MEK1/2).

4. Neurofibromatosis type 1: NF1.

5. NS-like syndromes: CBL-syndrome (CBL) and NS-like disorder with loose anagen hair (SHOC2).

6. Legius syndrome (NF-1-like syndrome): SPRED1.

Noonan syndrome (NS) is the most genetically diverse and most common RASopathy occurring in 1 of 1000 to 2500 births. NS is characterized by developmental disorders, short stature, a typical facial appearance (facial dysmorphism), congenital heart defects, and skeletal anomalies. So far, heterozygous mutations in nine genes (*PTPN11, SOS1, KRAS, NRAS, RAF1, BRAF, SHOC2, MEK1* and *CBL*) have been documented to underlie this disorder or clinically related phenotypes. Germline mutations in the *PTPN11* gene have been described in 50% of the Noonan syndrome cases. Somatically acquired JMML-associated PTPN11 mutations are not seen in NS. Somatic mutations differ from germline PTPN11 mutations which are predicted to result in a weaker gain-of-function than the somatic mutations [20].

The most common hematopoietic disorder in NS is a transient myeloproliferative disorder (MPD) estimated to occur in up to 10% of all children with NS. Nearly all patients with NS/MPD have mutations in *PTPN11*. The transient MPD in Noonan syndrome is diagnosed in the neonatal period or early infancy. In contrast to JMML, NS/MPD is thought to be of polyclonal origin. It generally resolves spontaneously over months or years. However, leukocytosis and tissue invasion by monocytes and immature myeloid cells can have deleterious effects. An estimated 10% of cases of NS/MPD acquire a cytogenetic abnormality and progress to JMML. Thus, NS/MPD is a tumor predisposition syndrome and affected patients should be followed closely. JMML in *PTPN11*-mutated NS seems to behave differently from sporadic JMML as it occurs at a very young age (infancy) and tends to regress spontaneously. Although the hematological picture can be indistinguishable from JMML in some cases, the myeloproliferation is polyclonal in most instances, and thus, the disorder has not been recognized by the World Health Organization (WHO) as a separate JMML category. Therefore, recognizing NS in a JMML patient is important in order to identify those patients who might benefit from a watch-and-wait strategy. Similar to *PTPN11*-mutated NS, a transient MPD was noted in some children with NS and *KRAS* or *NRAS* germline mutations.

NF1 gene is a negative modulator that normally restricts RAS activation. Loss of heterozygosity (LOH) with loss of the normal NF1 allele in leukemic cells leads to activation of RAS signaling pathway. In most cases, the diagnosis of NF1 can be established clinically by the presence of ≥6 caf'e au lait macules >0.5 cm in diameter. In addition, one-half of these children have a parent affected by NF1.The risk of developing JMML for the patient with NF1 is estimated 200- to 350-fold higher than in patients without NF1.

Germ line mutations of the *CBL* gene cause CBL syndrome characterized by a high frequency of neurologic features/vasculopathy, mild NS-like features, and a high risk of JMML. The germline mutation represents the first hit, with somatic LOH being the second hit positively selected in JMML cells. Indeed, all children with JMML and *CBL* mutations were found to have a germline *CBL* missense mutation on one allele and acquired LOH on the other allele in leukemic cells. The development of vasculopathies occurs in the second decade of life unless allogeneic HSCT is successful. The most frequently observed vasculopathies are optic atrophy, optic neuritis, hypertension, cardiomyopathy, and arteritis.

5.4 Cytogenetic studies

JMML cells show a normal karyotype in 65% of cases, sole monosomy 7 in about 25%, and other aberrations in 10%. A remarkable feature of many JMML cases with normal karyotype is a markedly increased synthesis of fetal hemoglobin (HbF). The likelihood of an abnormal karyotype is dependent on the genetic subtype, with monosomy 7 being noted most often in *KRAS*-mutated disease. Monosomy 7 is the most frequent chromosomal aberration in both MDS and JMML. It is likely that haploinsufficiency of genes located on chromosome 7 contributes to clonal evolution.

6. JMML genetic subtypes

Deregulated RAS signaling is the main driving event in JMML. The 5 canonical RAS pathway mutations (*PTPN11, KRAS, NRAS, CBL*, and *NF1* genes) represent five genetically and clinically distinct subtypes in JMML. Mutations in the respective genes can either occur as germline ("syndromic") or as somatic lesion in hematopoietic cells ("nonsyndromic"). *PTPN11-, NRAS-*, and *KRAS*-mutated JMML are characterized by heterozygous somatic gain-of-function mutations in nonsyndromic children, whereas JMML in neurofibromatosis type 1 and JMML in children with CBL syndrome are defined by germline RAS disease and acquired biallelic inactivation of the respective genes in hematopoietic cells. Their clinical features are presented in **Table 2**.

The concept that mutations associated with JMML are mutually exclusive within a given individual implies that a mutation in any one of these genes is sufficient to activate the signaling pathway and drive the proliferation of JMML cells. However, this does not mean that two or more genetic mutations cannot occur at the same time as one would comprehend from the term 'mutually exclusive'. In fact, coexisting mutations in *NRAS, KRAS, PTPN11, CBL and NF1* were found in 11% of JMML patients [21]. Analysis of single colonies for two patients with compound RAS pathway mutations demonstrated that both mutations occurred in the same colony. PTPN11 and NF1 lesions were the most frequent of these cooperative events. In addition, one patient harbored two *NRAS* lesions (p.G13D and p.Q61K).

The five JMML genetic subtypes are key determinants for treatment adaptation in patients with JMML. However, their use in a risk stratification algorithm is hindered by their failure to independently prognosticate the clinical outcome. In fact, the prognostic relevance is owned by the number of mutations at diagnosis rather than the type of mutation itself. Patients with JMML who harbor two or

Genetic subtype	Characteristics:
1- *NF1*-mutated JMML:	• Incidence: 5–10% of cases.
	• Higher platelet count.
	• Higher percentage of blasts in bone marrow.
	• More often diagnosed after the age of 5 years than other subtypes.
	• Although some of the younger children can initially enjoy a relatively unaffected clinical course, *NF1*-mutated JMML is invariably fatal unless allogeneic HSCT can successfully be performed.
2- *PTPN11*-mutated JMML:	• Incidence: 35% of cases.
	• A rapidly fatal disorder unless allogeneic HSCT can successfully be performed.
	• Significantly worse outcome with higher probability of relapse rates when compared with other subtypes.
	• Frequent acquisition of *NF1* haploinsufficiency.
	• The p.(Glu76Lys) is the most frequently observed *PTPN11* finding in JMML.
3- *NRAS*-mutated JMML:	• Incidence: 18% of cases.
	• A heterogeneous course.
	• A considerable percentage of patients relapse after HSCT (typically older children with high levels of HbF).
	• Some patients enjoy an indolent course with spontaneous regression (typically infants or cases with G12S mutation). Clinically, these children are well and show a normal or only slightly elevated HbF.
4- *KRAS*-mutated JMML:	• Incidence: 14% of cases.
	• Most children are diagnosed below the age of 1 year (i.e, infants). They often present with particularly severe disease.
	• Monosomy 7 is frequently noted in leukemic cells.
	• In some cases, an impressive treatment response to azacitidine has been observed.
	• Although Aggressive at presentation, *KRAS*-mutated JMML has a low relapse rate after allogeneic HSCT and may benefit from less intensive preparative regimens.
	• *KRAS*-mutated JMML shares many features with RALD.
5- *CBL*-mutated JMML:	• Incidence: 12 to 18% of cases.
	• Patients display several congenital anomalies that overlap with those observed in NF-1, NS, and Legius syndrome.
	• Self-limiting disease: most children experience spontaneous regression of their myeloproliferation despite the persistence of LOH of the CBL locus in hematopoietic cells.
	• Observation without therapeutic intervention is generally advised, but in some instances grossly enlarged spleens and thrombocytopenia require therapeutic intervention.
	• The value of allogeneic HSCT is uncertain.
	• Frequent occurrence of partial rejection with stable mixed chimerism after allogeneic HSCT.
	• The only recurrent variant is copy-neutral isodisomy (LOH) at 11q23.3 where CBL is located. No other concomitant mutations are found.

Table 2.
Clincal features of genetic subtypes of JMML.

Clinical risk factors:	**1- Age ≥ 2 years.**
	2- Platelet count ≤ 40 x 10⁹/L.
	3- Increased fetal hemoglobin (HbF) for age.
	4- Male sex (in some references).
Molecular risk factors:	**1- Two or more somatic mutations.**
	2- Secondary genetic mutations.
	3- DNA hypermethylation signature defines an aggressive JMML subgroup with high risk of relapse.
	4- *PTPN11* mutation.
	5- Monosomy 7.

Table 3.
Poor prognostic factors.

more somatic mutations at diagnosis have significantly worse event-free and overall survival rates than those with one or no event. In harmony with these findings, the known clinical risk factors predictive of poor outcome (**Table 3**) are only weakly associated with the type of index mutation but they would rather fit patients with two or more underlying somatic mutations.

In addition to the mutations in RAS pathway genes (*PTPN11, NRAS, KRAS, CBL, or NF1*), other driver mutations thought to be the initiating events of JMML have been recently identified such as *RRAS, RRAS2*, or *SH2B3* mutations. *RRAS* and *RRAS2* genes are both members of the RAS GTPase family and hence expanded the spectrum of RAS pathway mutations in JMML. Activating mutations in *RRAS* underlie a phenotype within the RASopathy spectrum. Children with *RRAS*-mutated JMML can have an atypical clinical course with rapid progression to AML [22]. Somatic *RRAS* mutations co-occurred with acquired *NRAS* lesions in atypical JMML characterized by late onset and rapid progression to AML as well.

7. Secondary genetic mutations in JMML

In addition to the initiating canonical RAS pathway mutations, secondary clonal abnormalities were detected in about one-half of the patients. The importance of these mutations relies in how secondary mutations alter the behavior of cells in contrast to cells harboring only the primary lesion. Secondary mutations are often subclonal and may be involved in disease progression rather than initiation of leukemia. It appears that such mutations characterize patients with the highest risk of progression and poor outcome. The acquisition of the second mutation would thus also explain the continuum between RALD and leukemia. The clone harboring the secondary event frequently expands at the time of relapse post HSCT. This phenomenon has important therapeutic implications. Combination of therapies with agents that target the RAS pathway as well as the secondary genetic event could prove more efficacious in the correct genetic context than monotherapy alone.

The secondary mutational events occur inside or outside the canonical RAS pathway axis. They include second hits targeting the RAS pathway (so-called 'RAS double mutants') as well as mutations in *SETBP1, JAK3, SH283*, components of the polycomb repressive complex 2 (like *EZH2* and *ASXL1*), and occasionally, spliceosome genes. Some authors linked differential expression of key regulatory noncoding RNAs, such as let-7100 or miR-150-5p,101 to the various genetic subgroups of JMML [23]. Secondary mutations of *SETBP1* and *JAK3* were the most frequent mutations (around 15% of children) and were presumed to be involved in tumor progression and poor clinical outcomes.

8. Epigenetic landscape of JMML

Aberrant DNA methylation was found to be an initiating event in JMML. This finding has instigated the research in the field of epigenetics and led to the landmark discovery of methylation classes in 2017. In addition, epigenetic modifications are implicated in JMML disease progression and together with established clinical and genetic markers fully recapitulate the clinical and biological heterogeneity of JMML. The genome-wide DNA methylation analysis of JMML patients identified three biologically distinct JMML subgroups [24]:

1. The high-methylation group (HM) was dominated by older children and cases with somatic *PTPN11* mutations and poor clinical outcome.

2. The intermediate methylation group (IM) showed enrichment for somatic *KRAS* mutations and monosomy 7.

3. The low methylation group (LM) is enriched for somatic *NRAS* and *CBL* mutations, as well as for Noonan patients, and has a good prognosis.

The results of all DNA methylome studies in JMML were exceptionally consistent with the fact that DNA hypermethylation is a recurrent feature of JMML cells that confers treatment resistance. The dysregulated genomic DNA methylation is a crucial component of RAS-driven malignant cell transformation proposing a possible functional links between RAS pathway mutational patterns and methylation classes. However, DNA hypermethylation was only weakly associated with the canonical genotypes or cytogenetic aberrations. Instead, it correlated strongly with the known clinical risk factors predictive of aggressive disease and poor outcome, especially older age and increased HbF level (**Table 3**). In fact, DNA methylation status is an independent prognostic factor and better predictor of clinical outcome than JMML genetic types. Frequent hypermethylation in 4 genes (*BMP4, CALCA, CDKN2B*, and *RARB*) were associated with a poor prognosis. Moreover, *RASA4* hypermethylation was related to poor prognosis and disease relapse after HSCT. DNA methylation could be used as a biomarker that can both identify patients who are predicted to fail HSCT as well as those who are most likely to experience spontaneous resolution and could be observed to avoid the acute and late side effects of HSCT [25].

9. Treatment

The heterogeneity of the disease is reflected by the varied clinical outcomes. Although the current standard of care for JMML is allogeneic HSCT, continued controversy exists about identifying those patients who need to be moved quickly to HSCT versus those rare patients who might be observed [26]. The majority of children with *CBL*-mutated JMML and some *NRAS*- mutated patients experience spontaneous disease regression. These children are clinically well with a low HbF. A careful watch-and-wait strategy may be indicated as the treatment of choice. On the other hand, JMML with somatic *PTPN11* mutations appear to represent cases with aggressive biology with a high risk of relapse even after HSCT.

Nevertheless, allogeneic HSCT remains the most effective means of stopping the uncontrolled production of monocytic cells in the majority of patients. If left untreated, survival for most children is less than one year. The predominant cause of JMML-related death is respiratory failure as a result of pulmonary infiltration by leukemic cells (blastic transformation is infrequent in JMML). In fact, HSCT early in the course of disease significantly improved the dismal prognosis of JMML patients. However, the 5-year event-free survival (EFS) rate after HSCT is only 44–53%. Disease recurrence is the most important cause of failure, occurring with a cumulative incidence of 35%. Of note, patients with JMML who transform into AML (defined as >20% blasts in bone marrow) generally have dismal outcomes following HSCT.

Pre-transplant chemotherapy for JMML had no benefit on EFS or overall survival. A variety of pre-HSCT treatments have been employed to control symptoms of JMML (such as high white blood cell count, pulmonary problems, and/or prominent organomegaly) as well as theoretically improve outcomes. However, none of these agents induced durable responses or reduced the relapse rate. The main aim of the pre-HSCT treatments remains to bridge HSCT. Given the current lack of convincing evidence for traditional myelosuppressive chemotherapy pre-HSCT, other treatment modalities has been sought. In particular, molecular classification of cancer based on DNA methylomes has revolutionized the diagnostic and prognostic parameters of JMML and aid our understanding of the mechanistic link between epigenetic dysregulation and resistance to treatment. A DNA methyltransferase–inhibiting azanucleoside is assumed to reverse the epigenetic dysregulation in malignant cells. This has led to a European protocol to employ DNA hypomethylating agents such as azacitidine for therapy in JMML [27]. The first case report of azacitidine for JMML before HSCT was published in 2009. The child achieved a complete clinical, hematologic, cytogenetic (monosomy 7) and molecular (*KRAS* index mutation) remission during eight monthly cycles of 5-day azacitidine. The reduction of *BMP4* promoter DNA methylation preceded the disappearance of leukemic cells, demonstrating the DNA-hypomethylating activity of azacitidine in JMML cells. Although azacytidine may induce complete clinical, cytogenetic and/or molecular remission before allogeneic HSCT, complete remission has not been sustained without transplant. On the other hand, the acceptable toxicity of low-dose azacitidine and its cytoreductive potential make it an attractive option as a bridging therapy before HSCT or as palliation after 1 or more transplants have failed [28].

10. Conclusion and future perspectives

JMML is a puzzling disease with blurring clinical presentation that can commonly mimic a wide variety of other diseases. Overall, the most consistent features of the JMML phenotype are young patient age, splenomegaly and increased synthesis of hemoglobin F (HbF). The molecular basis of JMML is closely linked to Rasopathies, a family of inherited cancer predisposition syndromes characterized by cardiac defects, defective growth, facial dysmorphism and variable cognitive deficits. Defining aberrant RAS signaling transduction pathway as the common denominator linking RASopathies to JMML and a transient JMML-like disease made JMML a fundamentally a disease of uncontrolled hyperactivation of RAS signaling. The identification of RAS pathway mutations in JMML has advanced the understanding of molecular mechanisms underlying the progression from cancer predisposition to neoplasia. Deciphering of the mutational spectrum had led to the classification of JMML into 5 genetic subtypes which have distinctive genotype–phenotype characteristics. However, the clinical outcome of JMML is not completely explained by the clinical and genetic markers which lent the epigenetic landscape of JMML a particular interest. There is hardly any pediatric oncology entity where research has benefited as much from epigenetics as JMML. Genome-wide interrogation of DNA methylation patterns has led to a classification of the disease into three distinct JMML subgroups that have clear pathogenetic and prognostic relationships. The DNA hypermethylation signature is associated with poor clinical outcome and increased risk for relapse following HSCT. Evidence suggests that DNA methylation changes could be used as a potential biomarker in a combined risk stratification algorithm in future clinical trials. Although the clinical activity of azacitidine as a DNA hypomethylating agent appears to be promising, it is unlikely that azacitidine alone have the potential to cure JMML [29]. However, azacitidine as monotherapy is safe and effective in controlling disease both in upfront and relapsed patients in order to proceed to HSCT [30]. In fact, azacitidine is currently the gold standard bridge to HSCT in JMML.

Despite the lack of associated mutations in the genes coding for the GMR, JMML is characterized by aberrant GMR signal transduction. This aberrant signaling is integral in the pathogenesis of JMML that underlines the dysregulated myelopoiesis of the disease. The resultant selective GM-CSF hypersensitivity was exploited as a diagnostic tool for JMML and it is especially useful for those diagnostically challenging cases with RAS pathway mutation-negative JMML. This entity represents the remaining 10% of cases where disease might be due to chromosomal translocations, other gene mutations, specific microRNAs (miRNA) or long non-coding RNAs (lncRNAs) [31]. GMR signal transduction is located upstream to both RAS signaling pathway and the JAK/STAT pathway. STAT5 is recruited to phosphorylated tyrosine residues on the activated β subunit of the GM-CSF receptor, indicating that STAT5 signaling profile reflects JMML hypersensitivity to GM-CSF. The p-STAT5 phospho-specific flowcytometry assay which largely replaced the traditional colony assay had also recently gained promising utility in monitoring the disease status. As disease worsens, a greater percentage of cells get hyper-responsive. Therefore, p-STAT5 phospho-flow signature could prove enticing as a marker of disease progression and indicator of relapse. As JMML lacks tractable markers, both DNA methylation and p-STAT5 phospho-flow signature are potential new armamentarium that could serve as futuristic checkpoints in order to promulgate uniform protocols designed to follow patients on therapy. Interestingly, the shared p-STAT5 phospho-flow signature in JMML, AML M4/M5 and CMML could explain the unique overlap of their clinical features.

So far HSCT represents the only therapy with a clear impact on the outcome of JMML patients. However, HSCT is replete with significant morbidities and deleterious late effects in this young population. The search for more effective and less toxic strategies coincided with advances in molecular oncology that opened up a realm of novel and targeted molecules capable of improving therapeutic tactics in JMML. In particular, scoping into the genetic basis of hyper-responsiveness in JMML could provide a means of assessing the efficacy of emerging kinase inhibitors such as those blocking the RAS (e.g., the oral MEK inhibitor trametinib) or JAK2-signaling pathways for the treatment of this disease. Notably, a combination of drugs targeting two different pathways might be more effective than a single drug. However, the choice of drugs used for treatment should be entirely based on patient's mutation status [32, 33].

Acknowledgements

I would like to express my deep gratitude for the following:

1. Dr. Bushra Mahmood Al-Abri (Hematopathologist) for her valuable contribution in illustrating and editing the peripheral blood and bone marrow figures.

2. Eng. Yasmin Adel (Architect) for designing the RAS pathway as a gear train.

Conflict of interest

The author declares no competing financial interests.

Abbreviations

KMT2A	Histone-lysine N-methyltransferase 2A
JAK	Janus-activated kinase
STAT	signal transducer and activator of transcription factor
p-STAT5	phospho-signal transducer and activator of transcription factor 5
PI 3-kinase	phosphatidylinositol-3 kinase
HSCT	Hematopoietic stem cell transplantation
GM-CSF	Granulocyte-macrophage colony-stimulating factor
GMR	GM-CSF receptor
CFA	hematopoietic colony formation assay
CFU-GM	colony-forming units -granulocyte/macrophage
CBL	Casitas B-lineage lymphoma
HHV-6	Human Herpesvirus 6
CMV	cytomegalovirus
CMML	chronic myelomonocytic leukemia
CML	Chronic myeloid leukemia

Author details

Ashraf Abdullah Saad
Pediatric Hematology, Oncology and HSCT Unit, Sultan Qaboos University Hospital (SQUH), Muscat, Oman

*Address all correspondence to: dr.ashraf123321@gmail.com

References

[1] Satwani P, Kahn J, Dvorak CC. Juvenile myelomonocytic leukemia. *Pediatr Clin North Am*. 2015;62(1):95-106. doi:10.1016/j.pcl.2014.09.003

[2] Ueda S, Sakata N, Muramatsu H, et al. Clinical course of juvenile myelomonocytic leukemia in the blast crisis phase treated by acute myeloid leukemia-oriented chemotherapy and allogeneic hematopoietic stem cell transplantation. *Int J Hematol*. 2014;100(5):502-506. doi:10.1007/s12185-014-1638-3

[3] Locatelli F, Niemeyer CM. How I treat juvenile myelomonocytic leukemia. *Blood*. 2015;125(7):1083-1090. doi:10.1182/blood-2014-08-550483

[4] Swerdlow SH, Campo E, Harris NL, Jaffe ES, Pileri SA, Stein H. *WHO classification of tumours of haematopoietic and lymphoid tissues, fourth edition.* Lyon, France: IARC; 2017

[5] Niemeyer CM. JMML genomics and decisions. *Hematology Am Soc Hematol Educ Program*. 2018;2018(1):307-312. doi:10.1182/asheducation-2018.1.307

[6] Kanayama T, Imamura T, Kawabe Y, et al. KMT2A-rearranged infantile acute myeloid leukemia masquerading as juvenile myelomonocytic leukemia. *Int J Hematol*. 2018;108(6):665-669. doi:10.1007/s12185-018-2522-3

[7] Czuchlewski DR, Reichard KK. Acute myeloid leukemia with t(9;11);MLLT3-KMT2A. In: Vasef M, Auerbach A, editor. Diagnostic Pathology: Molecular Oncology. Philadelphia:Elsev ier;2016:5-114.

[8] Saad AA, Beshlawi I, Zachariah M, Wali Y. KMT2A-MLLT3 AML Masquerading as JMML may Disguise Fatal Leukemia. *Oman Med J*. 2019;34(6):553-555. doi:10.5001/omj.2019.99

[9] Calvo KR, Price S, Braylan RC, et al. JMML and RALD (Ras-associated autoimmune leukoproliferative disorder): common genetic etiology yet clinically distinct entities. *Blood*. 2015;125(18):2753-2758. doi:10.1182/blood-2014-11-567917

[10] Ganapathi, K.A., Schafernak, K.T., Rao, V.K. *et al.* Pediatric myelodysplastic/myeloproliferative neoplasms and related diseases. *J Hematopathol* 8, 159-167 (2015).

[11] Chang TY, Dvorak CC, Loh ML. Bedside to bench in juvenile myelomonocytic leukemia: insights into leukemogenesis from a rare pediatric leukemia. *Blood*. 2014;124(16):2487-2497. doi:10.1182/blood-2014-03-300319

[12] de Vries AC, Zwaan CM, van den Heuvel-Eibrink MM. Molecular basis of juvenile myelomonocytic leukemia. *Haematologica*. 2010;95(2):179-182. doi:10.3324/haematol.2009.016865

[13] Hercus TR, Thomas D, Guthridge MA, et al. The granulocyte-macrophage colony-stimulating factor receptor: linking its structure to cell signaling and its role in disease. *Blood*. 2009;114(7):1289-1298. doi:10.1182/blood-2008-12-164004

[14] Guthridge MA, Stomski FC, Thomas D, et al. Mechanism of activation of the GM-CSF, IL-3, and IL-5 family of receptors. *Stem Cells*. 1998;16(5):301-313. doi:10.1002/stem.160301

[15] Gaipa G, Bugarin C, Longoni D, et al. Aberrant GM-CSF signal transduction pathway in juvenile myelomonocytic leukemia assayed by flow cytometric intracellular STAT5 phosphorylation measurement. *Leukemia*. 2009;23(4):791-793. doi:10.1038/leu.2008.265

[16] Hasegawa D, Bugarin C, Giordan M, et al. Validation of flow cytometric phospho-STAT5 as a diagnostic tool for juvenile myelomonocytic leukemia. *Blood Cancer J*. 2013;3(11):e160. Published 2013 Nov 15. doi:10.1038/bcj.2013.56

[17] Padron E, Painter JS, Kunigal S, et al. GM-CSF-dependent pSTAT5 sensitivity is a feature with therapeutic potential in chronic myelomonocytic leukemia. *Blood*. 2013;121(25):5068-5077. doi:10.1182/blood-2012-10-460170

[18] Kotecha N, Flores NJ, Irish JM, et al. Single-cell profiling identifies aberrant STAT5 activation in myeloid malignancies with specific clinical and biologic correlates. *Cancer Cell*. 2008;14(4):335-343. doi:10.1016/j.ccr.2008.08.014

[19] Niemeyer CM. RAS diseases in children. *Haematologica*. 2014;99(11):1653-1662. doi:10.3324/haematol.2014.114595

[20] Kratz CP, Niemeyer CM, Castleberry RP, et al. The mutational spectrum of PTPN11 in juvenile myelomonocytic leukemia and Noonan syndrome/myeloproliferative disease. *Blood*. 2005;106(6):2183-2185. doi:10.1182/blood-2005-02-0531

[21] Stieglitz E, Taylor-Weiner AN, Chang TY, et al. The genomic landscape of juvenile myelomonocytic leukemia [published correction appears in Nat Genet. 2015 Nov;47(11):1333] [published correction appears in Nat Genet. 2016 Jan;48(1):101]. *Nat Genet*. 2015;47(11):1326-1333. doi:10.1038/ng.3400

[22] Flex E, Jaiswal M, Pantaleoni F, et al. Activating mutations in RRAS underlie a phenotype within the RASopathy spectrum and contribute to leukaemogenesis. *Hum Mol Genet*. 2014;23(16):4315-4327. doi:10.1093/hmg/ddu148

[23] Niemeyer CM, Flotho C. Juvenile myelomonocytic leukemia: who's the driver at the wheel?. *Blood*. 2019;133(10):1060-1070. doi:10.1182/blood-2018-11-844688

[24] Lipka DB, Witte T, Toth R, et al. RAS-pathway mutation patterns define epigenetic subclasses in juvenile myelomonocytic leukemia. *Nat Commun*. 2017;8(1):2126. Published 2017 Dec 19. doi:10.1038/s41467-017-02177-w

[25] Stieglitz E, Mazor T, Olshen AB, et al. Genome-wide DNA methylation is predictive of outcome in juvenile myelomonocytic leukemia. *Nat Commun*. 2017;8(1):2127. Published 2017 Dec 19. doi:10.1038/s41467-017-02178-9

[26] Loh ML. Recent advances in the pathogenesis and treatment of juvenile myelomonocytic leukaemia. *Br J Haematol*. 2011;152(6):677-687. doi:10.1111/j.1365-2141.2010.08525.x

[27] Flotho C. Gene mutations do not operate in a vacuum: the increasing importance of epigenetics in juvenile myelomonocytic leukemia. *Epigenetics*. 2019;14(3):236-244. doi:10.1080/15592294.2019.1583039

[28] Cseh A, Niemeyer CM, Yoshimi A, et al. Bridging to transplant with azacitidine in juvenile myelomonocytic leukemia: a retrospective analysis of the EWOG-MDS study group. *Blood*. 2015;125(14):2311-2313. doi:10.1182/blood-2015-01-619734

[29] Dvorak CC, Loh ML. Juvenile myelomonocytic leukemia: molecular pathogenesis informs current approaches to therapy and hematopoietic cell transplantation. *Front Pediatr*. 2014;2:25. Published 2014 Mar 28. doi:10.3389/fped.2014.00025

[30] Marcu A, Colita A, Radu LE, et al. Single-Center Experience With Epigenetic Treatment for Juvenile Myelomonocytic Leukemia. *Front Oncol*. 2020;10:484. Published 2020 Apr 9. doi:10.3389/fonc.2020.00484

[31] Sonia Meynier and Frédéric Rieux-Laucat, Blood Reviews, https://doi.org/10.1016/j.blre.2020.100652

[32] Kong G, Wunderlich M, Yang D, Ranheim EA, Young KH, Wang J, et al. Combined MEK and JAK inhibition abrogates murine myeloproliferative neoplasm. J Clin Invest 2014;124(6):2762-73.

[33] Tasian SK, Casas JA, Posocco D, Gandre-Babbe S, Gagne AL, Liang G, et al. Mutation-specific signalling profiles and kinase inhibitor sensitivities of juvenile myelomonocytic leukemia revealed by induced pluripotent stem cells. Leukemia 2019;33(1):181-90.

Chapter 3

Reactive Oxygen Species and Metabolic Re-Wiring in Acute Leukemias

Andrew J. Robinson, Richard L. Darley and Alex Tonks

Abstract

Reactive oxygen species (ROS) is the collective term for several oxygen containing free radicals, such as hydrogen peroxide. ROS is important in innate immunity, protein folding in the endoplasmic reticulum and as a cell signalling molecule involved in cellular proliferation, survival, differentiation, and gene expression. ROS has been implicated in both hematopoietic stem cell quiescence and hematopoietic differentiation. Consequently, ROS is of considerable interest as a therapeutic target, with both pro-oxidant and anti-oxidant cellular modulation being explored. Recently, it has been established that increased ROS production in acute myeloid leukemia (AML) leads to increased glycolysis and metabolic reprogramming. It is often stated as a key tenet of the Warburg effect, that transformed cells, including AML, show increased aerobic glycolysis accompanied by increased cellular glucose uptake and lactate secretion. This review will summarize ROS state of the art in acute leukemia and how these reactive molecules re-wire metabolism in cancer cells. The review will focus on what are ROS? What are the sources of ROS in hematopoietic cells and their function and how this relates to the Warburg effect and regulation of metabolic pathways in acute leukemias.

Keywords: NADPH, NOX, ROS, hematopoiesis, HSC, AML

1. Introduction

To maintain hemostasis, new blood cells must be constantly generated to replace those lost through injury, disease, or age. Hematopoiesis, is the process where hematopoietic stem cells (HSC) differentiate into mature blood cells and is tightly regulated by the bone marrow (BM) micro-environment (or stem cell niche; reviewed in [1]), signal transduction pathways (reviewed in [2]), cytokines (reviewed in [3]), transcription factors (reviewed in [4]), epigenetics, (reviewed in [5]) and metabolic pathways (reviewed in [6]). HSCs are rare, constituting only 0.001% of peripheral blood (PB) and 0.05% of BM cells, but are responsible for producing a lifetime supply of blood cells. HSCs are cells that able to durably self-renew whilst also being multipotent. This differentiation is generally considered to occur via several intermediate progenitor cells, ultimately terminating in the specific mature blood cell through a process termed fate restriction or lineage commitment.

IntechOpen

The compartmentalization of HSC, their progenitors and terminally differentiated blood cells, into different stages of differentiation, is traditionally based on the expression of cell surface proteins (**Figure 1**). The recent emergence of single cell technologies such as fluorescent in situ hybridization, high-throughput single-cell quantitative PCR, single cell mass spectrometry and mass cytometry however, have led to re-analysis of these models of hematopoietic differentiation [7]. Discrete progenitor cell populations, as determined by cell surface markers, have been shown to consist of heterogenous populations with different fates [8]. Recently, a study by Velten *et al.*, 2017, using a combination of single cell technologies and xenotransplantation as functional validation, proposed that early hematopoiesis consists of, a cellular continuum of low-primed undifferentiated (CLOUD) hematopoietic stem progenitor cells (HSPC), with simultaneous lineage gene expression for multiple fates [9]. This study suggested that early discrete stable progenitors do not exist, with any lineage determination occurring further downstream than originally presumed.

Regardless of provenance, leukemogenesis is characterized by a block in differentiation and an accumulation of immature white blood cell blasts with a rapid increase in these blasts, characteristic of the acute leukemias. Acute lymphoblastic leukemia (ALL) and acute myeloid leukemia (AML) are heterogenous diseases with a block in lymphoid or myeloid differentiation, respectively. They occur due to one or more genetic insults. Whilst ALL is predominantly a disease of children (80%), with a greater than 90% 5 y survival rate [10], in adults long term survival stands at only 30–40% [11]. AML in contrast is primarily a disease of the elderly, and like adult ALL it's 5 y survival rate is around 30%, however this falls in the over

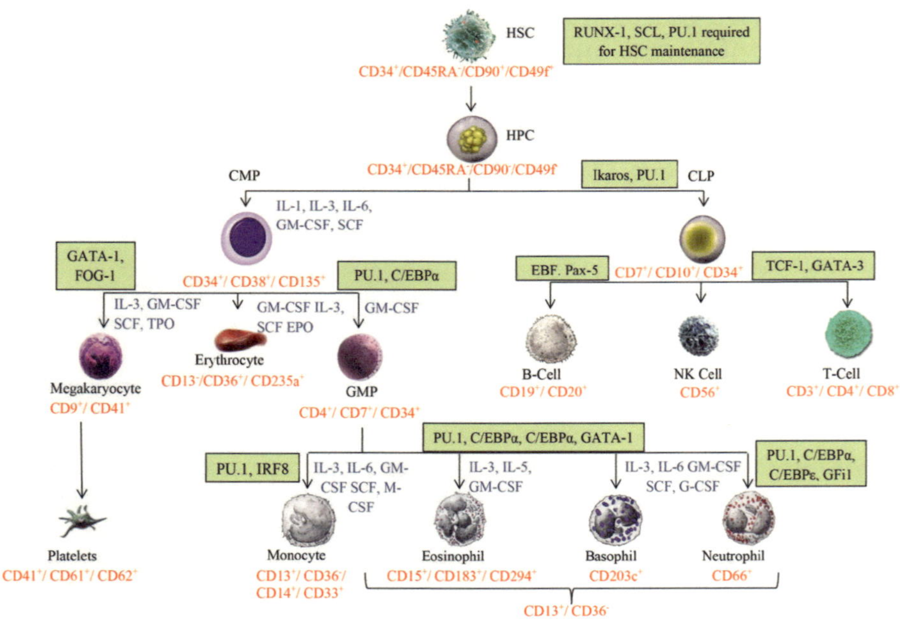

Figure 1.
Human hematopoiesis. Schematic diagram showing classical model of hematopoietic lineage commitment, with phenotypical cell surface markers (red), transcription factors determining differentiation (green box) and growth factors involved in myelopoiesis (blue). Hematopoietic stem cell (HSC), cluster of differentiation (CD), hematopoietic progenitor cell (HPC), common myeloid progenitor (CMP), common lymphoid progenitor (CLP), interleukin (IL), granulocyte macrophage (GM) colony-stimulating-factor (CSF), stem cell factor (SCF), thrombopoietin (TPO), erythropoietin (EPO), granulocyte myeloid progenitor (GMP), runt-related transcription factor 1 (RUNX1), transcription factor stem cell leukemia (SCL), ccaat enhancer binding proteins (C/EBP), friend of GATA protein 1 (FOG-1).

60's to a particularly bleak 10% [12]. In ALL, recent advances for example in the use of tyrosine kinase inhibitors and CAR-T cell therapy, have started to suggest improvements to overall survival [10]. However, in patients fit enough to tolerate chemotherapy, the standard treatment for AML since 1973 has been a seven-day continuous intravenous infusion of cytarabine (Ara-C) (100–200 mg/m^2) and 3 daily doses of daunorubicin (45–90 mg/m^2), sometimes followed by allogeneic or autologous stem cell transplantation, and despite some recent advances (reviewed in [13, 14]), current treatments appear to have reached their efficacious limits and new therapies are required.

One potential therapeutic opportunity involves exploiting the metabolic differences that exist between malignant and non-malignant cells [15]. Differences that, in AML at least, appear exacerbated by cellular levels of reactive oxygen species (ROS) [16].

2. Reactive oxygen species

ROS is the collective term for several oxygen containing free radicals and other reactive molecules, such as hydrogen peroxide (H_2O_2). Physiologically, ROS are initially generated via the univalent reduction of molecular oxygen which generates superoxide ($O2^{\bullet-}$). Superoxide (t1/2 = 1 μs) subsequently dismutates to H_2O_2 (t1/2 = 1 ms) [17], either spontaneously or via the catalytic action of the enzyme superoxide dismutase (SOD), or reacts with other ROS molecules, forming a variety of other ROS (**Figure 2**). Functionally, ROS is important in innate immunity,

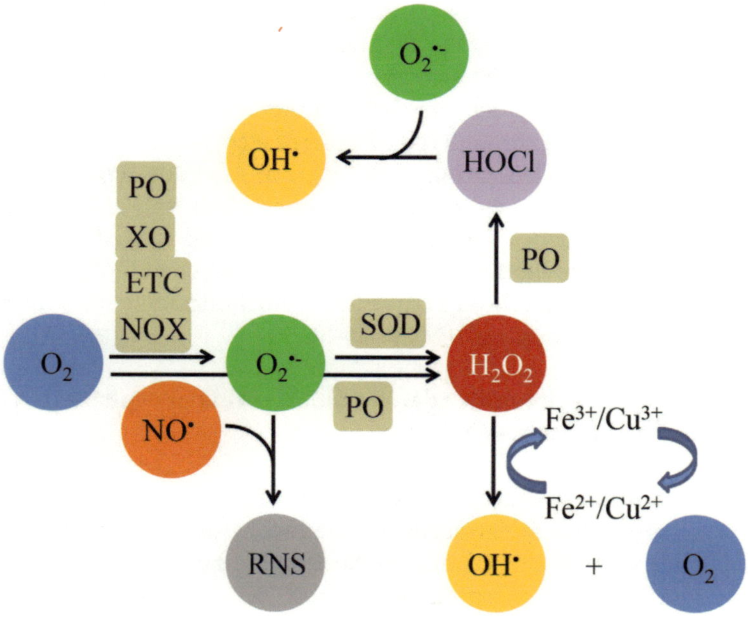

Figure 2.
Formation of reactive oxygen species (ROS). Diatomic oxygen (O_2) is univalently reduced by peroxisomes (PO), xanthine oxidase (XO), the electron transport chain (ETC), or NADPH oxidase (NOX) to generate superoxide ($O_2^{\bullet-}$). PO may also reduce O_2 directly to form H_2O_2. $O_2^{\bullet-}$ may then dismutate to H_2O_2 either spontaneously or through the enzymatic action of superoxide dismutase (SOD). Hydroxyl radicals ($OH^\bullet$) may then be formed from H_2O_2 via the formation of hypochlorous radical (HOCl) in the PO, or via Fenton chemistry. Reactive nitrogen species (RNS) may also be formed through the reaction of nitric oxide radical ($NO^\bullet$) with $O_2^{\bullet-}$.

protein folding in the endoplasmic reticulum and as a cell signalling molecule involved in cellular proliferation, survival, differentiation and gene expression [18].

There are several sources of cellular ROS, including the mitochondria, the nicotinamide adenine dinucleotide phosphate (NADPH) oxidase family of enzymes (NOX), the cytochrome P450 enzymes, peroxisomes and the metabolic enzyme xanthine oxidase (XO).

2.1 Sources of ROS: electron transport chain

Generation of ROS by the mitochondria is primarily a function of 'electron leakage' from the electron transport chain (ETC), however, mitochondrial ROS may also be generated as a result of numerous enzymes including monoamine oxidase, cytochrome b5 reductase, glycerol-3-phosphate dehydrogenase, aconitase, pyruvate dehydrogenase and α-ketoglutarate dehydrogenase (reviewed in [19]). Mitochondrial ROS production resulting from the ETC generates $O_2^{\bullet-}$, and is thought to occur as result of one of three mechanisms. The first mechanism is a consequence of a high NADH/NAD^+ ratio, and results from oxygen interacting with fully reduced FMN. Mitochondrial ROS generated by this mechanism has been observed due to mitochondrial mutation, physiological damage such as ischemia or aging, and only small amounts of ROS are thought to be generated via these mechanisms in normally respiring cells [20]. The second mechanism occurs when there is a high level of reduced co-enzyme Q (CoQH2) in complex II, which in the presence of a high proton motive force generated by the proton pump, force electrons back into complex I in a process known as reverse electron transport (RET). Whilst RET generated ROS has also been implicated in diseases such as ischemia, it is now also thought to be involved as a cell signalling molecule in metabolic adaptation, myeloid differentiation and response to bacterial infection [21]. The third mechanism of ROS generation by the ETC occurs at complex III and has also been implicated in ROS signalling. The formation of $O_2^{\bullet-}$ occurs at the ubiquinol oxidation centre (Qo) site of the cytochrome bc1 complex, in which fully oxidized CoQ supports formation of $O_2^{\bullet-}$, through the transfer of electrons from reduced heme b1 to molecular oxygen [22]. Generation of $O_2^{\bullet-}$ by complex I and II occurs exclusively in the mitochondrial matrix, whereas $O_2^{\bullet-}$ generated by complex III also occurs in the intermembrane space. $O_2^{\bullet-}$ generated in the mitochondrial matrix is rapidly converted to H_2O_2 by mitochondrial SOD (Mn-SOD), whereas $O_2^{\bullet-}$ generated in the intermembrane space travels through the outer mitochondrial membrane prior to conversion to H_2O_2 by cytosolic SOD (Cu/Zn-SOD).

2.2 Sources of ROS: nicotinamide adenine dinucleotide phosphate (NADPH) oxidase family of enzymes (NOX)

Whilst mitochondrial oxidative phosphorylation is a major source of intracellular ROS, the main source of extracellular ROS involves the nicotinamide adenine dinucleotide phosphate (NADPH) oxidase family of enzymes (NOX). The NOX family of enzymes comprise of seven members, NOX1–5 and dual oxidase (DUOX) 1 and 2. NOX enzymes are transmembrane proteins that transfer electrons from NADPH to molecular oxygen, generating $O_2^{\bullet-}$ (or H_2O_2), which can then be converted to other forms of ROS. Different NOX isoforms share conserved structural features comprising of six helical transmembrane domains (TM) (with helix III and helix V containing two heme-binding histidines), and a C-terminus cytosolic domain (DH), which allows binding of FAD and NADPH (**Figure 3**). Difficulties in obtaining suitable levels of NOX proteins mean that to date relatively little crystal structure data is available. However, a recently published report [23], has

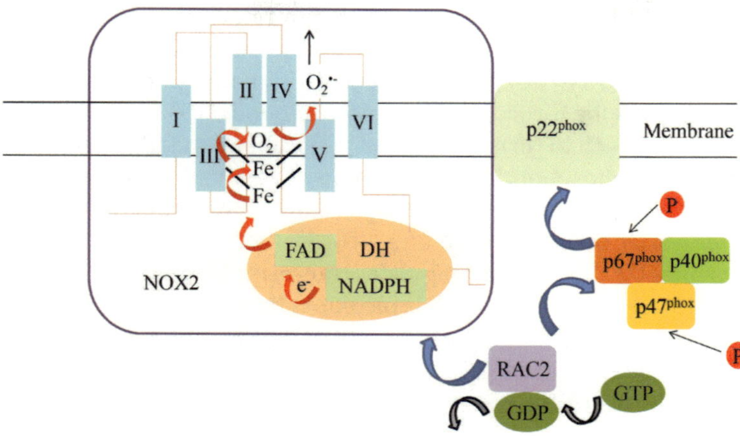

Figure 3.
Generation of superoxide ($O_2^{\bullet-}$) by NADPH Oxidase (NOX). Schematic diagram showing the major structural features of NOX2, it's activation by phosphorylation (P) of p67phoxand p47phox and the assembly of the major subunits of the NOX complex, and the generation of superoxide via electron transfer from NADPH to flavin adenine dinucleotide (FAD) to heme groups to diatomic oxygen. Guanosine triphosphate (GTP), guanosine diphosphate (GDP), homology domain (DH), RAS-related C3 botulinum toxin substrate 2 (Rac2).

elucidated the structure of the TM and DH domains (common to all NOX isoforms) of *Cylindrospermum stagnale* NOX5 in complex with FAD. In this structure, the six transmembrane helices of TM domain form a pyramidal shape with the base on the cytosolic side, a N-terminus α-helix runs parallel to the cytosolic side of the membrane and the heme groups sit in cavities formed by helices II–V, so that one is positioned near the cytosolic side of the membrane (heme 1) and the other on the outer side (heme 2). The DH domain, located on the cytosolic side, contains two pockets, one for FAD binding and one for NADPH binding. The FAD is positioned so that the flavin is in direct contact with heme 1 of the TM, to promote interdomain electron transfer. The proposed mechanism of electron transfer then involves NADPH donating its electron to FAD, which in turn donates an electron to heme 1 and then to heme 2 via Trp378 (equating to Phe 215 in human NOX2, Phe 200 in human NOX4 and Val 362 in human NOX5) of the loop between helix II and III of the TM, before reduction of molecular oxygen, via a final electron transfer step generates $O_2^{\bullet-}$ (**Figure 3**).

From a metabolic perspective, one source of NOX2 activation results when cells experience intermittent hypoxia. Under this condition activation of the metabolic enzyme XO, an enzyme important in the catabolism of purines and a major source of cellular ROS, occurs [24]. XO activation leads to increased ROS, which induces Ca^{2+} activation of protein kinase C, an enzyme important in cell signalling, migration of $p47^{phox}$ and $p67^{phox}$ to the cell membrane, resulting in activation of the NOX2 complex (**Figure 3**). Finally it is important to note, from a cell signalling perspective, that extracellular H_2O_2 (which is rapidly formed from $O_2^{\bullet-}$) is readily transported across the cell membrane via the transmembrane water permeable channel protein family of aquaporins [25, 26].

3. Role of ROS on normal hematopoiesis

ROS has been implicated in both HSC quiescence and hematopoietic differentiation. HSC reside in the bone marrow and their quiescence is known to be negatively regulated by ROS. Forkhead box O (FOXO) transcription factors are involved in cell-cycle arrest and apoptosis and are activated in response to oxidative stress whereupon they translocate to the nucleus [27]. Translocation of FOXO4 to the nucleus has been shown to be a function of redox signalling, where oxidation of cys-239 by ROS mediates the formation of disulphide bonds with nuclear import receptor transportin-1, which in turn allows nuclear localization [28]. FOXO deactivation occurs as a result of phosphorylation in response to activation of the regulatory cell cycle PI3K/AKT/mTOR pathway, resulting in their export from the nucleus and subsequent degradation in the cytoplasm [29]. Studies in murine HSC have shown that deletion of FOXO3a, which upregulates transcription of Mn-SOD [30], results in decreased HSC renewal [31] which is mediated by the tumor suppressor protein ataxia-telangiectasia mutated (ATM) and is accompanied by elevated ROS levels and myeloid lineage expansion [32]. Deletion of ATM in mice resulted in BM failure which was restored following treatment with antioxidants [33]. In a different study, isolation of murine HSC into ROS high and ROS low populations showed that the ROS low population maintained self-renewal capacity following serial transplantations, whilst the self-renewal capacity of the ROS high population was exhausted following the third serial transplantation. Treatment of the ROS high HSC with the antioxidant N-acetyl cysteine (NAC), the p38 inhibitor SB203508 or rapamycin (a mTOR inhibitor), restored self-renewal activity [34]. Interestingly, the ROS high population in this study also exhibited a decreased ability to adhere to cells containing calcium sensing receptors, whilst NOX generated ROS has additionally been implicated in osteoclast differentiation in human mesenchymal cells, further emphasizing a potential regulatory role of ROS, in the BM niche [35].

Whilst these increased ROS levels are associated with HSC losing quiescence, it has also been shown, in the human megakaryocytic cell line MO7e, that hematopoietic cytokines, such as granulocyte macrophage-colony stimulating factor, interleukin-3, stem cell factor and thrombopoietin all increase ROS levels [36]. In megakaryopoiesis, ROS has been shown to increase platelet production and maturation in the chronic myeloid leukemia (CML) cell line MEG-01 and primary human megakaryocytes [37], which in murine models is mediated by the transcription factor NF-E2 [38]. Following lineage commitment, megakaryocyte progenitors undergo endomitosis (chromosomal replication in the absence of cell division), which in murine cells is potentially mediated by NOX1-derived ROS [39]. In human HSC, NOX-derived ROS has also been shown to be crucial for megakaryocyte differentiation via activation of ERK, AKT and JAK2 signalling pathways [40], whilst another study revealed the importance of cytochrome P450 2E1-generated ROS in megakaryocyte differentiation in human HSC [41]. As noted above, increased ROS in HSC has been associated with expanded myelopoiesis. Interestingly, a recent study using murine CMP, showed that higher levels of ROS impeded megakaryopoiesis, instead directing differentiation of CMP into GMP [42]. Finally, ROS has also been shown to induce differentiation of the promonocytic cell line, U937, into macrophages [43], and the differentiation of primary human monocytes into dendritic cells [44].

4. Role of ROS on solid tumors and leukemia development

One of the first studies implicating ROS in carcinogenesis was performed in mice subcutaneously injected with C3H mouse fibroblasts, that had been previously cultured *in vitro* with neutrophils stimulated with 12-O-tetradecanoylphorbol-13-acetate (TPA) stimulated or unstimulated or with the ROS generating enzyme XO and hypoxanthine. In this study approximately 20% of mice treated with these cells developed tumors within 13–22 weeks compared to none of the control mice [45].

In 1991, analysis of H_2O_2 production in human melanoma, colon, pancreatic, neuroblastoma, breast and ovarian cancer cell lines, revealed constitutively active H_2O_2 production over a 4 h period, generating H_2O_2 levels similar to those observed in TPA stimulated neutrophils, suggesting increased ROS production may be a feature of transformation [46]. Later, studies in patients with liver disease suggested ROS plays a part in hepatocarcinogenesis [47], and levels of Cu/Zn-SOD are significantly lower in hepatoma tissue than normal human liver tissue [48]. Further, homozygous deletion of Cu/Zn-SOD in mice results in decreased lifespan, with 70% developing hepatocarcinoma or benign nodular hyperplasia [49], whilst homozygous deletion of Mn-SOD in mice is lethal within two weeks of birth [50]. In the same study, heterozygous deletion of Mn-SOD resulted in increased incidence of hemangioma and adenocarcinoma and significant increases in the incidence of lymphoma. Currently, elevated ROS levels have been reported in many solid tumors and the role they play in tumorigenesis is complex and multifaceted (reviewed in [51]).

In leukemia, a study which collected blood samples from ALL and CML patients samples and compared them with normal blood samples showed elevated levels of ROS in both ALL and CML patients [52], whilst elevated levels of NOX generated ROS, are observed, alongside increased proliferation in both AML models and AML patient samples when compared with healthy controls [53]. Reactions of ROS with DNA can generate numerous oxidised bases, including 8-hydroxy-2-deoxyguanosine (8-OHdG) which causes G:C to T:A DNA transversions (reviewed in [54]). Increased levels of 8-OHdG have been observed in patients with breast cancer [55], gastric carcinomas [56], lung cancer [57] and colorectal cancer [58]. In leukemia, a study of 116 Chinese children with either ALL or AML revealed significantly elevated levels of 8-OHdG, whilst 8-OHdG levels were also significantly elevated in relapsed AML adult patients [59].

As a signalling molecule, ROS can lead to hyperactivation of the PI3K pathway, a common feature of many cancers, resulting in increased cell survival, VEGF production, secretion of MMP (reviewed in [60]) and inactivation of FOXO [32]. In AML, constitutive activation of the PI3K/AKT pathway is frequently observed [61, 62], however the role of FOXO is less clear. A recent study revealed that FOXO1 expression in osteoblasts mediated β-catenin initiated AML [63], whilst a study of AML patient samples showed that 40% exhibited FOXO activation, that upon inhibition resulted in myeloid differentiation and AML cell death [64]. Additionally, in both CML and AML the BCR-ABL fusion protein and FMS-like tyrosine kinase receptor 3 internal tandem duplications (FLT3-ITD) have been shown to lead to phosphorylation of AKT resulting in increased activation of NOX, and increased ROS production (reviewed in [65]), which may in turn reinforce PI3K/AKT activation.

5. Metabolism and cancer

Broadly defined, cellular metabolism involves a series of catabolic or anabolic chemical reactions which generate or use energy as part of this process. In chemotrophs this energy is obtained through the oxidation of nutrients, with the energy typically stored in the form of ATP. Whilst in higher organisms a plethora of enzymatically catalyzed metabolic reactions occur, which are all part of different interconnecting metabolic pathways with multitudinous feedback mechanisms. These pathways are evolutionarily highly conserved with the citric acid cycle, for example, essentially a feature in all terrestrial life. There are three main classes of molecules involved in metabolism; carbohydrates, proteins and lipids that are either catabolized to generate energy or energy stores or used by anabolic pathways in the synthesis of, for example, nucleotides and structural molecules such as cell membranes. In mammals, a triumvirate of glycolysis, citric acid cycle and the ETC are central to the generation of ATP, with glycolysis and the citric acid cycle contributing 2 ATP molecules each and the ETC generating up to 34 ATP molecules in a process collectively termed aerobic respiration (reviewed in [66]).

Given the skew towards ATP production in the ETC, Otto Warburg's observation in 1956 that aerobic glycolysis was a hallmark feature of cancer cells [15], was initially attributed to being the result of defective mitochondria in malignant cells, and initially raised little interest. However, this hypothesis is now known in most cases to be incorrect (reviewed in [67]) and instead, it has been shown that mitochondrial respiration is often necessary in tumorigenesis [68]. However, given its ubiquity and despite its inefficiency when compared with ETC, it is clear that the phenomenon of increased aerobic glycolysis (eponymously titled 'The Warburg Effect'), must offer cancer cells some competitive advantage, although its exact ontology remains unclear. One hypothesis contends that whilst inefficient, aerobic glycolysis generates ATP at a rate 10–100 times faster than oxidative phosphorylation, therefore supplying cancer cells with energy at a faster rate. This increased glycolytic flux could then, potentially generate more nucleotides, amino acids and lipids for biosynthesis as well as generating the reducing agent NADPH, to deal with the increased levels of ROS common in many cancer cells [69]. Alternatively, increases in excreted lactate as a result of aerobic glycolysis would likely generate a more acidic microenvironment, breaking down stromal membrane structures and potentially increasing cancer cell motility and metastasis [70].

5.1 NADPH: a link between ROS and metabolism in cancer

It has been shown that activation of the tumor suppressor protein ATM by ROS promotes glucose-6-phosphate dehydrogenase (G-6-PD) activity, the first step of the pentose phosphate pathway (PPP), which in turn generates NADPH [71]. Given that major cellular antioxidant systems, ultimately rely on NADPH to provide their reducing power, it is perhaps not surprising that ROS in both normal and aberrant cellular processes is inextricably linked with metabolism. In the cytosol, NADPH is primarily generated through the PPP, whilst a number of mechanisms exist for mitochondrial NADPH generation [72], which include the serine synthesis pathway (SSP) (via the folate cycle) [73] and the action of the citric acid cycle enzyme isocitrate dehydrogenase (IDH). IDH1 and IDH2 are commonly mutated in AML [74], although in this context NADPH is consumed, and the D-2-hydroxyglutarate generated leads to stabilization of the hypoxia regulator, hypoxia inducible factor alpha (HIF-1α) [75].

HIF-1α as a target of ROS is controversial [76], however it is overexpressed in many cancers where it induces expression of numerous glycolytic genes. The ROS regulated transcription factor nuclear-related factor 2 (NRF2) has also been shown to modulate metabolism in lung cancer cell lines, through the upregulation of enzymes involved in the NADPH production, notably G-6-PD, IDH1 and malic enzyme 1 [77] and high NRF2 levels have previously been reported in AML [78]. Furthermore, the tumor suppressor protein TP53 is also important in regulating metabolism. Homozygous deletion of TP53 in mice results in decreased oxygen consumption arising from decreased mitochondrial respiration [79]. TP53 expression has been shown to inhibit, both glucose transporter (GLUT) 1 and 4 and the glycolytic enzyme phosphoglycerate mutase (PGAM) (reviewed in [80]) leading to decreased glycolysis and potentially increased metabolism via the PPP and SSP. Finally, TP53 also upregulates the apoptosis regulator (TIGAR) an enzyme which has an active domain similar to 6-Phosphofructo-2-kinase/fructoste-2,6-bisphosphatase

(PFKFB). TIGAR catalyzes the reaction of fructose-2,6-bisphosphate (F-2,6-BP) to fructose-6-phosphate (F-6-P), which inhibits glycolysis, redirects metabolites into the PPP, generating NADPH [81].

5.2 ROS regulation of metabolic pathways

Changes of cellular ROS levels in both normal signalling as well cell signalling following cellular transformation result in changes in numerous signalling pathways controlling multiple cellular functions including growth, proliferation and differentiation. A number of these signalling pathways, exercise regulatory control over various metabolic pathways, which in turn modulate ROS levels via several feedback mechanisms (**Figure 4**). In leukemia, mutations in the *RAS* gene are present in about 15% of hematological malignancies [82]. RAS activates the PI3K/AKT/mTOR pathway which promotes nucleotide biosynthesis and lipid synthesis (reviewed in [83]) as well as HIF-1α, which upregulate glycolysis via the activation of numerous glycolytic genes. In addition to HIF-1α, other ROS activated transcription factors are important in metabolic regulation such as STAT3, which has been shown to promote glycolysis in hepatocellular carcinoma cell lines [84], FOXO3A, which inhibits glycolysis via activation of tuberous sclerosis 1 protein [85] and NF-κB which was shown to upregulate GLUT3 in mouse embryonic fibroblasts [86].

Nuclear localization of the glycolytic enzyme pyruvate kinase muscle 2 (PKM2) is also ROS mediated, where it acts as a co-factor in the activation of the transcription factor, c-MYC. RAS also activates c-MYC which is overexpressed in greater than 50% of human cancers and c-MYC has been shown to activate glycolysis via the upregulation of GLUT, the glycolytic enzymes hexokinase (HK),

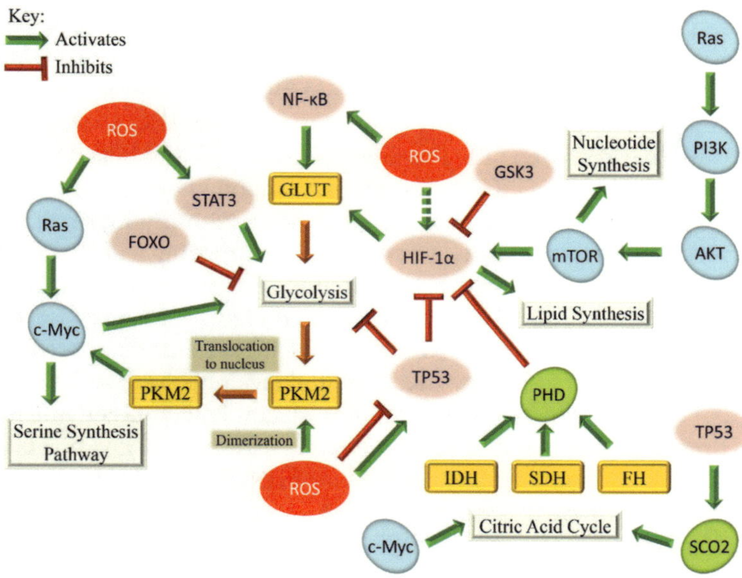

Figure 4.
Regulation of metabolic pathways. Schematic illustration outlining some of the regulatory mechanism involved in glycolysis and other key metabolic pathways. Transcription factors are in pink and signalling pathways in blue. Reactive oxygen species (ROS), forkhead box O (FOXO), pyruvate kinase muscle 2 (PKM2), signal transducer and activator of transcription (STAT), nuclear factor kappa-light-chain-enhancer of activated B-cells (NF-κB), glucose transporter (GLUT) hypoxia inducible factor-1 alpha (HIF-1α), tumour suppressor protein 53 (TP53), glycogen synthase kinase 3β (GSK-3β), isocitrate dehydrogenase (IDH), succinate dehydrogenase (SDH), fumarate hydratase (FH), protein kinase B (AKT), mammalian target of rapamycin (mTOR), phosphoinositide 3-kinase (PI3K), synthesis of cytochrome c oxidase 2 (SCO2) and prolyl-hydroxylase domain (PHD).

phosphoglucose isomerase (PGI), phosphofructokinase (PFK), glyceraldehyde-3-phosphate dehydrogenase (GAPDH), phosphoglycerate kinase (PGK), PKM2, as well as lactate dehydrogenase A (LDHA), pyruvate dehydrogenase kinase 1 (PDK1) and PFKFB3 (reviewed in [87]). Increased glutaminolysis is also a target of c-MYC, which upregulates the glutamine transporter ASCT2 and a key enzyme glutaminase. Additionally, c-MYC was shown to upregulate both phosphoglycerate dehydrogenase (PHGDH) which catalyzes the first step of the SSP, serine hydroxy-methyltransferase, part of the folate cycle as well as several genes involved in fatty acid metabolism and the citric acid cycle (reviewed in [67]). In contrast TP53 is known to inhibit glycolysis through inhibition of GLUT1, GLUT4 and PGAM and through activation of TIGAR and synthesis of cytochrome c oxidase 2 (SCO2). Inhibition of glycolysis also occurs due to the regulatory role of miRNA. For example, miR-195-5p inhibits GLUT3, miR-143 inhibits HK2 and miR-155 inhibits HIF-1α. Furthermore, TP53 induces miR-34a which suppresses HK1, HK2, GPI and PDK1, as well as sirtuin 1, which activates FOXO1, NF-κB and in a positive feedback loop TP53 (reviewed in [80]).

5.3 Metabolism and leukemia

Given the role that ROS plays in regulating metabolism, it is not surprising that expression of nearly all enzymes associated with glycolysis have been shown to be altered in solid tumors, a pattern also observed in leukemia. In ALL, micro-array analysis showed significant upregulation of PFK as well as the glucose transporters GLUT1 and GLUT4 in pediatric B-ALL samples [88], whilst deletion of GLUT1 in primary human B-ALL cells suppressed leukemic progression *in vivo* [89]. In AML, upregulation of *GLUT1* mRNA [90] and the fructose transporter *GLUT5* [91] have also been reported to be associated with poor outcome in AML patients. Furthermore, NOX generated ROS has previously been reported to modulate cellular glucose uptake through increased GLUT1 activity, in leukemic cell lines [92]. In Philadelphia$^+$ ALL (Ph$^+$ALL) GLUT5 has been found to be upregulated at both the mRNA and protein level [93]. Song *et al* have identified HK2 overexpression as a feature of AML patients who failed to show remission [90], whilst decreased proliferation in the AML cell line, KG-1, was observed upon knock-down of PGI with shRNA [94]. The HK inhibitors 2-deoxy-D-glucose and 3-bromopyruvate have both been shown to be cytotoxic in AML patient samples harboring a FLT3-ITD mutation both alone and in combination with sorafenib [90, 95]. In chronic lymphocytic leukemia (CLL), a study by Ryland et al., 2013 showed increased expression of glyceraldehyde phosphate dehydrogenase (GAPDH) in CLL patients compared to healthy controls [96]. Proteomic studies revealed elevated levels of aldolase A (ALDO(A)), ALDO(C) and enolase 1 (ENO1) in the chemoresistant leukemia cell line K562/A02 when compared with parental K562 cells and in the case of ENO1 this was confirmed by western blot [97]. Elevated levels of ENO2 have also been reported in patients with ALL where it is associated with lower overall survival [98], whilst PGAM is upregulated in both AML and CML patient samples [99]. LDH is a tetramer which exists as five isoforms, comprising of two subunits LDHA and LDHB in different combinations and encoded by the LDHA and LDHB genes [100], with LDHA strongly catalyzing pyruvate to lactate and LDHB preferentially catalyzing the reverse reaction. In B-ALL, mRNA expression levels of *LDHB* were shown to be decreased [88], suggesting increased lactate production, whilst more recently increased serum levels of LDH were found in patients with B-ALL in conjunction with increased levels of total oxidant status and decreased total anti-oxidant status [101]. Another recent study involving 204 patients with acute leukemia's also reported that LDH plasma levels were significantly elevated compared to healthy controls and were also increased in relapse patients compared to those in complete remission [102]. Recently, it was shown that ROS dependent proliferative increases observed in hematopoietic models [103] were also accompanied by increased glucose uptake and expression of the regulatory glycolytic enzyme PFKFB3 [53], whilst downregulation of this enzyme suppressed growth both *in vivo* and *in vitro* [16]. This study also reported that metabolomic analysis comparing AML patient samples with high/low levels of ROS, which showed significantly elevated levels of glucose, glucose-6-phosphate (G-6-P) and F-6-P in the ROS high patients. Another metabolomic study involving serum from 400 AML patients compared with 446 healthy controls, identified elevated levels of the glycolytic intermediates 3-phosphoglycerate (3-PG), pyruvate and lactate as conferring a poor prognosis for survival [104]. Interestingly, a recent study showed that the bromodomain and extra-terminal protein inhibitor JQ1, which has shown promise in ALL by targeting c-myc, downregulates expression of HK2, PKM2 and LDHA both at the transcriptional and protein level [105].

The citric acid cycle is a series of metabolic reactions involving oxidation/reduction reactions, which generate nicotinamide adenine dinucleotide (NAD)H and flavin adenine dinucleotide (FAD)H via the transfer of hydride ions, thus providing electrons for the ETC which is a major source of cellular ROS (reviewed in [106]). Mutations of IDH, which catalyzes the decarboxylation of isocitrate to alpha-ketoglutarate are frequently reported in AML (reviewed in [107]). Characterization of the inhibitor AG-221, which has been shown to inhibit mutant IDH2 in AML cells *in vitro* and *in vivo* and is currently undergoing phase I/II clinical trials [108], as is the IDH1 inhibitor, AG-120 [109]. A metabolomic study which examined a cohort of 183 patients with *de novo* AML matched with 232 healthy controls showed significant differences in citrate levels between AML patients and controls [110]. In pediatric ALL a recent metabolomic study revealed increased metabolites of glycolysis, the citric acid cycle and the PPP in patients testing positive for measurable residual disease compared to those testing negative [111]. Interestingly use of nicotinamide phosphoribosyltransferase (NAMPT) inhibitors on ALL cell lines and patient samples showed cytotoxicity *in vitro*. NAMPT is a key enzyme in the synthesis of the oxidizing agent NAD^+, in both glycolysis and the citric acid cycle.

The SSP branches from the glycolytic pathway at the glycolytic intermediate 3-PG, where it is converted into 3-phosphohydroxypyruvate by the enzyme PHGDH, followed by conversion to phosphoserine by phosphoserine aminotransferase 1 and finally to serine by the action of the enzyme phosphoserine phosphatase (reviewed in [73]). Regulation of the SSP is achieved through 2-phosphoglycerate (2-PG) which activates PHGDH whilst serine activates the tetrameric form of PKM2 leading to increased glycolysis and decreased levels of 2-PG. Importantly serine can enter the folate cycle, which provides another route for the generation of NADPH, which has been shown to contribute to tumor growth *in vivo* [112]. Whilst overexpression of PHGDH has been reported in melanomas, colorectal and breast cancers, little has been published from a leukemia perspective. Knock-down of PHGDH has been shown to inhibit the growth of the leukemia cell line, HL-60 [113], and in multiple myeloma increased expression of PHGDH led to increased SSP activity and antioxidant capacity in cells resistant to treatment with the proteasome inhibitor bortezomib [114].

The PPP generate nucleotides for biosynthesis and is a major source of cellular NADPH, an important cellular antioxidant. The first step involves the dehydrogenation of G-6-P to 6-phosphogluconolactone (6-PG) catalyzed by G-6-PD and the conversion of $NADP^+$ to [115]. Gluconolactonase catalyzes the hydrolysis of 6-PG to 6-phosphogluconate, which is then catalyzed by 6-phosphogluconate dehydrogenase (6-PGD) to ribulose-5-phosphate (Ru-5-P) alongside the generation of a second NADPH. Ru-5-P can then be converted into ribose-5-phosphate (R-5-P) by the enzymatic action of ribulose-5-phosphate isomerase. R-5-P can then be used in the synthesis of nucleotides. Alternatively, where redox homeostasis and not nucleotide synthesis is the major requirement of the cell Ru-5-P can be catalyzed by ribulose-5-phosphate epimerase, into xyulose-5-phosphate (X-5-P) and via a series of further metabolic reactions back into the glycolytic intermediates F-6-P and glyceraldehyde-3-phosphate. G-6-PD is the rate limiting step of the PPP and is regulated by the NADP+/NADPH ratio, RAS/PI3K signalling and phosphorylation by Src, whilst 6-PGD is inhibited by 3-PG [99]. In cancer, aberrant RAS signalling or activation of Src can promote activation of the PPP. In AML, a recent study showed upregulation of *G-6-PD* mRNA in approximately 60% of patients, although it was not correlated with overall survival or relapse [116]. Targeting of xenograft mice injected with the leukemic cell line K562, with the antimalarial drug dihydroartemisinin and the 6-PGD inhibitor Physicon resulted in decreased tumor growth, whilst primary leukemia cells isolated from the PB of AML patients showed significantly decreased viability, with no toxicity observed in hematopoietic cells isolated from healthy individuals [117]. A metabolomic study comparing primary AML samples with either high or low levels of ROS, have also shown increased levels of the PPP metabolites sedoheptulose-7-phosphate and Ru-5-P in the samples with higher ROS levels [16]. Another study, using both AML cell lines and patient material, showed increased glucose metabolism and increased flux through the PPP, alongside increased *G-6-PD* mRNA expression [118]. Importantly, this study showed that use of the G-6-PD inhibitor 6-aminonictoinamide (6-AN) in AML cell lines induced both *in vitro* and *in vivo* cytotoxicity, and induced apoptosis in primary AML cells but not normal HPCs. In B-ALL, redirection of carbon from the glycolytic pathway to the PPP by the serine/threonine-protein phosphatase 2A (PP2A), has been shown to occur to combat cellular oxidative stress. Synergistic inhibition of G-6-PD by 6-AN and PP2A inhibitor LB100 induced cell death in patient derived Ph$^+$ALL [119].

Lipid metabolism has also been shown to be dysregulated in both solid tumors and hematological malignancies (reviewed in [120]). Increased fatty acid oxidation (FAO) allows cancer cells to overcome metabolic and oxidative stress through the generation of ATP and NADPH. Significant changes to lipid metabolite levels are seen in AML patient samples with either high levels or low levels of ROS [16], whilst suppression of NOX2 has also been shown to increase FAO [121]. Furthermore, inhibition of the FAO using Avocatin B results in decreased NADPH levels and ROS dependent cell death in primary human AML samples but not normal mononuclear cells [122]. In ALL, use of L-asparaginase has been shown to increase FAO activity as a metabolic escape mechanism, however use of the FAO inhibitor etomoxir in combination with L-asparaginase has been shown to increase sensitivity of both leukemic cell lines and patient samples [123].

6. Conclusions

In the last twenty years, it has become increasingly clear that ROS play a significant role in cellular signalling, particularly pathways associated with growth, differentiation and survival, whilst its roles in HSC quiescence and normal hematopoiesis have started to be delineated. In many cancers including hematological malignancies, ROS levels have been shown to be elevated, leading to aberrant signalling in these pathways. Previously, arguments for both the use of anti-oxidant and pro-oxidant treatments in leukemia have been made (reviewed in [124]). Despite the transformation of survival rates in patients with acute promyelocytic leukemia using arsenic trioxide [125] cancer cells often upregulate the production of antioxidants, and downregulate pro-apoptotic pathways such as TP53, as a response to high ROS, allowing them to escape apoptosis. In addition, it has been shown that both cancer stem cells [126, 127] and leukemic stem cells [128] exhibit low ROS levels, suggesting that even if treatment with pro-oxidants eliminates the bulk of cancer cells, cancer/leukemic stem cells may survive and relapse occur. Conversely, studies involving the use of antioxidants in treatment and epidemiological studies of antioxidant use, have shown mixed results (reviewed in [129, 130]). Increasingly it is becoming apparent that increased levels of ROS are leading to changes in signalling pathways directly or indirectly controlling metabolism, as a mechanism for managing oxidative stress. Whilst, it has long been known that cancer cells exhibit greatly altered metabolism, only recently have the purposes behind this altered metabolism, started to be elucidated. Consequently, synergistic treatments involving the use of metabolic inhibitors, alongside classical treatments for leukemias are being explored. Future work, elucidating the intricate mechanisms governing the interplay between ROS and metabolism, alongside new and more specific metabolic inhibitors provide much promise for the future treatment of leukemia.

Acknowledgements

We are grateful to Blood Cancer UK for programmatic funding and to Tenovus Cancer Care for funding Andrew Robinson. We are grateful to Wellcome ISSF for funding aspects of ROS research. We are grateful for support from the NCRI AML trials cell bank and the AML patients for providing primary samples used in several of our studies.

Author details

Andrew J. Robinson, Richard L. Darley and Alex Tonks*
Department of Haematology, Division of Cancer and Genetics, Cardiff University, Cardiff, UK

*Address all correspondence to: tonksa@cf.ac.uk

References

[1] Ho MS, Medcalf RL, Livesey SA, Traianedes K. The dynamics of adult haematopoiesis in the bone and bone marrow environment. British Journal of Haematology. 2015;**170**:472-486

[2] Luis TC, Killmann NM, Staal FJ. Signal transduction pathways regulating hematopoietic stem cell biology: introduction to a series of Spotlight Reviews. Leukemia. 2012;**26**:86-90

[3] Tarasova A, Haylock D, Winkler D. Principal signalling complexes in haematopoiesis: structural aspects and mimetic discovery. Cytokine & Growth Factor Reviews. 2011;**22**:231-253

[4] Wolff L, Humeniuk R. Concise review: erythroid versus myeloid lineage commitment: regulating the master regulators. Stem Cells. 2013;**31**:1237-1244

[5] Alvarez-Errico D, Vento-Tormo R, Sieweke M, Ballestar E. Epigenetic control of myeloid cell differentiation, identity and function. Nature Reviews. Immunology. 2015;**15**:7-17

[6] Oburoglu L, Romano M, Taylor N, Kinet S. Metabolic regulation of hematopoietic stem cell commitment and erythroid differentiation. Current Opinion in Hematology. 2016;**23**:198-205

[7] Ye F, Huang W, Guo G. Studying hematopoiesis using single-cell technologies. Journal of Hematology & Oncology. 2017;**10**:27

[8] Cvejic A. Mechanisms of fate decision and lineage commitment during haematopoiesis. Immunology and Cell Biology. 2016;**94**:230-235

[9] Velten L, Haas SF, Raffel S, Blaszkiewicz S, Islam S, Hennig BP, et al. Human haematopoietic stem cell lineage commitment is a continuous process. Nature Cell Biology. 2017;**19**:271-281

[10] Samra B, Jabbour E, Ravandi F, Kantarjian H, Short NJ. Evolving therapy of adult acute lymphoblastic leukemia: state-of-the-art treatment and future directions. Journal of Hematology & Oncology. 2020;**13**:70

[11] Terwilliger T, Abdul-Hay M. Acute lymphoblastic leukemia: a comprehensive review and 2017 update. Blood Cancer Journal. 2017;7:e577

[12] Estey E, Gale RP. Acute myeloid leukemia therapy and the chosen people. Leukemia. 2017;**31**:269-271

[13] Tamamyan G, Kadia T, Ravandi F, Borthakur G, Cortes J, Jabbour E, et al. Frontline treatment of acute myeloid leukemia in adults. Critical Reviews in Oncology/Hematology. 2017;**110**:20-34

[14] Winer ES, Stone RM. Novel therapy in Acute myeloid leukemia (AML): moving toward targeted approaches. Ther Adv Hematol. 2019;**10**:2040620719860645

[15] Warburg O. On the origin of cancer cells. Science. 1956;**123**:309-314

[16] Robinson AJ, Hopkins GL, Rastogi N, Hodges M, Doyle M, Davies S, et al. Reactive Oxygen Species Drive Proliferation in Acute Myeloid Leukemia via the Glycolytic Regulator PFKFB3. Cancer Research. 2020;**80**:937-949

[17] Bienert GP, Schjoerring JK, Jahn TP. Membrane transport of hydrogen peroxide. Biochimica et Biophysica Acta. 1758;**2006**:994-1003

[18] Corcoran A, Cotter TG. Redox regulation of protein kinases. The FEBS Journal. 2013;**280**:1944-1965

[19] Angelova PR, Abramov AY. Functional role of mitochondrial reactive oxygen species in physiology. Free Radical Biology & Medicine. 2016;**100**:81-85

[20] Murphy MP. How mitochondria produce reactive oxygen species. The Biochemical Journal. 2009;**417**:1-13

[21] Scialo F, Fernandez-Ayala DJ, Sanz A. Role of Mitochondrial Reverse Electron Transport in ROS Signaling: Potential Roles in Health and Disease. Frontiers in Physiology. 2017;**8**:428

[22] Drose S, Brandt U. The mechanism of mitochondrial superoxide production by the cytochrome bc1 complex. The Journal of Biological Chemistry. 2008;**283**:21649-21654

[23] Magnani F, Nenci S, Millana FE, Ceccon M, Romero E, Fraaije MW, et al. Crystal structures and atomic model of NADPH oxidase. Proceedings of the National Academy of Sciences of the United States of America. 2017;**114**:6764-6769

[24] Nanduri J, Vaddi DR, Khan SA, Wang N, Makerenko V, Prabhakar NR. Xanthine oxidase mediates hypoxia-inducible factor-2alpha degradation by intermittent hypoxia. PLoS One. 2013;**8**:e75838

[25] Bertolotti M, Bestetti S, Garcia-Manteiga JM, Medrano-Fernandez I, Dal MA, Malosio ML, et al. Tyrosine kinase signal modulation: a matter of H2O2 membrane permeability? Antioxidants & Redox Signaling. 2013;**19**:1447-1451

[26] Miller EW, Dickinson BC, Chang CJ. Aquaporin-3 mediates hydrogen peroxide uptake to regulate downstream intracellular signaling. Proceedings of the National Academy of Sciences of the United States of America. 2010;**107**:15681-15686

[27] Essers MA, Weijzen S, de Vries-Smits AM, Saarloos I, de Ruiter ND, Bos JL, et al. FOXO transcription factor activation by oxidative stress mediated by the small GTPase Ral and JNK. The EMBO Journal. 2004;**23**:4802-4812

[28] Putker M, Madl T, Vos HR, de RH, Visscher M, van den Berg MC, et al. Redox-dependent control of FOXO/DAF-16 by transportin-1. Molecular Cell 2013;49:730-42.

[29] Brunet A, Bonni A, Zigmond MJ, Lin MZ, Juo P, Hu LS, et al. Akt promotes cell survival by phosphorylating and inhibiting a Forkhead transcription factor. Cell. 1999;**96**:857-868

[30] Kops GJ, Dansen TB, Polderman PE, Saarloos I, Wirtz KW, Coffer PJ, et al. Forkhead transcription factor FOXO3a protects quiescent cells from oxidative stress. Nature. 2002;**419**:316-321

[31] Miyamoto K, Araki KY, Naka K, Arai F, Takubo K, Yamazaki S, et al. Foxo3a is essential for maintenance of the hematopoietic stem cell pool. Cell Stem Cell. 2007;**1**:101-112

[32] Tothova Z, Kollipara R, Huntly BJ, Lee BH, Castrillon DH, Cullen DE, et al. FoxOs are critical mediators of hematopoietic stem cell resistance to physiologic oxidative stress. Cell. 2007;**128**:325-339

[33] Ito K, Hirao A, Arai F, Matsuoka S, Takubo K, Hamaguchi I, et al. Regulation of oxidative stress by ATM is required for self-renewal of haematopoietic stem cells. Nature. 2004;**431**:997-1002

[34] Jang YY, Sharkis SJ. A low level of reactive oxygen species selects for primitive hematopoietic stem cells that may reside in the low-oxygenic niche. Blood. 2007;**110**:3056-3063

[35] Huang H, Kim HJ, Chang EJ, Lee ZH, Hwang SJ, Kim HM, et al. IL-17 stimulates the proliferation and differentiation of human mesenchymal stem cells: implications for bone remodeling. Cell Death and Differentiation. 2009;**16**:1332-1343

[36] Sattler M, Winkler T, Verma S, Byrne CH, Shrikhande G, Salgia R, et al. Hematopoietic growth factors signal through the formation of reactive oxygen species. Blood. 1999;**93**:2928-2935

[37] O'Brien JJ, Spinelli SL, Tober J, Blumberg N, Francis CW, Taubman MB, et al. 15-deoxy-delta12,14-PGJ2 enhances platelet production from megakaryocytes. Blood. 2008;**112**:4051-4060

[38] Motohashi H, Kimura M, Fujita R, Inoue A, Pan X, Takayama M, et al. NF-E2 domination over Nrf2 promotes ROS accumulation and megakaryocytic maturation. Blood. 2010;**115**: 677-686

[39] McCrann DJ, Eliades A, Makitalo M, Matsuno K, Ravid K. Differential expression of NADPH oxidases in megakaryocytes and their role in polyploidy. Blood. 2009;**114**:1243-1249

[40] Sardina JL, Lopez-Ruano G, Sanchez-Abarca LI, Perez-Simon JA, Gaztelumendi A, Trigueros C, et al. p22phox-dependent NADPH oxidase activity is required for megakaryocytic differentiation. Cell Death and Differentiation. 2010;**17**:1842-1854

[41] Tang Y, Zhang G, Baird M, Racke F, Zhao W. A novel role of CYP2E1 in human megakaryocyte development. In Vivo. 2014;**28**:1077-1084

[42] Shinohara A, Imai Y, Nakagawa M, Takahashi T, Ichikawa M, Kurokawa M. Intracellular reactive oxygen species mark and influence the megakaryocyte-erythrocyte progenitor fate of common myeloid progenitors. Stem Cells. 2014;**32**:548-557

[43] Yamamoto T, Sakaguchi N, Hachiya M, Nakayama F, Yamakawa M, Akashi M. Role of catalase in monocytic differentiation of U937 cells by TPA: hydrogen peroxide as a second messenger. Leukemia. 2009;**23**:761-769

[44] Del Prete A, Zaccagnino P, Di PM, Saltarella M, Oliveros CC, Nico B, et al. Role of mitochondria and reactive oxygen species in dendritic cell differentiation and functions. Free Radical Biology & Medicine. 2008;**44**:1443-1451

[45] Weitzman SA, Weitberg AB, Clark EP, Stossel TP. Phagocytes as carcinogens: malignant transformation produced by human neutrophils. Science. 1985;**227**:1231-1233

[46] Szatrowski TP, Nathan CF. Production of large amounts of hydrogen peroxide by human tumor cells. Cancer Research. 1991;**51**:794-798

[47] Valgimigli M, Valgimigli L, Trere D, Gaiani S, Pedulli GF, Gramantieri L, et al. Oxidative stress EPR measurement in human liver by radical-probe technique. Correlation with etiology, histology and cell proliferation. Free Radical Research. 2002;**36**:939-948

[48] Liaw KY, Lee PH, Wu FC, Tsai JS, Lin-Shiau SY. Zinc, copper, and superoxide dismutase in hepatocellular carcinoma. The American Journal of Gastroenterology. 1997;**92**:2260-2263

[49] Elchuri S, Oberley TD, Qi W, Eisenstein RS, Jackson RL, Van RH, et al. CuZnSOD deficiency leads to persistent and widespread oxidative damage and hepatocarcinogenesis later in life. Oncogene. 2005;**24**:367-380

[50] Van Remmen H, Ikeno Y, Hamilton M, Pahlavani M, Wolf N, Thorpe SR, et al. Life-long reduction in MnSOD activity results in increased DNA damage and higher incidence of cancer but does not accelerate aging. Physiological Genomics. 2003;**16**:29-37

[51] Galadari S, Rahman A, Pallichankandy S, Thayyullathil F.

Reactive oxygen species and cancer paradox: To promote or to suppress? Free Radical Biology & Medicine. 2017;**104**:144-164

[52] Devi GS, Prasad MH, Saraswathi I, Raghu D, Rao DN, Reddy PP. Free radicals antioxidant enzymes and lipid peroxidation in different types of leukemias. Clinica Chimica Acta. 2000;**293**:53-62

[53] Hole PS, Zabkiewicz J, Munje C, Newton Z, Pearn L, White P, et al. Overproduction of NOX-derived ROS in AML promotes proliferation and is associated with defective oxidative stress signaling. Blood. 2013;**122**:3322-3330

[54] Cooke MS, Evans MD, Dizdaroglu M, Lunec J. Oxidative DNA damage: mechanisms, mutation, and disease. The FASEB Journal. 2003;**17**:1195-1214

[55] Matsui A, Ikeda T, Enomoto K, Hosoda K, Nakashima H, Omae K, et al. Increased formation of oxidative DNA damage, 8-hydroxy-2′-deoxyguanosine, in human breast cancer tissue and its relationship to GSTP1 and COMT genotypes. Cancer Letters. 2000;**151**:87-95

[56] Borrego S, Vazquez A, Dasi F, Cerda C, Iradi A, Tormos C, et al. Oxidative Stress and DNA Damage in Human Gastric Carcinoma: 8-Oxo-7′8-dihydro-2′-deoxyguanosine (8-oxo-dG) as a Possible Tumor Marker. International Journal of Molecular Sciences. 2013;**14**:3467-3486

[57] Gackowski D, Kowalewski J, Siomek A, Olinski R. Oxidative DNA damage and antioxidant vitamin level: comparison among lung cancer patients, healthy smokers and nonsmokers. International Journal of Cancer. 2005;**114**:153-156

[58] Obtulowicz T, Swoboda M, Speina E, Gackowski D, Rozalski R, Siomek A, et al. Oxidative stress and 8-oxoguanine repair are enhanced in colon adenoma and carcinoma patients. Mutagenesis. 2010;**25**:463-471

[59] Zhou FL, Zhang WG, Wei YC, Meng S, Bai GG, Wang BY, et al. Involvement of oxidative stress in the relapse of acute myeloid leukemia. The Journal of Biological Chemistry. 2010;**285**:15010-15015

[60] Gao X, Schottker B. Reduction-oxidation pathways involved in cancer development: a systematic review of literature reviews. Oncotarget. 2017;**8**:51888-51906

[61] Altomare DA, Testa JR. Perturbations of the AKT signaling pathway in human cancer. Oncogene. 2005;**24**:7455-7464

[62] Xu Q, Simpson SE, Scialla TJ, Bagg A, Carroll M. Survival of acute myeloid leukemia cells requires PI3 kinase activation. Blood. 2003;**102**:972-980

[63] Kode A, Mosialou I, Manavalan SJ, Rathinam CV, Friedman RA, Teruya-Feldstein J, et al. FoxO1-dependent induction of acute myeloid leukemia by osteoblasts in mice. Leukemia. 2016;**30**:1-13

[64] Sykes SM, Lane SW, Bullinger L, Kalaitzidis D, Yusuf R, Saez B, et al. AKT/FOXO signaling enforces reversible differentiation blockade in myeloid leukemias. Cell. 2011;**146**:697-708

[65] Jayavelu AK, Moloney JN, Bohmer FD, Cotter TG. NOX-driven ROS formation in cell transformation of FLT3-ITD-positive AML. Experimental Hematology. 2016;**44**:1113-1122

[66] Mikawa T, LLeonart ME, Takaori-Kondo A, Inagaki N, Yokode M, Kondoh H. Dysregulated glycolysis as an oncogenic event. Cellular and Molecular Life Sciences. 2015;**72**:1881-1892

[67] DeBerardinis RJ, Chandel NS. Fundamentals of cancer metabolism. Science Advances. 2016;**2**:e1600200

[68] Weinberg F, Hamanaka R, Wheaton WW, Weinberg S, Joseph J, Lopez M, et al. Mitochondrial metabolism and ROS generation are essential for Kras-mediated tumorigenicity. Proceedings of the National Academy of Sciences of the United States of America. 2010;**107**:8788-8793

[69] Liberti MV, Locasale JW. The Warburg Effect: How Does it Benefit Cancer Cells? Trends in Biochemical Sciences. 2016;**41**:211-218

[70] Han T, Kang D, Ji D, Wang X, Zhan W, Fu M, et al. How does cancer cell metabolism affect tumor migration and invasion? Cell Adhesion & Migration. 2013;**7**:395-403

[71] Cosentino C, Grieco D, Costanzo V. ATM activates the pentose phosphate pathway promoting anti-oxidant defence and DNA repair. The EMBO Journal. 2011;**30**:546-555

[72] Ciccarese F, Ciminale V. Escaping Death: Mitochondrial Redox Homeostasis in Cancer Cells. Frontiers in Oncology. 2017;**7**:117

[73] Yang M, Vousden KH. Serine and one-carbon metabolism in cancer. Nature Reviews. Cancer. 2016;**16**:650-662

[74] Dang L, Jin S, Su SM. IDH mutations in glioma and acute myeloid leukemia. Trends in Molecular Medicine. 2010;**16**:387-397

[75] Zhao S, Lin Y, Xu W, Jiang W, Zha Z, Wang P, et al. Glioma-derived mutations in IDH1 dominantly inhibit IDH1 catalytic activity and induce HIF-1alpha. Science. 2009;**324**:261-265

[76] Hagen T. Oxygen versus Reactive Oxygen in the Regulation of HIF-1alpha: The Balance Tips. Biochemistry Research International. 2012;**2012**:436981

[77] Mitsuishi Y, Taguchi K, Kawatani Y, Shibata T, Nukiwa T, Aburatani H, et al. Nrf2 redirects glucose and glutamine into anabolic pathways in metabolic reprogramming. Cancer Cell. 2012;**22**:66-79

[78] Rushworth SA, MacEwan DJ. HO-1 underlies resistance of AML cells to TNF-induced apoptosis. Blood. 2008;**111**:3793-3801

[79] Matoba S, Kang JG, Patino WD, Wragg A, Boehm M, Gavrilova O, et al. p53 regulates mitochondrial respiration. Science. 2006;**312**:1650-1653

[80] Zhao L, Mao Y, Zhao Y, Cao Y, Chen X. Role of multifaceted regulators in cancer glucose metabolism and their clinical significance. Oncotarget. 2016;**7**:31572-31585

[81] Bensaad K, Tsuruta A, Selak MA, Vidal MN, Nakano K, Bartrons R, et al. TIGAR, a p53-inducible regulator of glycolysis and apoptosis. Cell. 2006;**126**:107-120

[82] Prior IA, Lewis PD, Mattos C. A comprehensive survey of Ras mutations in cancer. Cancer Research. 2012;**72**:2457-2467

[83] Efeyan A, Zoncu R, Sabatini DM. Amino acids and mTORC1: from lysosomes to disease. Trends in Molecular Medicine. 2012;**18**:524-533

[84] Li M, Jin R, Wang W, Zhang T, Sang J, Li N, et al. STAT3 regulates glycolysis via targeting hexokinase 2 in hepatocellular carcinoma cells. Oncotarget. 2017;**8**:24777-24784

[85] Khatri S, Yepiskoposyan H, Gallo CA, Tandon P, Plas DR. FOXO3a regulates glycolysis via transcriptional control of tumor suppressor TSC1.

The Journal of Biological Chemistry. 2010;**285**:15960-15965

[86] Kawauchi K, Araki K, Tobiume K, Tanaka N. p53 regulates glucose metabolism through an IKK-NF-kappaB pathway and inhibits cell transformation. Nature Cell Biology. 2008;**10**:611-618

[87] Hsieh AL, Walton ZE, Altman BJ, Stine ZE, Dang CV. MYC and metabolism on the path to cancer. Seminars in Cell & Developmental Biology. 2015;**43**:11-21

[88] Boag JM, Beesley AH, Firth MJ, Freitas JR, Ford J, Hoffmann K, et al. Altered glucose metabolism in childhood pre-B acute lymphoblastic leukaemia. Leukemia. 2006;**20**:1731-1737

[89] Liu T, Kishton RJ, Macintyre AN, Gerriets VA, Xiang H, Liu X, et al. Glucose transporter 1-mediated glucose uptake is limiting for B-cell acute lymphoblastic leukemia anabolic metabolism and resistance to apoptosis. Cell Death & Disease. 2014;**5**:e1470

[90] Song K, Li M, Xu X, Xuan LI, Huang G, Liu Q. Resistance to chemotherapy is associated with altered glucose metabolism in acute myeloid leukemia. Oncology Letters. 2016;**12**:334-342

[91] Chen WL, Wang YY, Zhao A, Xia L, Xie G, Su M, et al. Enhanced Fructose Utilization Mediated by SLC2A5 Is a Unique Metabolic Feature of Acute Myeloid Leukemia with Therapeutic Potential. Cancer Cell. 2016;**30**:779-791

[92] Prata C, Maraldi T, Fiorentini D, Zambonin L, Hakim G, Landi L. Nox-generated ROS modulate glucose uptake in a leukaemic cell line. Free Radical Research. 2008;**42**:405-414

[93] Zhao P, Huang J, Zhang D, Zhang D, Wang F, Qu Y, et al. SLC2A5 overexpression in childhood philadelphia chromosome-positive acute lymphoblastic leukaemia. British Journal of Haematology. 2018;**183**:242-250

[94] You ZM, Zhao L, Xia J, Wei Q, Liu YM, Liu XY, et al. Down-regulation of phosphoglucose isomerase/autocrine motility factor enhances gensenoside Rh2 pharmacological action on leukemia KG1alpha cells. Asian Pacific Journal of Cancer Prevention. 2014;**15**:1099-1104

[95] Ju HQ, Zhan G, Huang A, Sun Y, Wen S, Yang J, et al. ITD mutation in FLT3 tyrosine kinase promotes Warburg effect and renders therapeutic sensitivity to glycolytic inhibition. Leukemia. 2017;**31**:2143-2150

[96] Ryland LK, Doshi UA, Shanmugavelandy SS, Fox TE, Aliaga C, Broeg K, et al. C6-ceramide nanoliposomes target the Warburg effect in chronic lymphocytic leukemia. PLoS One. 2013;**8**:e84648

[97] Shi SY, Lu SY, Sivasubramaniyam T, Revelo XS, Cai EP, Luk CT, et al. DJ-1 links muscle ROS production with metabolic reprogramming and systemic energy homeostasis in mice. Nature Communications. 2015;**6**:7415

[98] Liu CC, Wang H, Wang JH, Wang L, Geng QR, Chen XQ, et al. Serum neuron-specific enolase levels are upregulated in patients with acute lymphoblastic leukemia and are predictive of prognosis. Oncotarget. 2016;**7**:55181-55190

[99] Hitosugi T, Zhou L, Elf S, Fan J, Kang HB, Seo JH, et al. Phosphoglycerate mutase 1 coordinates glycolysis and biosynthesis to promote tumor growth. Cancer Cell. 2012;**22**:585-600

[100] McCleland ML, Adler AS, Deming L, Cosino E, Lee L, Blackwood EM, et al. Lactate dehydrogenase B is required

for the growth of KRAS-dependent lung adenocarcinomas. Clinical Cancer Research. 2013;**19**:773-784

[101] Tahir IM, Iqbal T, Jamil A, Saqib M. Association of BCL-2 with oxidative stress and total antioxidant status in pediatric acute lymphoblastic leukemia. Journal of Biological Regulators and Homeostatic Agents. 2017;**31**:1023-1027

[102] Hu W, Wang X, Yang R. Evaluation of D-dimer and lactate dehydrogenase plasma levels in patients with relapsed acute leukemia. Oncology Letters. 2016;**12**:591-596

[103] Hole PS, Pearn L, Tonks AJ, James PE, Burnett AK, Darley RL, et al. Ras-induced reactive oxygen species promote growth factor-independent proliferation in human CD34+ hematopoietic progenitor cells. Blood. 2010;**115**:1238-1246

[104] Chen WL, Wang JH, Zhao AH, Xu X, Wang YH, Chen TL, et al. A distinct glucose metabolism signature of acute myeloid leukemia with prognostic value. Blood. 2014;**124**:1645-1654

[105] Zhang MY, Liu SL, Huang WL, Tang DB, Zheng WW, Zhou N, et al. Bromodomains and Extra-Terminal (BET) Inhibitor JQ1 Suppresses Proliferation of Acute Lymphocytic Leukemia by Inhibiting c-Myc-Mediated Glycolysis. Medical Science Monitor. 2020;**26**:e923411

[106] Wallace DC. Mitochondria and cancer. Nature Reviews. Cancer. 2012;**12**:685-698

[107] Naoe T, Kiyoi H. Gene mutations of acute myeloid leukemia in the genome era. International Journal of Hematology. 2013;**97**:165-174

[108] Yen K, Travins J, Wang F, David MD, Artin E, Straley K, et al. AG-221, a First-in-Class Therapy Targeting Acute Myeloid Leukemia Harboring Oncogenic IDH2 Mutations. Cancer Discovery. 2017;**7**:478-493

[109] DiNardo C, Botton S, Pollyea D, Stein E, Fathi A, Roboz G, et al. Molecular Profiling and Relationship with Clinical Response in Patients with IDH1 Mutation-Positive Hematologic Malignancies Receiving AG-120, a First-in-Class Potent Inhibitor of Mutant IDH1, in Addition to Data from the Completed Dose Escalation Portion of the Phase 1 Study. Blood. 2015;**126**:1306

[110] Wang Y, Zhang L, Chen WL, Wang JH, Li N, Li JM, et al. Rapid diagnosis and prognosis of de novo acute myeloid leukemia by serum metabonomic analysis. Journal of Proteome Research. 2013;**12**:4393-4401

[111] Schraw JM, Junco JJ, Brown AL, Scheurer ME, Rabin KR, Lupo PJ. Metabolomic profiling identifies pathways associated with minimal residual disease in childhood acute lymphoblastic leukaemia. eBioMedicine. 2019; **48**:49-57

[112] Ye J, Fan J, Venneti S, Wan YW, Pawel BR, Zhang J, et al. Serine catabolism regulates mitochondrial redox control during hypoxia. Cancer Discovery. 2014;**4**:1406-1417

[113] Polet F, Corbet C, Pinto A, Rubio LI, Martherus R, Bol V, et al. Reducing the serine availability complements the inhibition of the glutamine metabolism to block leukemia cell growth. Oncotarget. 2016;**7**:1765-1776

[114] Zaal EA, Wu W, Jansen G, Zweegman S, Cloos J, Berkers CR. Bortezomib resistance in multiple myeloma is associated with increased serine synthesis. Cancer Metab. 2017;**5**:7

[115] Patra KC, Hay N. The pentose phosphate pathway and cancer.

Trends in Biochemical Sciences. 2014;**39**:347-354

[116] Chen Y, Xu Q, Ji D, Wei Y, Chen H, Li T, et al. Inhibition of pentose phosphate pathway suppresses acute myelogenous leukemia. Tumour Biology. 2016;**37**:6027-6034

[117] Elf S, Lin R, Xia S, Pan Y, Shan C, Wu S, et al. Targeting 6-phosphogluconate dehydrogenase in the oxidative PPP sensitizes leukemia cells to antimalarial agent dihydroartemisinin. Oncogene. 2017;**36**:254-262

[118] Poulain L, Sujobert P, Zylbersztejn F, Barreau S, Stuani L, Lambert M, et al. High mTORC1 activity drives glycolysis addiction and sensitivity to G6PD inhibition in acute myeloid leukemia cells. Leukemia. 2017;**31**:2326-2335

[119] Xiao G, Chan LN, Klemm L, Braas D, Chen Z, Geng H, et al. B-Cell-Specific Diversion of Glucose Carbon Utilization Reveals a Unique Vulnerability in B Cell Malignancies. Cell. 2018;**173**:470-484

[120] Starkova J, Hermanova I, Hlozkova K, Hararova A, Trka J. Altered Metabolism of Leukemic Cells: New Therapeutic Opportunity. International Review of Cell and Molecular Biology. 2018;**336**:93-147

[121] Adane B, Ye H, Khan N, Pei S, Minhajuddin M, Stevens BM, et al. The Hematopoietic Oxidase NOX2 Regulates Self-Renewal of Leukemic Stem Cells. Cell Reports. 2019;**27**:238-254

[122] Lee EA, Angka L, Rota SG, Hanlon T, Mitchell A, Hurren R, et al. Targeting Mitochondria with Avocatin B Induces Selective Leukemia Cell Death. Cancer Research. 2015;**75**:2478-2488

[123] Hermanova I, Arruabarrena-Aristorena A, Valis K, Nuskova H, Alberich-Jorda M, Fiser K, et al. Pharmacological inhibition of fatty-acid oxidation synergistically enhances the effect of l-asparaginase in childhood ALL cells. Leukemia. 2016;**30**:209-218

[124] Hole PS, Darley RL, Tonks A. Do reactive oxygen species play a role in myeloid leukemias? Blood. 2011;**117**:5816-5826

[125] McCulloch D, Brown C, Iland H. Retinoic acid and arsenic trioxide in the treatment of acute promyelocytic leukemia: current perspectives. Oncotargets and Therapy. 2017;**10**:1585-1601

[126] Diehn M, Cho RW, Lobo NA, Kalisky T, Dorie MJ, Kulp AN, et al. Association of reactive oxygen species levels and radioresistance in cancer stem cells. Nature. 2009;**458**:780-783

[127] Kim HM, Haraguchi N, Ishii H, Ohkuma M, Okano M, Mimori K, et al. Increased CD13 expression reduces reactive oxygen species, promoting survival of liver cancer stem cells via an epithelial-mesenchymal transition-like phenomenon. Annals of Surgical Oncology. 2012;**19**(Suppl 3):S539-S548

[128] Lagadinou ED, Sach A, Callahan K, Rossi RM, Neering SJ, Minhajuddin M, et al. BCL-2 inhibition targets oxidative phosphorylation and selectively eradicates quiescent human leukemia stem cells. Cell Stem Cell. 2013;**12**:329-341

[129] Poprac P, Jomova K, Simunkova M, Kollar V, Rhodes CJ, Valko M. Targeting Free Radicals in Oxidative Stress-Related Human Diseases. Trends in Pharmacological Sciences. 2017;**38**:592-607

[130] Yasueda A, Urushima H, Ito T. Efficacy and Interaction of Antioxidant Supplements as Adjuvant Therapy in Cancer Treatment: A Systematic Review. Integrative Cancer Therapies. 2016;**15**:17-39

Chapter 4

The Key Role of the Phosphatase PP2A in the Development of Acute Myeloid Leukemia

Javier Marco, Irene Peris, Carmen Vicente and Elena Arriazu

Abstract

Acute myeloid leukemia (AML) is a heterogeneous malignant disorder of hematopoietic progenitor cells characterized by the accumulation of several genetic and epigenetic mutations. Despite the progressive understanding of the molecular heterogeneity of the disease, the survival rate of patients older than 60 years old remains poor. Therefore, it is necessary to develop an effective treatment strategy for those patients in order to beat the disease and improve life quality. Reversible phosphorylation has been widely studied over the last years, and the deregulation of kinases and phosphatase have been verified to have a huge impact in leukemogenesis. Inactivation of the tumor-suppressor protein phosphatase 2A (PP2A) is frequent in AML patients, constituting a promising target for cancer therapy. There are several PP2A inactivation mechanisms. However, overexpression of SET or cancerous inhibitors of PP2A, both endogenous inhibitors of PP2A, are recurrent events in AML patients, leading to the inactivation of the phosphatase PP2A. Preclinical studies show that PP2A reactivation using PP2A-activating drugs (PADs) manage to stop the development of the disease, and its combination with conventional chemotherapy and tyrosine kinase inhibitors have a synergistic cytotoxic effects. Recent studies have demonstrated that specifically activation of PP2A subunits, target crucial pathogenic drivers, increasing the efficacy of conventional treatments and opening new possibilities for personalized treatment in AML patients, especially in cases of PP2A deregulation. Here, we review the role of PP2A in AML as well as its drugable options.

Keywords: AML, PP2A, SET, PADs, FTY720, CM-1231

1. Introduction

Acute myeloid leukemia (AML) is a heterogeneous clonal disorder characterized by the accumulation of poorly differentiated cells, derived from the differentiation blockage of myeloid hematopoietic progenitors in the bone marrow (BM) [1]. As consequence, immature cells called "blast" displace other cell populations invading the BM and other tissues [2, 3].

AML is a malignant disorder of the bone marrow characterized by the clonal expansion and differentiation arrest of myeloid progenitor cells. Incidence increases with age, with 68 years being the median age at diagnosis. AML is the most common form of acute leukemia in adults and has the shortest survival. Effective therapies, including intensive chemotherapy and allogeneic stem cell transplantation, are generally applicable to young patients, while treatment options for older patients (≥65 years), which are the largest group, have historically been limited to DNA methyltransferase inhibitors (i.e. azacitidine and decitabine) and low doses of cytarabine, and have only provided a modest benefit [1, 4, 5]. Besides, treatment is often ineffective in both groups due to drug resistance and relapse, particularly in patients with FMS-like tyrosine kinase 3 (FLT3)-internal tandem duplication (ITD), that represent ~25% of all AML cases, and have poor outcome, with high risk of relapse and low cure rates [1–6]. The AML treatment landscape has changed substantially since 2017. New targeted drugs have emerged, including midostaurin and gilteritinib to target FLT3, and venetoclax to target BCL-2 [1]. This has created novel treatment options, especially in older as well as in refractory/relapsed patients. The natural history of FLT3-mutated AML is changing after the approval of midostaurin for frontline therapy and gilteritinib for relapsed or refractory patients. Nevertheless, despite initial clinical responses to FLT3 kinase inhibitors (FKIs), patients eventually relapse. Mechanisms of resistance include the acquisition of secondary FLT3 mutations and protective stromal signaling within the bone marrow niche [2–4]. In the same way, venetoclax combined with hypomethylating agents or low-dose cytarabine is an effective therapy for older or unfit patients with AML, which represents most of the cases. However, it is now clear that multiple resistant sub-clones evolving contemporaneously during therapy can occur in AML and act as a barrier to the long-term success of targeted therapies. Studies about the molecular determinants of outcome with clinical relevance to patients with AML show that FLT3-ITD mutations or TP53 loss conferred cross-resistance to both venetoclax and cytotoxic-based therapies [5]. Besides, even with these and other potent targeted therapies, the disease persists within the bone marrow microenvironment, mainly due to activating parallel signaling pathways that maintain pro-survival factors. Therefore, acquired resistance to these targeted drugs remains a challenge and provides a rationale for combining either FLT3 inhibitors or venetoclax with other therapies, both conventional and investigational [6]. Reversible phosphorylation of proteins is a post-translational modification that regulates all aspect of life through the antagonistic action of kinases and phosphatases. Protein kinases are popular drug targets and are well characterized, but protein phosphatases have been relatively neglected [7]. In this chapter, we will focus on the role of protein phosphatase 2A (PP2A), inactivation of which is a recurrent event in AML, as a druggable tumor suppressor.

2. Protein phosphatase 2A

PP2A, a ubiquitously expressed protein serine/threonine phosphatase in mammalian cells, is a tumor suppressor that regulates essential cell processes and counteracts most of kinases-driven intracellular signaling pathways [7–11]. Recent evidences indicate that PP2A inactivation arises in several solid and hematological tumors causing the prolong activation of survival pathways or the inhibition of apoptotic pathways, pointing out its relevance in leukemogenesis [9, 12–14]. The use of okadaic acid (OA), a potent tumor promoter that inhibits PP2A activity, has greatly contributed to the understanding of the phosphatase functions [15].

PP2A appear in two different forms: a dimeric and a trimeric form [9, 16]. The dimer, known as the core enzyme, consists of a structural A subunit (PP2A-A) and a catalytic C subunit (PP2A-C), whereas the trimeric form, is comprised by a structural A subunit, a catalytic C subunit and a regulatory B subunit (PP2A-B). Interestingly, the function of the scaffold subunit varies depending on the PP2A complex. In the heterotrimeric form, PP2A-A mediates the interaction between the catalytic subunit with the regulatory subunit, while in the dimeric form, it acquires a regulatory function changing the catalytic specificity. Furthermore, each subunit is encoded by different genes, which further generate distinct isoforms. PP2A-A (PPP2R1/Aα and PPPR1B/Aβ) and PP2A-C (PPP2CA/Cα and PPP2CB/Cβ) are more conserve, whereas in PP2A-B four families of genes (B/PR55/B55, B′/PR61/B56, B″/PR72, B‴/The striatins, STRN) have been recognized including 23 different alternative transcript and spliced forms, which determine the substrate specificity and intracellular localization of PP2A (**Figures 1** and **2**) [12, 14, 17, 18]. Therefore, the actual challenge is not only to identify deregulation of PP2A functions in AML patients, but also to recognize the subunit affected with the goal to develop efficient target therapies [19].

The precise mechanism of PP2A active complex assembly remains obscure, but there are evidence that determine that post-translational modifications of PP2A-C residues, such as methylation and phosphorylation, plays an essential role in modulating the formation of active PP2A holoenzym. For instance, the methylation of PP2A-C subunit in leucine 309 (L09) by leucine carboxyl methyltransferase I is crucial for PR55/B55 binding, being not an essential requisite for other B families subunits [20–22]. However, post-translational modifications not only have an activating role, but also inhibitor since phosphorylation of tyrosine 307 (Y307) impairs the interaction of PP2A-C with the PR55/B55 and PR61/B56 subunits [20]. Interestingly, both cell lines and AML patient samples show an increase of Y307 phosphorylation [23]. On the

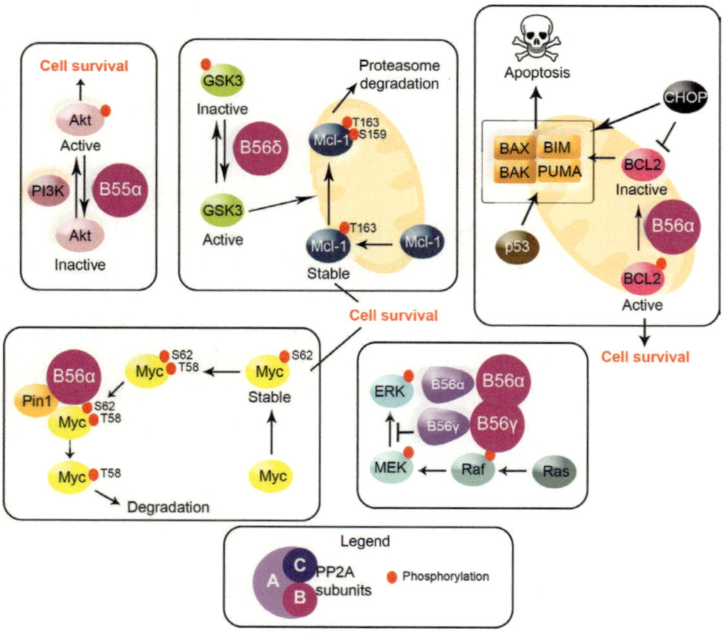

Figure 1.
*Signaling pathways involving PP2A in AML. Scheme showing some of the molecular pathways regulated by PP2A complexes. Different isoforms of PP2A regulatory subunits are shown. The regulatory subunit B55α regulates the Akt pathway by dephosphorylating and inactivating Akt, which is the responsible of GSK3 phosphorylation and inactivation. On the other hand, B56δ PP2A regulatory subunit dephosphorylates and activates GSK3. Active GSK3 can phosphorylate MCl-1 in S159 (previous phosphorylation in T163 by ERK), leading to MCL-1 proteasome degradation and contributing to apoptosis. Active GSK3 can also phosphorylate Myc in T58 (previous phosphorylation in S62 by ERK), leading to the binding of B56α PP2A regulatory subunit, which dephosphorylates Myc in S62, leaving T58 phosphorylation that generates Myc instability and proteasome degradation. B56α can also dephosphorylate and inactivate BCL-2, activating the caspase dependent apoptosis. B56γ and B56α PP2A regulatory subunits control the MEK/ERK pathway, which is responsible of MCL-1 and Myc stability. *B regulatory PP2A subunits are exemplified in representation of PP2A enzyme, which is represented in the legend. Red dots are symbolized as phosphate groups.*

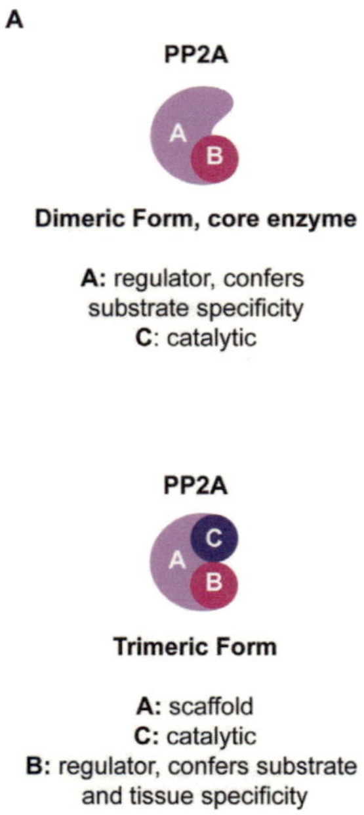

B

Subunit	Isoform	Gene name	Other names
A	α	PPP2R1A	PR65α
	β	PPP2R1B	PR65β
C	α	PPP2CA	PPP2cα
	β	PPP2CB	PPP2Acβ
B	α	PPP2R2A	B55α, PR55α
	β	PPP2R2B	B55β, PR55β
	γ	PPP2R2C	B55γ, PR55γ
	δ	PPP2R2D	B55δ, PR55δ
B'	α	PPP2R5A	B56α, PR56/61α
	β	PPP2R5B	B56β, PR56/61β
	γ	PPP2R5C	B56γ, PR56/61γ
	δ	PPP2R5D	B56δ, PR56/61δ
	ε	PPP2R5E	B56ε, PR56/61ε
B''	α	PPP2R3A	PR72, B''α2
	β	PPP2R3B	PR70, PR48, B''β
	γ	PPP2R3C	G5PR, G4-1
	δ	PPP2R3D	PR59, B''δ
B'''		STRN	Startin, PR110
		STRN3	SG2NA
		STRN4	
		PPP2R4	PTPA, PR53

Figure 2.
PP2A subunits. (A) Schematic representation of PP2A subunits and their functions. (B) all different isoforms of every subunit of PP2A.

other hand, post-translational modifications of PP2A-B can also affect the localization of the holoenzyme, complicating its targeting [24].

We and others have determined that PP2A deregulation is a common event in AML patients, and the restoration of PP2A activity with PP2A activating drugs (PADs), such as FTY720, has potent antileukemic effects in AML cells, preventing cell growth and inducing caspase-dependent apoptosis [12, 13, 23, 26–28]. However, FTY720 induces cardio-toxicity at the anti-neoplastic dose. Hence, we develop a novel non-phosphorylable FTY720 analogue called CM-1231, which has a great antileukemic potential without inducing secondary effects [28]. Furthermore, we have shown that PADs can be used in combination with kinase inhibitors or chemotherapy agents, suggesting that PP2A activity restoration could have a huge therapy potential in AML patients [23, 25, 27, 29–32].

2.1 Mechanism of PP2A inactivation in AML

Several somatic mutations have been described in PP2A subunits in different types of tumors such as melanoma, colon, lung and breast cancers [19, 33–39]. Mutations in PP2A-Aα or PP2A-Aβ subunits cause defective binding of B and C subunits, inhibiting PP2A active holoenzyme and favoring a malignant cell transformation [36, 37]. However, the frequency of PP2A inactivation due to mutations is low, with PPP2R1A subunit owning the highest mutational percentage rate (1,17%), and it seems to be an uncommon mechanism in AML. Likewise, our analysis of the genome of 250 patients with leukemia from the Cancer Genome Atlas Research Network (https://tcga-data.nci.nih.gov/tcga), show that only one patient has somatic mutations in PPP2R2B, which encode for PR55β subunit [14, 40].

Thus, the main mechanism that employs cancer cells to evade PP2A-mediated tumor suppression is through the overexpression of proteins that mediate PP2A post-translational modifications or molecules that inactivates the holoenzyme function [41–43].

2.2 SET/I2PP2A

The SET oncoprotein, also known as I2PP2A (Inhibitor 2 of PP2A), TAF-1β or PHAP1, is a potent endogenous PP2A inhibitor that plays an essential role in myeloid leukemias (**Figure 3**) [44]. Firstly, SET was identified as an oncogene fused with nucleoporin NUP214 (CAN) in undifferentiated leukemias [45], to later be considered as a PP2A inhibitor [46]. This protein is mostly located in the nucleus, and is implicated in a wide range of cell processes such as DNA replication, gene transcription, chromatin remodeling [47, 48], DNA repair [49], cell differentiation [50], migration [51] and cell-cycle regulation [52]. SET is up-regulated in hematological and solid tumors, including breast cancer [53] and colorectal cancer [54]. Its role has been studied in depth in chronic myeloid leukemia (CML). Interestingly, patients with BCR-ABL1 gene fusion, which constitutively activates tyrosine kinase activity, essential for CML emergence, maintenance and progression, have SET overexpression [55]. The expression of BCR-ABL1 allows recruitment and activation of JAK2, which enhance β-catenin activity and induce SET-mediated inactivation of PP2A [56].

Likewise, SET overexpression is also an important event in AML. We performed a quantification of SET expression in AML patients, observing that SET overexpression is a recurrent event (60/214, 28%) associated with poor survival in AML. Furthermore, the protein overexpression has a prognostic impact in patients with

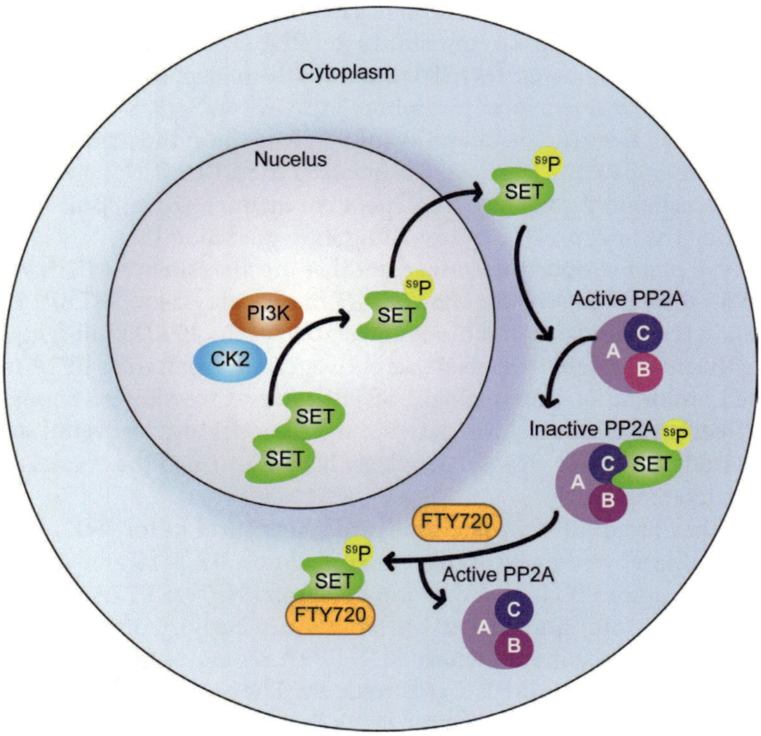

Figure 3.
PP2A inactivation by SET in AML. PI3K and CK2 can phosphorylate SET at serine 9 (S9), located in the nuclear localization signal. This phosphorylation translocates SET to the cytosol and impairs its return to the nucleus, increasing its ability to bind to the catalytic subunit of PP2A (PP2A-C), and inactivating PP2A. Treatment with FTY720 disrupts SET–PP2A interaction, allowing PP2A activation [57].

normal karyotype, defining a subgroup of patients with worse outcome. Additional observations reveals that SET overexpression is associated with other adverse prognostic markers such as monosomy 7, SET binding protein a (SETBP1) overexpression and EVI1 overexpression, suggesting that this oncoprotein could cooperate with other additional aberrations in leukemogenesis program. Our analysis by western blot confirmed that SET is overexpressed at protein levels in both AML cell lines and patients samples [29].58.

In addition, we observed that SET promote cell survival by inhibiting PP2A activity through its binding to PP2A-C, forming an inhibitory complex that prevent phosphatase activity (**Figure 3**) [30]. That is the main reason why the use of PADs such as FTY720, OP449 or its analogues, show potent antileukemic effects, since prevent the interaction between SET and PP2A, recovering the antitumoral activity of PP2A [27, 28, 30]. Nevertheless, despite the importance of SET overexpression and its prognostic impact in hematological tumors, little is known about the mechanism involved in SET regulation, constituting a barrier to the development of new PP2A activating drugs.

Recent studies have described mechanism of post-translational regulation of SET that modulate the inhibitory activity against PP2A [58, 57]. Using genetic and pharmacological approaches, we found that p38β has a dual role in SET regulation in AML. We found that p38β up-regulation, but not p38α, is a common event in AML that contributes to SET-mediated PP2A inactivation [57]. It has been reported that p38 form complexes with PP2A [59–66]. However, their connection can vary depending on the cellular context. Upon TNF-induced stress conditions in endothelium-derived cell lines, p38 positively regulates PP2A activity [63], whereas under hypoxia and survival conditions, PP2A negatively regulates p38 activity [65]. Nevertheless, the regulatory mechanism has not been discovered until now. We show for the first time that p38β contributes to PP2A inactivation via SET regulation through two mechanisms: (i) p38β promotes the phosphorylation of the casein kinase 2 (CK2) which active form phosphorylates SET on Ser9, located in a nuclear localization signal, favoring the retention of SET into the cytoplasm and consequence inhibition of PP2A. Thus, p38β is involved in SET trafficking to the cytosol and PP2A inactivation through a CK2-dependent manner. (ii) p38β also binds to SET stabilizing the oncoprotein and avoiding its degradation [57].

Similarly, it had previously described another mechanism in AML that impairs PP2A activity through the stabilization of SET in the cytoplasm. SETBP1 is a protein located in the cytoplasm that binds and stabilizes the 39 kDa full-length SET, protecting the oncoprotein from protease cleavage, and facilitating PP2A inactivation and cell proliferation. Interestingly, SETBP1 overexpression is a common event in AML, affecting the 28% of AML patients and diminishing the overall survival [29]. Later studies in other myeloid neoplasm have confirmed the crucial role of SETBP1 in leukemogenesis.

On the other hand, SET is also implicated in natural killer (NK) cell cytotoxicity. Upon cytokine stimulation (Interlukin-12, −18 and − 15), SET up-regulation impairs IFN-γ production in human NK via PP2A inactivation, limiting the anti-tumor and/or anti-inflammatory activity of the NK cells [67]. Trotta *et al.* described a model where SET/PP2A regulates granzyme B expression which leads to determine NK cytotoxicity. They observed that SET knockdown inhibited the expression of granzyme B at mRNA and protein levels, limiting NK cytotoxicity [68].

Others have reported SET as an inhibitor of the DNAse activity of the tumor-suppressor NM23-H1; a promoter of AP-1 activity; or an activator of MAPK signaling. These data suggest that SET not only induce the inactivation of PP2A but also promotes other signaling pathways ensure tumor growth.

2.3 Cancerous inhibitor of PP2A (CIP2A)

Another endogenous PP2A inhibitor is cancerous inhibitor of PP2A (CIP2A) [69], an oncoprotein that controls oncogenic cellular signals by inhibiting PP2A activity through the stabilization of c-MYC [21, 69–71], which play an important role in AML [72].

CIP2A is expressed in very few tissues in normal conditions but it is overexpressed in a wide variety of human cancers, where it is associated with an aggressive clinical behavior [70, 71, 73–76]. However, few studies have focused on AML. Wang et al. using conventional PCR found that 77.4% of AML patients [55 of 84] overexpressed CIP2A, confirming their results at protein levels, however, they did not provide quantitative data to support that [77]. Recently, our group using quantitative real-time RT-PCR studied the prevalence of this oncoprotein in a series of 203 normal karyotype AML patients. We reported that CIP2A overexpression is a recurrent event in this subgroup of the disease (51/203, 25%), and is associated with a very poor prognostic impact in the overall survival of normal karyotype AML patients. Our results indicate that CIP2A knockout downregulates c-MYC, leading to a reduction of the cell proliferation, supporting the malignant role of CIP2A and c-MYC in leukemogenesis [31].

In addition, cancerous inhibitor of PP2A has been extensively studied in CML. Similarly, high levels of CIP2A were found in CML patients at diagnosis being significantly associated with risk of progression to blast crisis. Therefore, CIP2A protein levels have been postulated as a biomarker of disease progression in Imatinib-treated CML patients [78]. Furthermore, as indicated above with SET, high levels of CIP2A are associated with an up-regulation of c-MYC and BCR-ABL1 tyrosine kinase activity [78]. However, second-generation tyrosine kinase inhibitors (TKI) manage the disruption of CIP2A/c-MYC/E2F1 loop, preventing the malignant progression and constituting a promising therapeutic strategy [79]. These data support that CIP2A inhibits PP2A activity, stabilizing E2F1, and creating a CIP2A/c-MYC/E2F1 positive feedback loop, which imatinib cannot overcome [78]. However, greater efforts are need to elucidate the exact role of CIP2A in leukemias.

2.4 PP2A-activating drugs

The increased number of studies pointing to the crucial role of PP2A inactivation in cancer growth has led to the development of drugs that favors PP2A reactivation [12, 80]. The most widely studied drugs are FTY720 and OP449, but its limitations have encouraged the search of new drugs that have greater efficacy and clinical applicability.

FTY720, an oral sphingosine analog derived from myriocin, is a metabolite isolated from fungus Isaria Sinclairii that has been approved for the treatment of patients with relapse multiple sclerosis, but recently it has been studied for its potential antitumoral properties [81]. FTY720 is administrated as a pro-drug, which needs an activation by phosphorylation through sphingosine kinase 2, binding the active form to one of the sphingosine-1-phosphate receptors (S1P1, S1P3, S1P4 or S1P5). The phosphorylated form does not prevent T-lymphocyte or B-lymphocyte activation, but does interfere with the immune cell trafficking from the lymphoid organs to the peripheral blood [82]. Likewise, FTY720 is a potent inhibitor of tumor growth and angiogenesis, being attractive its use in the treatment of both solid and hematological tumors. Interestingly, the anticancer activity of the drug depends on the ability to act as a PP2A activator [83], inducing apoptosis by interfering with Bcl-2, and suppressing mitogenic and survival signals, and inhibiting the ERK and PI3K/AKT pathways [13, 84].

Mechanistically, FTY720 binds to globular amphipathic domain of the C-terminal hydrophobic pocket of SET [85], preventing the formation of the SET/PP2A-C inhibitory complex and reactivating PP2A functionality [12, 29–32]. Our group has confirmed these results in AML, showing that FTY720 binds to SET within the last 100 amino acids of the C-terminal fragment, producing a destabilization of the SET/PP2A-C inhibitory complex, which promote PP2A reactivation and a reduction of AML cell viability [30]. Several reports back it up pointing out the efficacy of FTY720 in vitro and in vivo models of AML, suggesting that PP2A restoration decreases clonogenicity and induces a suppression of the disease [12, 29–32]. Moreover, FTY720 perturbs the sphingolipid metabolism pathway, favoring the accumulation of ceramide, a pro-apoptotic second messenger, mostly in the mitochondria, leading to the death of AML cells [86]. In the same way as in AML, the effects induced by FTY720 are well characterized in Ph positive and negative leukemias. In CML and Ph-positive B-ALL progenitors, the drug promotes the BCR-ABL1 inactivation and degradation, leading to the inhibition of survival factors such as JAK2, AKT and ERK1/2, which results in apoptosis of CD34+ progenitors in patients with TKI sensitive and TKI-resistant CML [12, 55, 84]. In addition, a recent study provide new evidences for the use of FTY720 as an oral therapeutic agent in AML, highlighting that FTY720 lipid nanoparticles were more effective in vitro and in vivo models than FTY720 solutions because are able to increase the bioavailability of the free drug [32]. However, the main problem of the usage of FTY720 continues due to the induction of cardiotoxicity at the anti-neoplastic dose by the phosphorylated form. So, it has been proposed FTY720 analogues that are not targets for phosphorylation by SPHK2 [28].

Our group has recently revealed a novel non-phosphorylable FTY720 analogue called CM-1231, which reactivates PP2A activity by preventing the formation of the SET/PP2A-C inhibitory complex, inhibiting cell proliferation and promoting apoptosis in AML cell lines and primary patient samples. Importantly, CM-1231 does not induce cardiotoxicity in zebrafish models, maintaining its anti-leukemic potential in zebrafish xenograft models [28].

Other molecules have been tested to activate PP2A in AML, such as OP449 [87]. OP449 is a small physiological stable and cell-penetrating peptide, which binds specifically to SET leading to PP2A reactivation. It has been shown that OP449 treatment suppress tumor growth, enhance apoptosis and impairs clonogenicity of CML and AML cell lines and primary samples [87, 88]. Furthermore, the combination of OP449 with chemotherapy or specific TKI in AML and CML cell lines and primary patient samples have a synergistic effect [27]. However, OP449 like others PADs are unable to activate specific PP2A complexes against the exact pathogenic driver of the disease.

The ability of PP2A to dephosphorylate hundreds of proteins is mediated by over 40 specificity-determining B subunit, which competes for the assembly and activation of PP2A heterogeneous complex [89–91]. Therefore, it is essential to identify which regulatory isoform is deregulated in order to selectively reactivate it and direct PP2A against pathogenic drivers [92–94]. DT-061, a SMAP (small molecules that activate the phosphatase PP2A), selectively binds and stabilizes a PP2A complex containing a single B-subunit, B56α, which promote the dephosphorylation of selective PP2A substrates such as c-Myc. Stabilization of the PP2A-B56α complex by DT-061 has shown potent anti-leukemic effect, and their combination with TKI have improve anti-tumor effects while provide an opportunity to decrease kinase inhibitors related toxicities in some malignancies such as lung adenocarcinoma [95]. Interestingly, Kauko *et al.* determined that PP2A inactivation is a mechanism of kinase inhibitor resistance in cancer, thus the use of DT-061 could overcome the initial therapeutic resistance [96]. These observations raise the question on the appropriate temporal application of the drug: before the appearance of the resistance or upon its arrival. Whatever the answer, the important fact is that developing drugs against specific B regulatory subunits is a key event to face crucial pathogenic drivers [95].

Similarly, a class of small-molecules iHAPs (improved heterocyclic activators of PP2A) facilitate the assembly of the holoenzyme PP2R1A-B56ε-PPP2CA, which dephosphorylates MYBL2 transcription factor in Ser241, causing irreversible arrest of leukemic cells in the prometaphase [97]. Thus, the use of these molecules to target deregulated PP2A subunits; facilitate the activation/deactivation of specific molecular targets deregulated by PP2A inactivation in the tumoral scenario, reducing the toxicity induced by general activation of PP2A.

These findings open new possibilities to establish innovative therapeutic approach that targets PP2A in order to improve therapeutic options in AML patients.

3. Conclusion

Despite cytogenetic heterogeneity in AML was discovered 30 years ago, it was not until 15 years ago when the molecular heterogeneity of the disease began to be studied in depth. However, the general therapeutic strategy in AML patients has not changed substantially and high dose of chemotherapy continues to be the standard one. Consequently, the outcome for most patients, especially elder patients, remains poor. Thus, many new drugs targeting a variety of pathological cellular processes have been developed over the last years for the treatment of AML, although few have been translated into clinical practice. The reason is that they are used as single agents instead of following a combinatory therapy, decreasing its effectiveness. The Cancer Genome Atlas Research Network confirmed the molecular heterogeneity of the disease and organized important mutated genes in AML into a functional category, pointing out the importance of developing new compound against specific cancer pathways. In this regard, the tumor-suppressor PP2A has emerged as an important promising therapeutic target because its anti-proliferative function is inactivated in a large part of patients with AML.

PP2A inactivation is a recurrent event in AML patients. PP2A reactivation by PADs has shown important antileukemic effects in both KIT-positive and KIT-negative AML cells. Preclinical studies show that pharmacological restoration of PP2A tumor-suppressor activity by PADs (FTY720, OP499 or CM-1231) prevents the growth of tumor cells, increasing the cell death ratio. Furthermore, the combination of these drugs with both conventional chemotherapy and tyrosine kinases has synergistic cytotoxic effects in AML cells, decreasing the appearance of side effects. However, recently, have been developed small molecules that are capable of activating specific PP2A complexes that target particular disease-causing pathogenic pathways. The importance on knowing which B subunit is deregulated to applied a specific compound that reactivates this subunit opens new possibilities for personalize medicine, or personalized treatment, which improve the overall survival of patients with hematopoietic and non-hematopoietic malignancies.

Acknowledgements

This work was supported by grants from the ISCIII and Spanish Ministry of Economy and Competiveness (grants PI14/02073 and PI17/02272) (M.D.O.) and by CIBERONC (CB16/12/00489, CB16/12/00369, CB19/07/00031) (M.D.O., D.A.)

(Co-financed with FEDER funds), Department of Health of the Government of Navarra (29/2015) (M.D.O.), Department of Industry of the Government of Navarra (0011-1365-2016-000294) (M.D.O.).

Conflict of interest

The authors declare no conflict of interest.

Abbreviations

AML	acute myeloid leukemia
BM	bone marrow
CIP2A	cancerous inhibitor of PP2A
CK2	casein kinase 2
CML	chronic myeloid leukemia
iHAPs	improved heterocyclic activators of PP2A
NK	natural killer
OA	okadiac acid
PADs	PP2A-activating drugs
PP2A	protein phosphatase 2A
SETBP1	SET binding protein 1
TKI	tyrosine kinase inhibitors

Author details

Javier Marco[1,2], Irene Peris[2,3], Carmen Vicente[1,2,3] and Elena Arriazu[1,2,4]*

1 Centro de Investigación Médica Aplicada (CIMA), University of Navarra, Pamplona, Spain

2 Biochemistry and Genetics Department, University of Navarra, Pamplona, Spain

3 IdiSNA, Instituto de Investigación Sanitaria de Navarra, Pamplona, Spain

4 CIBERONC, Instituto de Salud Carlos III, Madrid, Spain

*Address all correspondence to: earriazu@unav.es

References

[1] DiNardo CD, Wei AH. How I treat acute myeloid leukemia in the era of new drugs. Blood. 2020;**135**:85-96

[2] Perl AE. Availability of FLT3 inhibitors: how do we use them? Blood. 2019;134:741-45.

[3] Smith CC. The growing landscape of FLT3 inhibition in AML. Hematology Am Soc Hematol Educ Program. 2019;2019:539-47.

[4] Antar AI, Otrock ZK, Jabbour E, Mohty M, Bazarbachi A. FLT3 inhibitors in acute myeloid leukemia: ten frequently asked questions. Leukemia. 2020. Published 2020 Jan 9.

[5] DiNardo CD, Tiong IS, Quaglieri A, et al. Molecular patterns of response and treatment failure after frontline venetoclax combinations in older patients with AML. Blood. 2020. Published 2020 Jan 13.

[6] Daver N, Schlenk RF, Russell NH, Levis MJ. Targeting FLT3 mutations in AML: review of current knowledge and evidence. Leukemia. 2019;33:299-312.

[7] Fowle H, Zhao Z, Graña X. PP2A holoenzymes, substrate specificity driving cellular functions and deregulation incancer. Adv Cancer Res. 2019;144:55-93

[8] Bertolotti A. The split protein phosphatase system. Biochem J. 2018;475:3707-3723.

[9] Mumby M. PP2A: Unveiling a Reluctant Tumor Suppressor. Cell. 2007 Jul;130(1):21-4.

[10] Westermarck J, Hahn WC. Multiple pathways regulated by the tumor suppressor PP2A in transformation. Trends Mol Med. 2008 Apr;14(4):152-60.

[11] Low ICC, Loh T, Huang Y, Virshup DM, Pervaiz S. Ser70 phosphorylation of Bcl-2 by selective tyrosine nitration of PP2A-B56δ stabilizes its antiapoptotic activity. Blood. 2014 Oct 2;124(14):2223-34.

[12] Perrotti D, Neviani P. Protein phosphatase 2A: a target for anticancer therapy. Lancet Oncol. 2013 May;14(6):e229-38.

[13] Neviani P, Harb JG, Oaks JJ, Santhanam R, Walker CJ, Ellis JJ, et al. PP2A-activating drugs selectively eradicate TKI-resistant chronic myeloid leukemic stem cells. J Clin Invest. 2013 Oct 1;123(10):4144-57.

[14] Arriazu E, Pippa R, Odero MD. Protein Phosphatase 2A as a Therapeutic Target in Acute Myeloid Leukemia. Front Oncol. 2016 Apr 6;6.

[15] Schönthal AH. Role of serine/threonine protein phosphatase 2A in cancer. Cancer Lett. 2001 Sep;170(1):1-13.

[16] Haesen D, Sents W, Lemaire K, Hoorne Y, Janssens V. The Basic Biology of PP2A in Hematologic Cells and Malignancies. Front Oncol. 2014 Dec 11;4.

[17] Eichhorn PJA, Creyghton MP, Bernards R. Protein phosphatase 2A regulatory subunits and cancer. Biochim Biophys Acta - Rev Cancer. 2009 Jan;1795(1):1-15.

[18] Lambrecht C, Haesen D, Sents W, Ivanova E, Janssens V. Structure, Regulation, and Pharmacological Modulation of PP2A Phosphatases. In 2013. p. 283-305.

[19] Sablina AA, Hector M, Colpaert N, Hahn WC. Identification of PP2A Complexes and Pathways Involved in

Cell Transformation. Cancer Res. 2010 Dec 15;70(24):10474-84.

[20] Janssens V, Longin S, Goris J. PP2A holoenzyme assembly: in cauda venenum (the sting is in the tail). Trends Biochem Sci. 2008 Mar;33(3):113-21.

[21] Leulliot N, Quevillon-Cheruel S, Sorel I, de La Sierra-Gallay IL, Collinet B, Graille M, et al. Structure of Protein Phosphatase Methyltransferase 1 (PPM1), a Leucine Carboxyl Methyltransferase Involved in the Regulation of Protein Phosphatase 2A Activity. J Biol Chem. 2004 Feb 27;279(9):8351-8.

[22] Longin S, Zwaenepoel K, Louis J V., Dilworth S, Goris J, Janssens V. Selection of Protein Phosphatase 2A Regulatory Subunits Is Mediated by the C Terminus of the Catalytic Subunit. J Biol Chem. 2007 Sep 14;282(37):26971-80.

[23] Cristóbal I, Garcia-Orti L, Cirauqui C, Alonso MM, Calasanz MJ, Odero MD. PP2A impaired activity is a common event in acute myeloid leukemia and its activation by forskolin has a potent anti-leukemic effect. Leukemia. 2011 Apr 14;25(4):606-14.

[24] Bononi A, Agnoletto C, De Marchi E, Marchi S, Patergnani S, Bonora M, et al. Protein Kinases and Phosphatases in the Control of Cell Fate. Enzyme Res. 2011;2011:1-26.

[25] Roberts KG, Smith AM, McDougall F, Carpenter H, Horan M, Neviani P, et al. Essential Requirement for PP2A Inhibition by the Oncogenic Receptor c-KIT Suggests PP2A Reactivation as a Strategy to Treat c-KIT + Cancers. Cancer Res. 2010 Jul 1;70(13):5438-47.

[26] Ramaswamy K, Spitzer B, Kentsis A. Therapeutic Re-Activation of Protein Phosphatase 2A in Acute Myeloid Leukemia. Front Oncol. 2015 Feb 2;5.

[27] Agarwal A, MacKenzie RJ, Pippa R, Eide CA, Oddo J, Tyner JW, et al. Antagonism of SET Using OP449 Enhances the Efficacy of Tyrosine Kinase Inhibitors and Overcomes Drug Resistance in Myeloid Leukemia. Clin Cancer Res. 2014 Apr 15;20(8):2092-103.

[28] Vicente C, Arriazu E, Martínez-Balsalobre E, Peris I, Marcotegui N, García-Ramírez P, et al. A novel FTY720 analogue targets SET-PP2A interaction and inhibits growth of acute myeloid leukemia cells without inducing cardiac toxicity. Cancer Lett. 2020 Jan;468:1-13.

[29] Cristobal I, Garcia-Orti L, Cirauqui C, Cortes-Lavaud X, Garcia-Sanchez MA, Calasanz MJ, et al. Overexpression of SET is a recurrent event associated with poor outcome and contributes to protein phosphatase 2A inhibition in acute myeloid leukemia. Haematologica. 2012 Apr 1;97(4):543-50.

[30] Pippa R, Dominguez A, Christensen DJ, Moreno-Miralles I, Blanco-Prieto MJ, Vitek MP, et al. Effect of FTY720 on the SET–PP2A complex in acute myeloid leukemia; SET binding drugs have antagonistic activity. Leukemia. 2014 Sep 30;28(9):1915-8.

[31] Barragan E, Chillon MC, Castello-Cros R, Marcotegui N, Prieto MI, Hoyos M, et al. CIP2A high expression is a poor prognostic factor in normal karyotype acute myeloid leukemia. Haematologica. 2015 May 1;100(5):e183-5.

[32] de Mendoza AE-H, Castello-Cros R, Imbuluzqueta E, Cirauqui C, Pippa R, Odero MD, et al. Lipid Nanosystems Enhance the Bioavailability and the Therapeutic Efficacy of FTY720 in Acute Myeloid Leukemia. J Biomed Nanotechnol. 2015 Apr 1;11(4):691-701.

[33] Sangodkar J, Farrington CC, McClinch K, Galsky MD, Kastrinsky DB, Narla G. All roads lead

to PP2A: exploiting the therapeutic potential of this phosphatase. FEBS J. 2016 Mar;283(6):1004-24.

[34] Wang SS. Alterations of the PPP2R1B Gene in Human Lung and Colon Cancer. Science (80-). 1998 Oct 9;282(5387):284-7.

[35] Calin GA, di Iasio MG, Caprini E, Vorechovsky I, Natali PG, Sozzi G, et al. Low frequency of alterations of the α (PPP2R1A) and β (PPP2R1B) isoforms of the subunit A of the serine-threonine phosphatase 2A in human neoplasms. Oncogene. 2000 Feb 7;19(9):1191-5.

[36] Ruediger R, Pham HT, Walter G. Alterations in protein phosphatase 2A subunit interaction in human carcinomas of the lung and colon with mutations in the Aβ subunit gene. Oncogene. 2001 Apr;20(15):1892-9.

[37] Ruediger R, Pham HT, Walter G. Alterations in protein phosphatase 2A subunit interaction in human carcinomas of the lung and colon with mutations in the Aβ subunit gene. Oncogene. 2001 Apr;20(15):1892-9.

[38] Esplin ED, Ramos P, Martinez B, Tomlinson GE, Mumby MC, Evans GA. The glycine 90 to aspartate alteration in the Aβ subunit of PP2A (PPP2R1B) associates with breast cancer and causes a deficit in protein function. Genes, Chromosom Cancer. 2006 Feb;45(2):182-90.

[39] Kalla C, Scheuermann MO, Kube I, Schlotter M, Mertens D, Döhner H, et al. Analysis of 11q22–q23 deletion target genes in B-cell chronic lymphocytic leukaemia: Evidence for a pathogenic role of NPAT, CUL5, and PPP2R1B. Eur J Cancer. 2007 May;43(8):1328-35.

[40] Genomic and Epigenomic Landscapes of Adult De Novo Acute Myeloid Leukemia. N Engl J Med. 2013 May 30;368(22):2059-74.

[41] Hwang J, Lee JA, Pallas DC. Leucine Carboxyl Methyltransferase 1 (LCMT-1) Methylates Protein Phosphatase 4 (PP4) and Protein Phosphatase 6 (PP6) and Differentially Regulates the Stable Formation of Different PP4 Holoenzymes. J Biol Chem. 2016 Sep 30;291(40):21008-19.

[42] Sontag J-M, Nunbhakdi-Craig V, Sontag E. Leucine Carboxyl Methyltransferase 1 (LCMT1)-dependent Methylation Regulates the Association of Protein Phosphatase 2A and Tau Protein with Plasma Membrane Microdomains in Neuroblastoma Cells. J Biol Chem. 2013 Sep 20;288(38):27396-405.

[43] Tsai M-L, Cronin N, Djordjevic S. The structure of human leucine carboxyl methyltransferase 1 that regulates protein phosphatase PP2A. Acta Crystallogr Sect D Biol Crystallogr. 2011 Jan 1;67(1):14-24.

[44] Li M, Makkinje A, Damuni Z. The Myeloid Leukemia-associated Protein SET Is a Potent Inhibitor of Protein Phosphatase 2A. J Biol Chem. 1996 May 10;271(19):11059-62.

[45] Adachr Y, Pavlakis GN, Copeland TD. Identification of in vivo phosphorylation sites of SET, a nuclear phosphoprotein encoded by the translocation breakpoint in acute undifferentiated leukemia. FEBS Lett. 1994;340(3):231-5.

[46] Saito S, Miyaji-Yamaguchi M, Nagata K. Aberrant intracellular localization of SET-CAN fusion protein, associated with a leukemia, disorganizes nuclear export. Int J Cancer. 2004 Sep 10;111(4):501-7.

[47] Seo S, McNamara P, Heo S, Turner A, Lane WS, Chakravarti D. Regulation of Histone Acetylation and Transcription by INHAT, a Human Cellular Complex Containing

the Set Oncoprotein. Cell. 2001 Jan;104(1):119-30.

[48] Kutney SN, Hong R, Macfarlan T, Chakravarti D. A Signaling Role of Histone-binding Proteins and INHAT Subunits pp32 and Set/TAF-Iβ in Integrating Chromatin Hypoacetylation and Transcriptional Repression. J Biol Chem. 2004 Jul 16;279(29):30850-5.

[49] Kalousi A, Hoffbeck A-S, Selemenakis PN, Pinder J, Savage KI, Khanna KK, et al. The Nuclear Oncogene SET Controls DNA Repair by KAP1 and HP1 Retention to Chromatin. Cell Rep. 2015 Apr;11(1):149-63.

[50] Kandilci A, Mientjes E, Grosveld G. Effects of SET and SET-CAN on the differentiation of the human promonocytic cell line U937. Leukemia. 2004 Feb 4;18(2):337-40.

[51] ten Klooster JP, Leeuwen I v, Scheres N, Anthony EC, Hordijk PL. Rac1-induced cell migration requires membrane recruitment of the nuclear oncogene SET. EMBO J. 2007 Jan 24;26(2):336-45.

[52] Canela N, Rodriguez-Vilarrupla A, Estanyol JM, Díaz C, Pujol MJ, Agell N, et al. The SET Protein Regulates G 2 /M Transition by Modulating Cyclin B-Cyclin-dependent Kinase 1 Activity. J Biol Chem. 2003 Jan 10;278(2):1158-64.

[53] Cristobal I, Rincon R, Manso R, Carames C, Zazo S, Madoz-Gurpide J, et al. Deregulation of the PP2A Inhibitor SET Shows Promising Therapeutic Implications and Determines Poor Clinical Outcome in Patients with Metastatic Colorectal Cancer. Clin Cancer Res. 2015 Jan 15;21(2):347-56.

[54] Janghorban M, Farrell AS, Allen-Petersen BL, Pelz C, Daniel CJ, Oddo J, et al. Targeting c-MYC by antagonizing PP2A inhibitors in breast cancer. Proc Natl Acad Sci. 2014 Jun 24;111(25):9157-62.

[55] Neviani P, Santhanam R, Trotta R, Notari M, Blaser BW, Liu S, et al. The tumor suppressor PP2A is functionally inactivated in blast crisis CML through the inhibitory activity of the BCR/ABL-regulated SET protein. Cancer Cell. 2005 Nov;8(5):355-68.

[56] Perrotti D, Jamieson C, Goldman J, Skorski T. Chronic myeloid leukemia: mechanisms of blastic transformation. J Clin Invest. 2010 Jul 1;120(7):2254-64.

[57] Arriazu E, Vicente C, Pippa R, Peris I, Martínez-Balsalobre E, García-Ramírez P, et al. A new regulatory mechanism of protein phosphatase 2A activity via SET in acute myeloid leukemia. Blood Cancer J. 2020 Jan 8;10(1):3.

[58] Cristóbal I, Blanco FJ, Garcia-Orti L, Marcotegui N, Vicente C, Rifon J, et al. SETBP1 overexpression is a novel leukemogenic mechanism that predicts adverse outcome in elderly patients with acute myeloid leukemia. Blood. 2010 Jan 21;115(3):615-25.

[59] Igea A, Nebreda AR. The Stress Kinase p38 as a Target for Cancer Therapy. Cancer Res. 2015 Oct 1;75(19):3997-4002.

[60] Zhong W, Zhu H, Sheng F, Tian Y, Zhou J, Chen Y, et al. Activation of the MAPK11/12/13/14 (p38 MAPK) pathway regulates the transcription of autophagy genes in response to oxidative stress induced by a novel copper complex in HeLa cells. Autophagy. 2014 Jul 29;10(7):1285-300.

[61] Beenstock J, Ben-Yehuda S, Melamed D, Admon A, Livnah O, Ahn NG, et al. The p38β Mitogen-activated Protein Kinase Possesses an Intrinsic Autophosphorylation Activity, Generated by a Short Region Composed of the α-G Helix and MAPK Insert. J Biol Chem. 2014 Aug 22;289(34):23546-56.

[62] del Barco Barrantes I, Coya JM, Maina F, Arthur JSC, Nebreda AR. Genetic analysis of specific and redundant roles for p38 and p38 MAPKs during mouse development. Proc Natl Acad Sci. 2011 Aug 2;108(31):12764-9.

[63] Grethe S, Pörn-Ares MI. p38 MAPK regulates phosphorylation of Bad via PP2A-dependent suppression of the MEK1/2-ERK1/2 survival pathway in TNF-α induced endothelial apoptosis. Cell Signal. 2006 Apr;18(4):531-40.

[64] Junttila MR, Li S, Westermarck J. Phosphatase-mediated crosstalk between MAPK signaling pathways in the regulation of cell survival. FASEB J. 2008 Apr 26;22(4):954-65.

[65] Lin S-P, Lee Y-T, Wang J-Y, Miller SA, Chiou S-H, Hung M-C, et al. Survival of Cancer Stem Cells under Hypoxia and Serum Depletion via Decrease in PP2A Activity and Activation of p38-MAPKAPK2-Hsp27. Koritzinsky M, editor. PLoS One. 2012 Nov 20;7(11):e49605.

[66] Guillonneau M, Paris F, Dutoit S, Estephan H, Bénéteau E, Huot J, et al. Oxidative stress disassembles the p38/NPM/PP2A complex, which leads to modulation of nucleophosmin-mediated signaling to DNA damage response. FASEB J. 2016 Aug 3;30(8):2899-914.

[67] Trotta R, Ciarlariello D, Col JD, Allard J, Neviani P, Santhanam R, et al. The PP2A inhibitor SET regulates natural killer cell IFN-γ production. J Exp Med. 2007 Oct 1;204(10):2397-405.

[68] Trotta R, Ciarlariello D, Dal Col J, Mao H, Chen L, Briercheck E, et al. The PP2A inhibitor SET regulates granzyme B expression in human natural killer cells. Blood. 2011 Feb 24;117(8):2378-84.

[69] Junttila MR, Puustinen P, Niemelä M, Ahola R, Arnold H, Böttzauw T, et al. CIP2A Inhibits PP2A in Human Malignancies. Cell. 2007 Jul;130(1):51-62.

[70] Niemelä M, Kauko O, Sihto H, Mpindi J-P, Nicorici D, Pernilä P, et al. CIP2A signature reveals the MYC dependency of CIP2A-regulated phenotypes and its clinical association with breast cancer subtypes. Oncogene. 2012 Sep 16;31(39):4266-78.

[71] Khanna A, Pimanda JE, Westermarck J. Cancerous Inhibitor of Protein Phosphatase 2A, an Emerging Human Oncoprotein and a Potential Cancer Therapy Target. Cancer Res. 2013 Nov 15;73(22):6548-53.

[72] Luo H, Li Q, O'Neal J, Kreisel F, Le Beau MM, Tomasson MH. c-Myc rapidly induces acute myeloid leukemia in mice without evidence of lymphoma-associated antiapoptotic mutations. Blood. 2005 Oct 1;106(7):2452-61.

[73] Come C, Laine A, Chanrion M, Edgren H, Mattila E, Liu X, et al. CIP2A Is Associated with Human Breast Cancer Aggressivity. Clin Cancer Res. 2009 Aug 15;15(16):5092-100.

[74] Khanna A, Böckelman C, Hemmes A, Junttila MR, Wiksten J-P, Lundin M, et al. MYC-Dependent Regulation and Prognostic Role of CIP2A in Gastric Cancer. JNCI J Natl Cancer Inst. 2009 Jun;101(11):793-805.

[75] Dong Q-Z, Wang Y, Dong X-J, Li Z-X, Tang Z-P, Cui Q-Z, et al. CIP2A is Overexpressed in Non-Small Cell Lung Cancer and Correlates with Poor Prognosis. Ann Surg Oncol. 2011 Mar 15;18(3):857-65.

[76] Xue Y, Wu G, Wang X, Zou X, Zhang G, Xiao R, et al. CIP2A is a predictor of survival and a novel therapeutic target in bladder urothelial cell carcinoma. Med Oncol. 2013 Mar 30;30(1):406.

[77] WANG J, LI W, LI L, YU X, JIA J, CHEN C. CIP2A is over-expressed in acute myeloid leukaemia and associated with HL60 cells proliferation and differentiation. Int J Lab Hematol. 2011 Jun;33(3):290-8.

[78] Lucas CM, Harris RJ, Giannoudis A, Copland M, Slupsky JR, Clark RE. Cancerous inhibitor of PP2A (CIP2A) at diagnosis of chronic myeloid leukemia is a critical determinant of disease progression. Blood. 2011 Jun 16;117(24):6660-8.

[79] Lucas CM, Harris RJ, Holcroft AK, Scott LJ, Carmell N, McDonald E, et al. Second generation tyrosine kinase inhibitors prevent disease progression in high-risk (high CIP2A) chronic myeloid leukaemia patients. Leukemia. 2015 Jul 13;29(7):1514-23.

[80] Ciccone M, Calin GA, Perrotti D. From the Biology of PP2A to the PADs for Therapy of Hematologic Malignancies. Front Oncol. 2015 Feb 16;5.

[81] Cohen JA, Barkhof F, Comi G, Hartung H-P, Khatri BO, Montalban X, et al. Oral Fingolimod or Intramuscular Interferon for Relapsing Multiple Sclerosis. N Engl J Med. 2010 Feb 4;362(5):402-15.

[82] Martin R. Anti-CD25 (daclizumab) monoclonal antibody therapy in relapsing–remitting multiple sclerosis. Clin Immunol. 2012 Jan;142(1):9-14.

[83] Oaks JJ, Santhanam R, Walker CJ, Roof S, Harb JG, Ferenchak G, et al. Antagonistic activities of the immunomodulator and PP2A-activating drug FTY720 (Fingolimod, Gilenya) in Jak2-driven hematologic malignancies. Blood. 2013 Sep 12;122(11):1923-34.

[84] Neviani P, Santhanam R, Oaks JJ, Eiring AM, Notari M, Blaser BW, et al. FTY720, a new alternative for treating blast crisis chronic myelogenous leukemia and Philadelphia chromosome–positive acute lymphocytic leukemia. J Clin Invest. 2007 Sep 4;117(9):2408-21.

[85] Arnaud L, Chen S, Liu F, Li B, Khatoon S, Grundke-Iqbal I, et al. Mechanism of inhibition of PP2A activity and abnormal hyperphosphorylation of tau by I 2 PP2A /SET. FEBS Lett. 2011 Sep 2;585(17):2653-9.

[86] Chen L, Luo L-F, Lu J, Li L, Liu Y-F, Wang J, et al. FTY720 Induces Apoptosis of M2 Subtype Acute Myeloid Leukemia Cells by Targeting Sphingolipid Metabolism and Increasing Endogenous Ceramide Levels. Siskind LJ, editor. PLoS One. 2014 Jul 22;9(7):e103033.

[87] Christensen DJ, Chen Y, Oddo J, Matta KM, Neil J, Davis ED, et al. SET oncoprotein overexpression in B-cell chronic lymphocytic leukemia and non-Hodgkin lymphoma: a predictor of aggressive disease and a new treatment target. Blood. 2011 Oct 13;118(15):4150-8.

[88] Switzer CH, Cheng RYS, Vitek TM, Christensen DJ, Wink DA, Vitek MP. Targeting SET/I2PP2A oncoprotein functions as a multi-pathway strategy for cancer therapy. Oncogene. 2011 Jun 7;30(22):2504-13.

[89] Wlodarchak N, Guo F, Satyshur KA, Jiang L, Jeffrey PD, Sun T, et al. Structure of the Ca2+–dependent PP2A heterotrimer and insights into Cdc6 dephosphorylation. Cell Res. 2013 Jul 11;23(7):931-46.

[90] Xu Y, Xing Y, Chen Y, Chao Y, Lin Z, Fan E, et al. Structure of the Protein Phosphatase 2A Holoenzyme. Cell. 2006 Dec;127(6):1239-51.

[91] Xu Y, Chen Y, Zhang P, Jeffrey PD, Shi Y. Structure of a Protein Phosphatase 2A Holoenzyme: Insights into

B55-Mediated Tau Dephosphorylation. Mol Cell. 2008 Sep;31(6):873-85.

[92] Arnold HK, Sears RC. A tumor suppressor role for PP2A-B56α through negative regulation of c-Myc and other key oncoproteins. Cancer Metastasis Rev. 2008 Jun 2;27(2):147-58.

[93] Letourneux C, Rocher G, Porteu F. B56-containing PP2A dephosphorylate ERK and their activity is controlled by the early gene IEX-1 and ERK. EMBO J. 2006 Feb 22;25(4):727-38.

[94] Casado P, Rodriguez-Prados J-C, Cosulich SC, Guichard S, Vanhaesebroeck B, Joel S, et al. Kinase-Substrate Enrichment Analysis Provides Insights into the Heterogeneity of Signaling Pathway Activation in Leukemia Cells. Sci Signal. 2013 Mar 26;6(268):rs6-rs6.

[95] Leonard D, Huang W, Izadmehr S, O'Connor CM, Wiredja DD, Wang Z, et al. Selective PP2A Enhancement through Biased Heterotrimer Stabilization. Cell. 2020;181(3):688-701.e16.

[96] Kauko O, O'Connor CM, Kulesskiy E, Sangodkar J, Aakula A, Izadmehr S, et al. PP2A inhibition is a druggable MEK inhibitor resistance mechanism in KRAS-mutant lung cancer cells. Sci Transl Med. 2018 Jul 18;10(450):eaaq1093.

[97] Morita K, He S, Nowak RP, Wang J, Zimmerman MW, Fu C, et al. Allosteric Activators of Protein Phosphatase 2A Display Broad Antitumor Activity Mediated by Dephosphorylation of MYBL2. Cell. 2020 Apr;181(3):702-715.e20.

Chapter 5

Melanin, from an Evolutionary Remnant to the Myeloid Lineage Cell's Main Energy Source. The Unsuspected Intrinsic Property of Melanin to Dissociate the Molecule from Water. Possible Implications in the Context of Acute Leukemias

Arturo Solís Herrera, Ruth I. Solís Arias and Luis F. Torres Solís

Abstract

Melanin is one of the most stable substances known. The study of the ink bags of fossilized squid that died 160 million years ago has found it in good condition. Its extraordinary stability is what had prevented, to date; assign a relevant role in biology. Sir Everard Holmes' proposal in London; in the eighteenth century, about the role of melanin as a simple sunscreen, it has permeated to this day, especially among dermatologists. Despite the unique physical–chemical qualities of melanin, its biological role as a simple sunscreen that protects us from the dangerous UV rays remained immutable. Our circumstantial discovery during an observational study that lasted 12 years (1990–2002) and which included the ophthalmologic studies of 6000 patients, about the relationship between the vessels of the optic nerve and the three main causes of blindness (Macular degeneration, diabetes, and glaucoma) allowed us to discern the unexpected and surprising true role of melanin in Biology as an energy transducer. The unsuspected intrinsic property of melanin to transform light into chemical energy through water dissociation, like chlorophyll in plants; opens a new era in Biology and therefore in Medicine. And Acute Leukemias are no exception.

Keywords: energy, mitochondria, melanin, water, hydrogen, oxygen, ATP

1. Introduction

Wasserman described the accidental discovery of lymphocytes containing melanin granules in humans since 1963 [1]. Through the reaction to a non-immune Antigen (Egg white), Wasserman found in all the 46 non-White subjects' investigation of the hourly preparations revealed that melanin became discernible in neutrophils as well as in the subsequent mononuclear phase. The same pattern of events was observed in all these experiments, differing only in the time of appearance and number of pigmented leukocytes present. Theoretically was thought that Neutrophils, as microphages, phagocytose small particles of melanin, and by shrinkage, prior to the stage of lymphocytic influx, condense these particles to clearly discernible granules.

Pigmented leukocytes could be demonstrated in blood from Amphibians and Reptiles, as reported by several previous investigators [2]. The pigment could be identified as melanin in the ease of amphibians by the highly specific ferrous iron technic of Lillie. More pigmented leukocytes were found in those amphibians suffering from the active skin- and subcutaneous infection than in normal animals.

It is not easy to demonstrate melanin inside cells, especially when cytoplasm is scarce, it had been described the following techniques in this regard:

Mop-Gruenwald-Giemsa -—Formed cutaneous melanin present a green-black color when stained by this procedure. This color was noted in several studies describing melanin-containing cells in the bone-marrow either as melanin-laden macrophages [3].

Distaining Procedure. —May-Gruenwald- Giemsa stained preparations may be distained by immersion in absolute methyl alcohol. In skin- window preparations it was confirmed that the dc-stained melanin granule had the same brown appearance as before any staining procedure was carried out. In freshly stained preparations, the granule loses its green-black color before the nucleus of the cell is decolorized, and this facilitates localization of pigment-containing cells and identification of cell-type.

Dope staining. —Though carried out on blood smears by the method of Laidlaw and Blackberg [4], the nonspecific nature of the reaction is of no practical use in determining the nature of the pigment.

Ferrous Iron Uptake (Lillie). - Gives a dark green color with melanin, while lipofuscins do not stain. The specificity of this reaction for melanin is high [5].

2. Melanin in the bone marrow

Since melanin is the energy source par excellence of eukaryotic cells, it is present in all cell lineages, being its main location in perinuclear space in the form of melanosomes. And its presence in the bone marrow solves the conundrum about the energy source of the yellow bone marrow, which has no blood vessels despite being the most metabolically active part.

Melanin may be easily overlooked in routine histological sections, as it resembles hemosiderin and its presence should be confirmed by Masson-Fontana silver impregnation [6]. Melanocytes may be present even in the apparent absence of melanin [7] and can be recognized by electron microscopy [8] and immunohistochemistry for S-100 protein [9], melanoma-associated antigen [10], or HMB-45 antigen [11]. In fact, all cells require melanin to generate the energy they need to function and preserve form. Some cells contain melanin in greater quantity depending on their location and function (**Figure 1**).

The most used staining in histology is hematoxylin and eosin (H & E), but it does not allow differentiation between melanin and hemosiderin.

Hemosiderin comes from aging erythrocytes, so there must be the history of erythrocyte diapedesis that mainly occur in acute stages of inflammation. Hemosiderin appears to be both intra and extracellular [12]. The abnormal presence of hemosiderin is explained by extravasation and lysis of red blood cells, followed by decomposition of hemoglobin into hemosiderin [13].

Melanin is always intracellular because is easily metabolized by the organism to cysteinyl-dopa, which can be found as a urinary metabolite. However, inside the cell, is a quite important component due to bioenergetic role.

The melanin observed with different wavelengths tends to preserve its dark brown hue. It is a practical way to differentiate it without touching tissue samples (**Figure 2**).

Perl's stain is currently used for the detection of hemosiderin granules because it detects the presence of ferric ions ($Fe3^+$) in the tissue due to the production of ferric ferrocyanide which results from the reaction of ferric ions with ferrocyanide [14].12Haemosiderin was visible as granules (siderosomes) within macro-phages (siderophages). These granules appeared brownish or black in H & E sections and blue in Perl's stain (**Figure 3**).

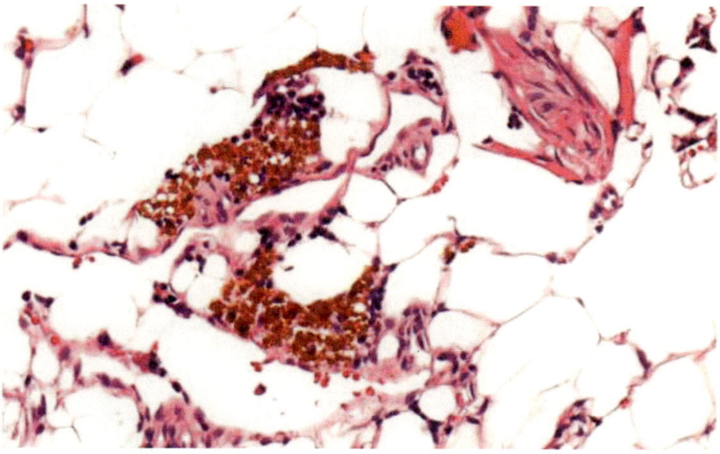

Figure 1.
Melanin in the bone marrow. Melanin appeared as brown, brownish-black, or black granules co-located within cells.

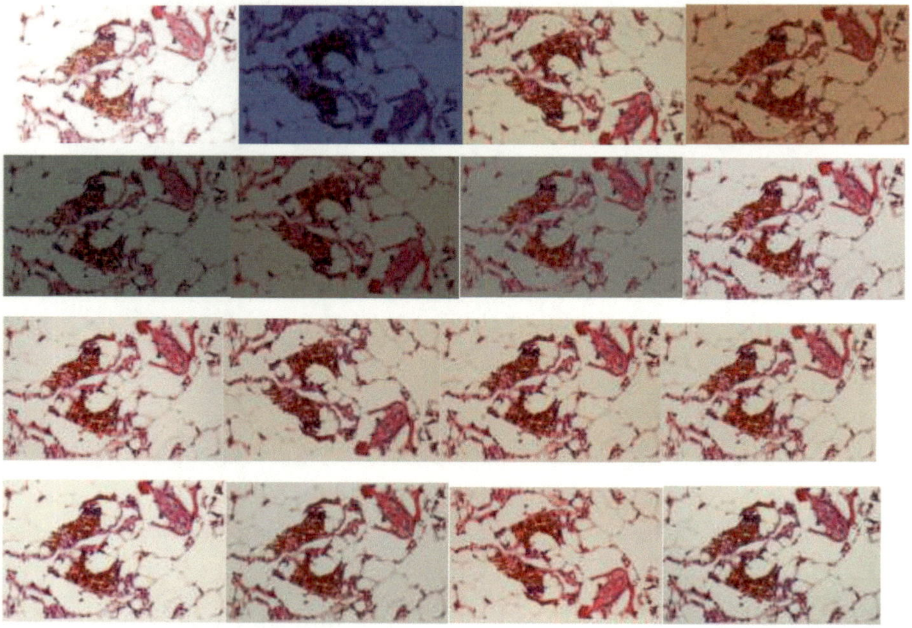

Figure 2.
Melanin observed with different wavelengths.

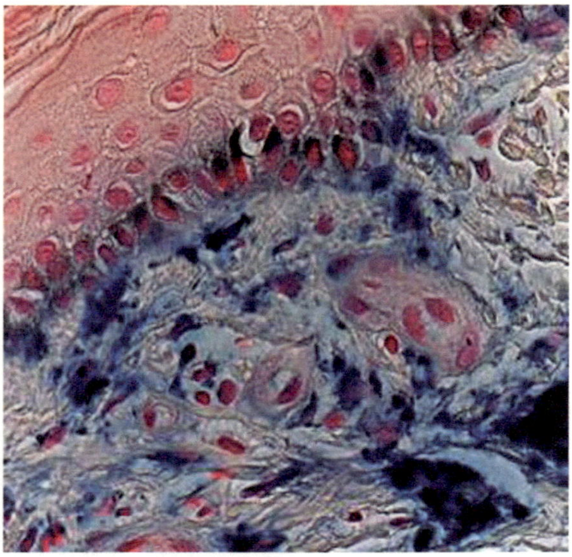

Figure 3.
Perl's stain. Hemosiderin is seen as deep blue. Excess hemosiderin accumulates in the liver and spleen causing impaired organ function culminating in death. Iron poisons melanin itself.

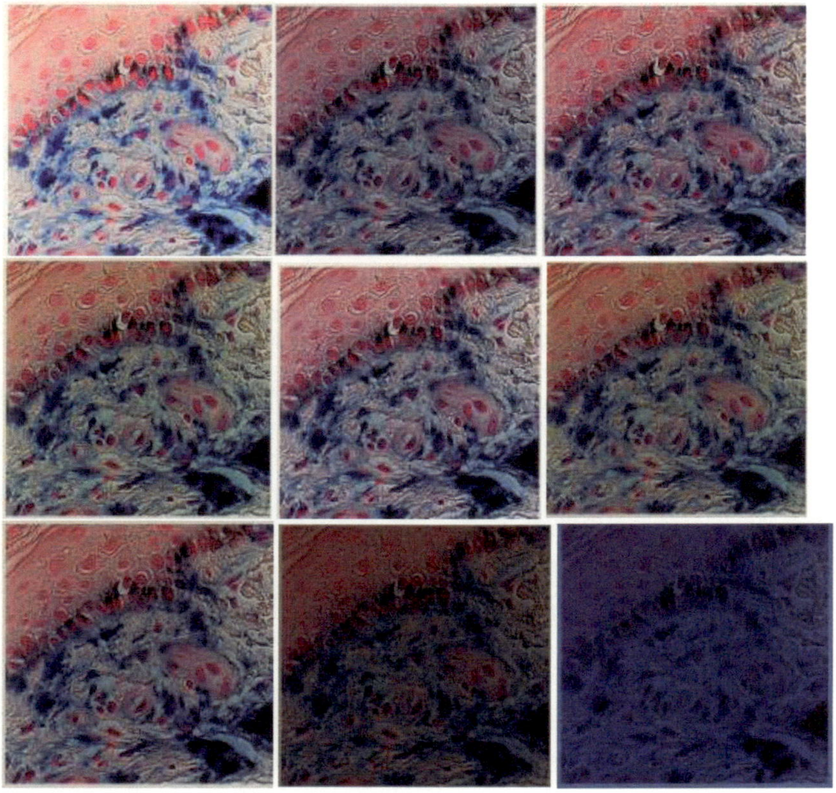

Figure 4.
*The same tissue in **Figure 3** observed with different wavelengths, allows us to identify the dark brown color characteristic of melanin happens with any wavelength.*

Hemoglobin is a conjugated protein found in erythrocytes, that stains vividly with acid (anionic) dyes such as eosin. Hemoglobin breaks down into two parts: globin (protein that is returned to the amino acid pool) and heme (iron-containing pigment part). The heme portion splits again into iron (hemosiderin) and bile pigments (biliverdin). Hemosiderin (stored ferric iron) is a breakdown product of hemoglobin; if the iron is not needed immediately to produce new hemoglobin, hemosiderin is stored in bone marrow and splenic red pulp. If the production and destruction of red blood cells is not balanced, there may be increased deposition of hemosiderin in tissues. Hemosiderin is differentiated from other yellow to brown pigments with the Prussian blue reaction which detects ferric ($Fe3^{+}$) iron.

Observation of tissue sections with different wavelengths, allow us to differentiate reasonable the presence of melanin from hemosiderin without the need to add different chemical compounds to the tissues (**Figure 4**).

The distinction between hemosiderin and melanin pigmentation is difficult in routine histological examination. Excessive amounts of splenic hemosiderin are seen when erythropoiesis is reduced (less demand for iron) or from the rapid destruction of erythrocytes in hemolytic anemias (increased stores of iron), such as those caused by immune-mediated hemolytic anemias or hemotropic parasites. Excess splenic hemosiderin may also occur in conditions such as chronic heart failure or injections of iron dextran or as focal accumulations at the sites of old hematomas, infarcts, or trauma-induced hemorrhages. The precise reason for deposition of iron is not always clear. Aniline and related agents may also increase splenic iron content.

3. Energy plays a fundamental role in all processes of the body

Energy is defined as everything that produces a change. Metabolism means continuous change. Therefore, our body requires energy constantly, all the time, day, and night. Glucose is the universal precursor to any organic matter in plants and animals, but it cannot provide the energy that its own metabolism needs.

Our body takes the necessary energy from light, dissociating the molecule from water, such as chlorophyll in plants. A reliable test is that two of the most active metabolic areas - the layer of cones and rods in the retina and the yellow bone marrow - do not have blood vessels.

Being the beginning of everything, events that alter the generation and distribution of energy from melanin, cause important effects on health depending on the nature of the physical, chemical, and/or biological agent.

The generation and distribution of energy from melanin is an astonishingly accurate process and has not changed since the beginning of time. The energy requirements of the bone marrow are incessant, day and night. Only in this way does the balance between mass and energy happen properly so that the bone marrow produces 2 to 3 million blood cells per second.

Therefore, there are physical factors (electrical trauma, extreme temperatures, ionizing radiation, etc.) and chemical factors such as contaminated water, contaminated air, pesticides, herbicides, fertilizers, metals, plastics, solvents, industrial waste, solvents, alcohol, addictive drugs, anesthetic agents, etc., which alter the process, resulting in the balance between mass and energy being disturbed and the body, or in this case, the bone marrow is disorganized and cannot perform its functions efficiently, as it has millions of years ago.

For clarity purposes, we will refer especially to water, for two reasons: 1) water is the perfect substrate for melanin and 2) any type of contamination eventually reaches the water.

When water becomes contaminated, the first thing it loses is viscosity and then other characteristics, and as the physicochemical properties of water are altered by contaminants, efficiency and accuracy in that melanin dissociates and re-associates the water molecule is disturbed resulting in intracellular biochemical processes beginning to disorganize.

In any system, when the problem is power, the failure is widespread, and the bone marrow is no exception. Several histological alterations must occur almost simultaneously for acute leukemia to manifest.

Therefore, contaminated water can produce all kinds of diseases, mainly because it affects the generation and distribution of energy from melanin.

4. Melanin in leukocytes

Pigmented leukocytes are considered rare so far, but now that we are aware of the importance of bioenergetic role of melanin in cell biology, we think it is rather the difficulty in identifying the microscopic melanin granules (**Figure 5**).

Until today, it is abnormal to have a greater number of pigmented leukocytes, for instance more than two percent [15] and frequently there is also histiocytes in the peripheral blood with massive amounts of pigment granules.

There was an impression about that the abdominal vein and renal portal vein transported more melanin, the abdominal vein and renal portal vein often had cells densely packed with melanin granules. The pigment in large cells, and present in large amounts, was shown to be mostly melanin. In some of these cells only a positive Schmorl reaction was obtained, and such pigment may be lipofuscins rather than melanin.

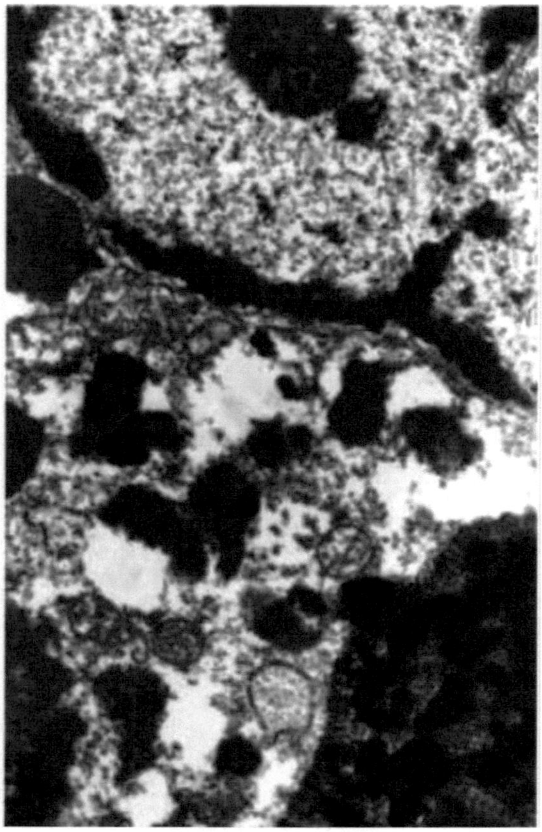

Figure 5.
The cytoplasm of macrophage loaded with melanin. X 10000.

In some cells a few black granules were seen but could not be identified as melanin. Most of the pigmented leukocytes were mononuclear cell types. The neutrophils of amphibians contain none or only a few specific granules, and it is impossible to decide on the actual nature of some very dark, slightly larger granules in some neutrophils.

Some cells with a basophilic cytoplasm but a nucleus resembling a granulocytic nucleus should probably be classified as a monocytic cell type rather than granulocytic. But it would be difficult to conceive how such granules of melanin reached the blood.

The organs most heavily laden with melanin are the liver, the spleen, and the lung approximately in this order, but the kidney and myocardium also contain some melanin. These melanin deposits are not P.A.S.-positive, a reaction obtained from phagocytosed melanin in macrophages, but the granules vary in size, which does suggest phagocytized melanin. All cells in your body have the necessary genetic information to synthesize melanin. Wandering cells require an energy source, so it is not uncommon for synthetize and carrying it with them, for instance histiocytes.

Cells that form in the bone marrow have unique characteristics since their generation, starting with the central part of the bone marrow (**Figure 6**), the area of greatest metabolic activity; and paradoxically has no blood vessels at all. According to the current dogma, glucose has a double paper (theory), a) universal precursor of 99% of organic matter and b) the energy source par excellence of the eukaryotic cell.

Glucose carbon chains are the building blocks of any organic matter, but glucose cannot provide the energy that its own metabolism requires.

Bone fluorescence is a known phenomenon, and occurs when short-wavelength photons, such as ultraviolet; are absorbed by some molecule containing a fluorophore and is re-emitted at longer wavelengths (**Figure 7**). Hemoglobin from the blood vessels that cover the periosteum absorb this emission. Since hemoglobin and chlorophyll are remarkably similar molecules, it is perfectly possible that hemoglobin also dissociates the molecule from water, transforming luminous energy into chemical energy, such as chlorophyll in plants. The energy that is released by

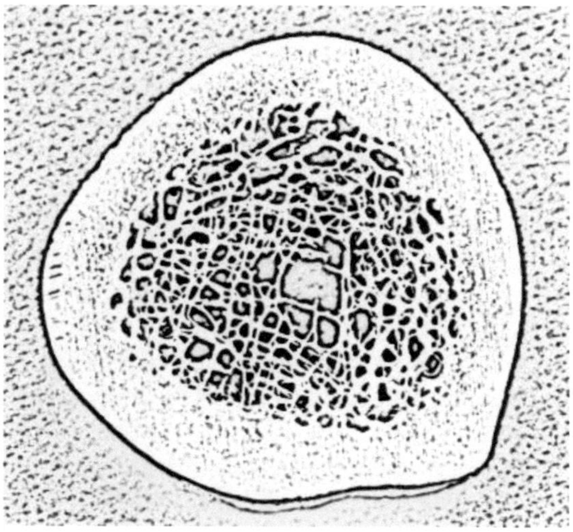

Figure 6.
The bone marrow has a part called a red bone marrow because it contains blood vessels and bone spicules (spongy bone) that function as a vessel supporter. The other part called yellow bone marrow that does not contain vessels or spicules and is the most metabolically active part. It is surrounded by a compact outer shell located in the medullary cavity of the diaphysis. The periosteum (membrane covering bone) is richly vascularized.

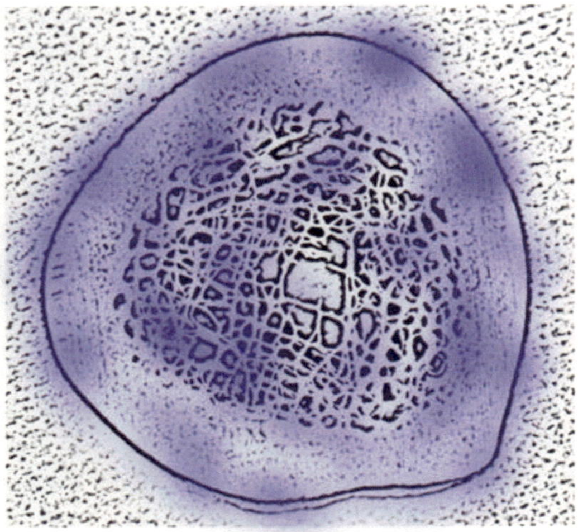

Figure 7.
Bone fluorescence (violet) when illuminated with wavelengths close to UV-A. the absorbed energy is re-emitted at different wavelengths. Erythrocyte hemoglobin completely absorbs UV wavelengths, and hemoglobin dissipates absorbed energy by dissociating the water molecule.

breaking down the water molecule is transported by hydrogen, the energy carrier par excellence in the entire universe. Oxygen is actually a necessary evil, a waste of reaction, this is: a byproduct.

Bone marrow is a relatively hypoxic microenvironment. Oxygen tensions fluctuate through the medullary cavity and along the endosteal and periosteal surfaces [16]. Despite being a highly vascularized tissue, the bone is a particularly hypoxic environment. Oxygen tension in most normal tissues falls between 2% and 9% (14–65 mm Hg) [17], however, in the bone it is widely accepted that oxygen levels range from <1–6% (~7 mm Hg – 43 mm Hg) [18] like in the umbilical artery.. Oxygen tension in the bone is likely determined by the level of cellularity and oxygen consumption rate in particular regions of the bone [19], however, the body's cells cannot take and do not require oxygen from the blood. The main reason is that oxygen is not used as we have so far believed, this is to combine it with glucose and obtain energy, because our body takes energy from light directly; and the second reason is all the body's cells have the ability to dissociate the molecule from the water by means of the pigments they possess, that is: the cells of the organism are able to produce their own oxygen by dissociating the molecule from the water, such as chlorophyll in plants.

In fact, we must consider oxygen as an indirect indicator of the molecular hydrogen levels of tissues, because by dissociating water, our body obtains hydrogen and oxygen at the same time, but the really valuable is hydrogen since it is the energy hauler per excellence in the entire universe (**Figure 8**).

Therefore, low oxygen levels are not caused by high cellular consumption, but by the low light conditions of the microenvironment of the bone marrow, and because hemoglobin and chlorophyll are not as efficient as melanin to dissociate the molecule from water. What goes according to the significant differences in hematological parameters [20] and in the prevalence and incidence of blood diseases between the different skin phototypes, as well as their geographical location according to the amount of sunlight [21]. The absolute oxygen concentration around blood stem cells was indeed low, despite an exceptionally large density of the blood vessels. The marrow is extremely densely populated by various cell types (not just hematopoietic stem cells or HSCs), so that the oxygen concentration drops steeply just microns away from feeding capillaries, but this is not due to an higher oxygen consumption, but oxygen, like any other gas; is not combined with water and is far from easily crossing the different barriers between blood vessels and tissues. It is reported that oxygen does not cross the blood/brain barrier [22].

On the other hand, just as the umbilical artery has a saturation similar to that of the bone marrow, about 40%, and elevated oxygen levels in the region in question, regardless of where they came from, would have toxic effects on surrounding tissues. The fundamental processes of the body are astonishingly accurate.

The analysis of peripheral blood values and bone marrow cell populations in newly born and young infants is particularly suited for the detection of racial differences. Such subjects have experienced limited impact from extrauterine factors that might be responsible for environmentally induced differences in hemopoietic cell distributions. American black infants have a consistently lower hemoglobin level than their American white counterparts. This lower hemoglobin level in black infants is compatible with the relative erythroid hyperplasia of their bone marrow. This 0.5–1.0 gm difference in hemoglobin levels has been found at all ages, even when corrected for sex, dietary intake, socioeconomic status, and place of residence. There are reports of a higher 2–3 DPG level in healthy black males and females [23]. Racial differences in peripheral blood leukocyte counts have also been well documented [24]. As in the older individuals, this population of black infants had consistently lower total leukocyte and total neutrophil values. The racial differences in peripheral blood leukocyte counts were not reflected in the prevalence of bone marrow myeloid or small lymphocyte cell compartments. So far, it is

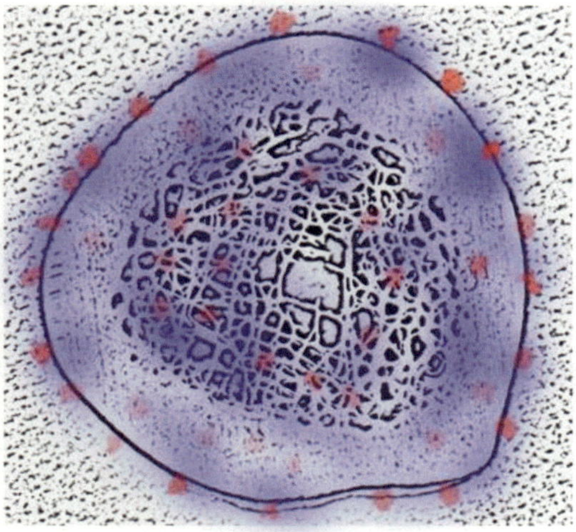

Figure 8.
The red dots repress the hemoglobin present in the periosteum, in the cortex, in the endosteum, and in the compact and spongy bone. Hemoglobin well absorbs wavelengths close to 300 μm, and the energy absorbed by hemoglobin is dissipated by dissociating the water molecule, transforming photonic energy into chemical energy, which is transported by diatomic hydrogen (H_2). Cells and tissues use this energy in many ways.

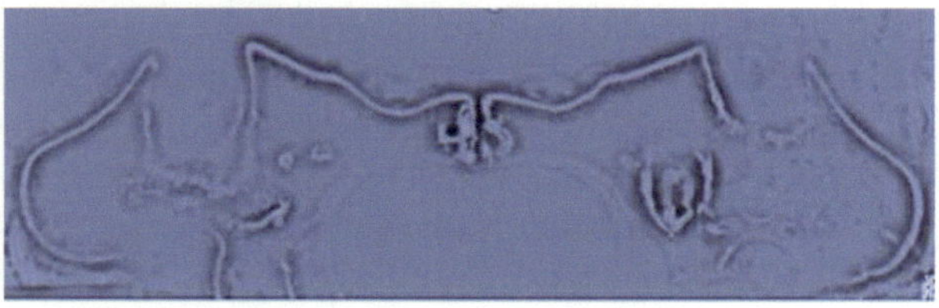

Figure 9.
Fluorescence of bone is a well-known phenomenon. Furthermore, is used to identify and differentiate healthy from necrotic bone tissue during resection surgeries [25].

not possible to explain this discrepancy, except if we consider that the higher the amount of melanin, the greater the proportion of water dissociation and therefore greater energy availability in tissues (**Figure 9**).

5. Melanin, considered for a long time an evolutionary remnant, participate substantively in energetic cell's metabolism

The synthesis of melanin is a multistep and highly regulated pathway, and so far, considered as a simple sunscreen that protect against UV-induced damage [26]. Although some research had shown that the presence of melanin pigment affected the elastic properties of the cells as well as the transmigration abilities, they concluded that inhibitory effect being mechanical in nature [27].

Theoretically, melanin granules can attenuate the movement of cells due to mechanical (physical) effect of loading. However, the induction of melanogenesis is accompanied by the dramatic changes in cyto-architecture such as round morphology which correlates positively with the melanin content of the cell [28]. Interestingly, SKMMEL – 188 cells, supplemented with L-tyrosine, increase melanin content, and can easily detach from the culture substratum, which contrasts with the amelanotic cells cultured in Ham's F10 medium [29].

This significant change in adhesiveness and form due to the presence of melanin, include a complex and reciprocal interactions that are context dependent and are nonlinear in nature with multitude of regulatory pathways/factors operating in a form that cannot be explained in a reductionistic form. We must keep in mind that melanin presence induces dramatic changes in the metabolic status of the cells and their behavior both on biochemical and on molecular levels **Figure 10**.

6. Leukocytes are wandering cells that require an energy source at its own

The dynamic functions of peripheral blood leukocytes (Eosinophils, Basophils, Neutrophils, monocyte, Erythrocytes, T-cells, B-cells) and platelets require an integrated metabolic machinery to meet energetic demand during normal physiology which is likely (theoretically) to involve both glycolysis and mitochondrial oxidative phosphorylation. The role of both these important ATP generating pathways in supporting supposedly the biological function of platelets and leukocytes has been postulated but have not been integrated into an overall understanding of these cell types in human subjects.

The myeloid lineage supports the greatest variety of differentiated circulating cells which include erythrocytes, platelets, neutrophils, basophils, eosinophils, and monocytes (**Figure 7**). Two stages of some cells are described once they are secreted by the bone marrow: M1 or pro-inflammatory and M2 or anti-inflammatory. The difference that is handled relates undoubtedly to energy levels.

Thus, the metabolic programs of monocyte/macrophage populations are highly plastic and adapt to facilitate the changing function of these cells in the inflammatory process. However, the possibility of detecting these important changes through current laboratory methodology is not clear. Typically, differentiation of the M1/M2 macrophages occurs at the site of inflammation not in the circulation.

From the translational perspective the pre-differentiated monocyte is the dominant form in the circulation. What there is no doubt about is that energy levels are what make the difference. Supposedly, there is something like a switch to a metabolic phenotype with an increase in both glycolytic function and mitochondrial

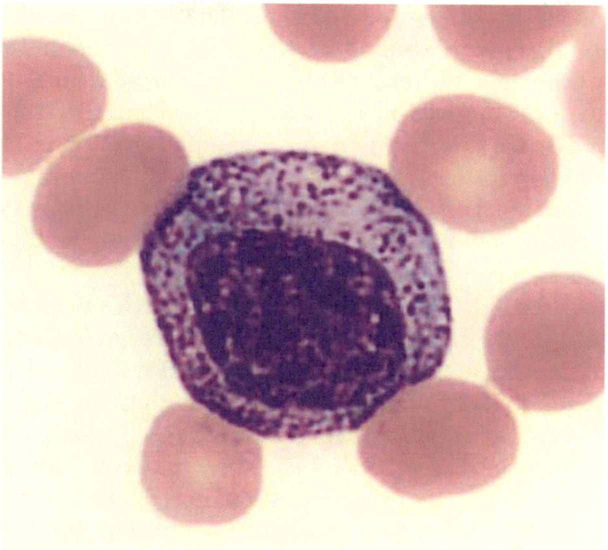

Figure 10.
Typical aspect of a myelocyte. The usual stains do not demonstrate or rule out the presence of melanin, which on the other hand is something that seems to be of no interest to researchers.

oxygen consumption, which is essential for their diverse immunological functions, which includes clonal expansion and the production of cytokines and antibodies. It should be noted that mitochondria are not proper organelles that produce energy, their resemblance to the heat sinks of electronic circuits leads us to think that they are rather temperature regulators, and on the other hand, animal species that require exposure to the sun to start moving, characteristically have a very small number of mitochondria.

Thereby, the relationship of bioenergetics with the disease processes associated with inflammation still has numerous mysteries. For instance, Neutrophils have very few mitochondria which do not play a role in energy metabolism, by other side, the space available in the mitochondrial matrix calls into question the existence and location of enzymes required by their supposed energetic function.

Hereby, it is argued that the energy required for neutrophil chemotaxis and activity is derived from glycolysis with very few mitochondria, which is paradoxical. It is interesting that patients with septic shock demonstrated a strong association between decreased mitochondrial function, specifically loss of ATP synthase activity in peripheral blood mononuclear cells and increased mortality. But we must keep in mind that mitochondria are not an energy-autonomous organelle. Mitochondria requires energy to perform its function, requiring energy even to preserve form.

The ATP synthase enzyme does not use ATP to perform its function, but that does not mean that it does not require energy, because of course it requires it, because any chemical reaction needs it. Whether in the form of activation energy, or termination, or reaction support, whatever you want to call it. Enzymes that do not use ATP to perform their function use another form of power that is not yet determined by the orthodox science; however, it is accepted. By the way, energy is defined as everything that causes a change.

It has also been shown that platelets from patients with type 2 diabetes have lower mitochondrial membrane potential and higher ATP content compared to controls, which does not make sense. Furthermore, a normal mitochondrial membrane potential requires energy, and regulation of ATP content requires energy also.

A study of mononuclear cells in type 2 diabetes showed that the mitochondrial mass was decreased and that the mitochondria were hyperpolarized; but in any system, when the energy decreases, the mass tends to disappear, so we can think that the energy source of the mitochondria is compromised and therefore the mass is tending to disappear, like in any system; and hyperpolarization would be explained simply because the normal electronic behavior of the mitochondria requires adequate levels of energy, and if it is disturbed, then changes happen that are not compatible with the normal functional balance of the organelle. This is: the balance of charges requires energy.

It has been reported that leukocytes from patients with leukemia have higher numbers of circular dimer mitochondrial DNA compared to healthy controls, which is surprising, because the number of circular dimers of mitochondrial DNA is a process strictly regulated by millions of years of evolution, but such controls require the right energy, we could say accurate in time and form. Just as melanin generates and distributes it from the dissociation of the water molecule, such as chlorophyll in plants. It is an astonishingly accurate process, which is the same since the beginning of time, and after millions of years of evolution has not changed, it is not going to change, it cannot change.

But it is disturbed by contaminated water, with polluted air, with pesticides, herbicides, fertilizers, metals, plastics, solvents, industrial waste, alcohol, abuse drugs, anesthetic agents, etc.

It is therefore not surprising that leukemias are significantly more common in populations exposed to such pollutants. Because when the generation and distribution of energy from melanin is disturbed by the aforementioned factors, the whole organism begins to disorganize until, eventually, some sicknesses appear, which are nothing more than a manifestation of imbalance between mass and energy from melanin, not glucose.

7. Melanin laden macrophages in CSF

Vogt- Koyanagi- Harada Syndrome (VKH) is suspected to be systemic immunological reactions in various organs containing melanocytes [30], suggesting that the cell mediated immune process involving melanocytes plays an important role in the pathogenesis of VKH [31]. Supporting this idea, Nakamura et al., reported the existence of melanin laden macrophages (MLMs) in the cerebrospinal fluid of VKH patients [32]. Few months later, Nakamura et al. reported a VKH patient whose CSF examination reported pleocytosis (cell counts 273 X 10^6/L) and a large number of MLMS (**Figure 5**) [33] and after three months of initial administration of corticosteroid, visual acuity recovered and cell counts in the CSF had decreased (cell count 13 X 106/L), to within normal range, but MLMS were still present and after fourth months ophthalmologic manifestations recurred (**Figure 11**).

Pleocytosis in VKH is considered a sign of the focal immune response against melanocytes in meninges. Although lymphocytes are predominantly observed in the CSF and uveal tract of the eye in patients with VKH, a small number of macrophages are detected.

It has been reported that patient with melanin granules in the cytoplasm of macrophages in CSF of patients with VKH that appears in early stage and disappear after steroid treatment have, supposedly, a better prognosis. However, small melanin granules are not routinely looking for. Thereby, we could think that macrophages that are "activated" requires more energy to carry out their function, and therefore synthesize melanin more than phagocyte it. An errant cell, such as the

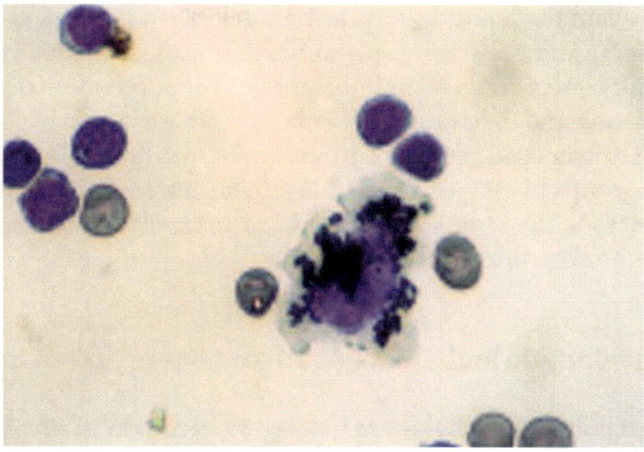

Figure 11.
Morphological characteristics of a melanin laden macrophage (May-Grünwald staining, original magnification × 400) in CSF from the VKH patient obtained 2 weeks after the initial corticosteroid therapy was started. Melanin pigments are identified as basophilic granules in the cytoplasm of a macrophage. (Takayuki Takeshita et al. Br J Ophthalmol 1997; 81: 1113 reprinted with permission, license number: 4852140023803).

macrophage, requires carrying its energy source with it, because the proximity to the supposed source of energy (glucose carried by the blood vessels) is not usual.

8. Biological characteristics of acute leukemias and its relationship to the energy of melanin

They were 13, 780 new cases of acute myeloid leukemia (AML) and 6050 new cases of acute lymphocytic leukemia (ALL) in the United States in 2012 [34]. Supposedly, acute leukemia is the result of a series of mutational events occurring in an early hematopoietic precursor that theoretically prevents the progeny of that precursor from maturing normally. Although advanced age, white ancestry, and family history of hematologic malignancies are risk factors, the etiology of acute leukemias is unknown. This explanation only takes structural issues into account but does not mention at any time the energy needed or where it comes from.

Patient with at least one affected relative is considered "familial" [35], which means that more than hereditary, they are groups of people exposed to similar toxics. Familial cases have an earlier age of onset than sporadic cases [36]. This leads us to think that exposure to environmental pollutants is more marked in family cases, and therefore develop alterations to minor age and therefore at a shorter time of exposure than sporadic that require longer exposure time. The generation and distribution of energy that comes from melanin is an astonishingly accurate process that has not changed since the beginning of time, because the components of the process: light, melanin and water, in order of abundance in the universe, are extremely stable, because they do not show even the minimum data suggesting evolution.

There is no consistent pattern of illness that can be explained by a simple mode of genetic transmission [37]. Strong familial aggregation favored the relatives sharing environmental risk factors. For example, relatives of patients with colon cancer are at increased risk for developing colon cancer. An astonishingly accurate process (water dissociation by melanin) is easily disturbed by contaminated water, contaminated air, pesticides, herbicides, fertilizers, metals, plastics, solvents, industrial waste, etc. And when the liquid–gas cycle is altered, then the tissues of the organism begin to disorganize and eventually appear what we call sick, which do not actually exist as such, it all comes down to an imbalance of the fundamental process of life that is the generation and distribution of energy from melanin.

And in colon cancer as in acute or chronic leukemias labeled as familial disease, what we see are groups of people exposed to similar toxics, because they lived in the same house, they took the same water, they had the same habits, the same air, the same soil, the same environment, etc.

9. Acute promyelocytic leukemia (APL) and energy from melanin

Few thousand people worldwide are diagnosed each year of Acute Promyelocytic Leukemia (APL). Once considered the most malignant human leukemia as well as the one associated with the worst prognosis, APL has been transformed in the past few decades into the most frequently curable one.

"Most outstanding feature was its very rapidly downhill course of few weeks' duration, a white blood cell picture dominated by promyelocytes and severe bleeding caused mainly by fibrinolysis" [38]; it was the description of Hillestad, in 1957, about acute promyelocytic leukemia (APL). J Bernard, in 1959; reported a series of 20 patients, with the full definition of the disease and its association with promyelocytic proliferation, hyperacute onset and catastrophic hemorrhagic events [39].

The life-threatening coagulopathy was recognized as the defining clinical feature of APL accounting for most deaths at presentation and during initial cytotoxic treatment, with most fatal events being intracranial and pulmonary hemorrhages. The hemostatic abnormalities were attributed to a disseminated intravascular coagulopathy in which fibrinolysis and procoagulant activity triggered by APL blasts played a major role, and hematologic remission resulted in the resolution of the coagulopathy [40].

The impressive improvement in outcome achieved after the advent of all-trans retinoic acid (ATRA) (**Figure 12a** and **b**) the early death rate in APL has remained elevated even in recent years, mostly because many patients die even before they can start treatment [41], and older age remains a prominent negative prognostic factor [42].

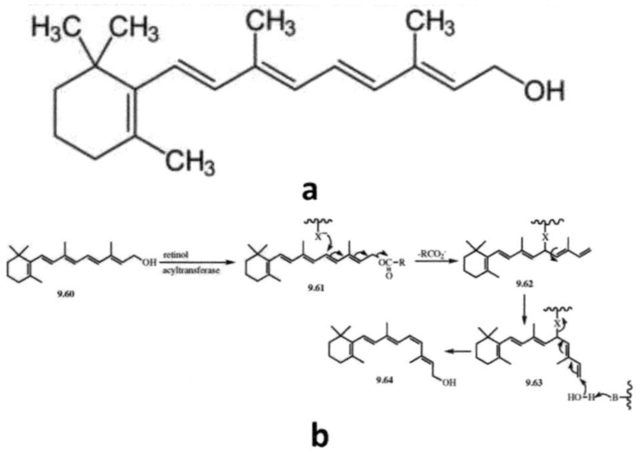

Figure 12.
(a) Structure of all-trans retinol. (b) Proposed mechanism for the reaction catalyzed by retinol isomerase. Note two things: (a) the scheme is theoretical and (b) does not mention energy flow at all. Retrieved in June 122,020 from: https://www.sciencedirect.com/science/article/pii/B978008051336250005X

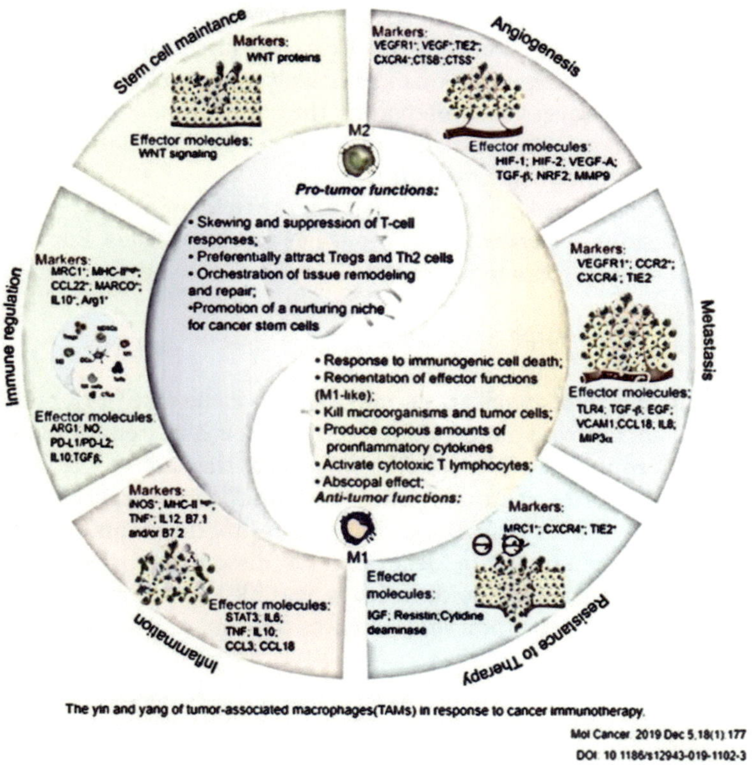

Figure 13.
Literature is abundant in terms of structures, processes, and sequences; but it is silent about the energy required by each chemical reaction that incessantly happens inside each cell.

All *trans*-retinol is converted (energy required) to 11-*cis*-retinol by retinol isomerase (enzymes also require energy) in a covalent catalytic process [43]. Control of retinoic acid levels is maintained (energy required) by a suite of proteins that control synthesis and degradation of retinoic acid (**Figure 13**) Again, the control of retinoic acid levels requires energy, in several ways (suite of proteins that control synthesis) and degradation of retinoic acid.

10. Energy production, the true role of melanin in biology

Einstein said it is easier to break the atom and break a prejudice. Therefore, breaking the dogma so rooted that glucose and ATP are the energy source of the eukaryotic cell is not an easy challenge. Given the space limitations we will only mention a few demonstrative examples.

Glucose is the universal precursor of any organic compound of the organism, its carbon chains are the fundamental basis of the anabolic processes of cell synthesis that culminates in a myriad of extraordinary complex compounds. But it is not possible for glucose to provide the energy that your own metabolism requires. Therefore, the double role assigned to glucose since centuries ago should be discarded.

Our body takes glucose, from food; the building blocks, the precursors, with which it builds, rebuilds, and replaces those molecules that continually wear out throughout the day, but the energy needed for such metabolic activities is taken from light.

The passage of carbon chains in the body's metabolism ends with the formation of CO_2 (O=C=O), the most oxidized form of carbon, suggesting that our body uses the carbon chains present in food exhaustively, oxidizing them to their lowest expression. And said process uses intensively the energy that comes from light, but it must first be transformed into chemical energy by dissociating the water molecule, which happens inside melanin.

The dissociation of water is a process that requires a lot of energy, in the laboratory we require heating the water to two thousand degrees Celsius. But melanin and chlorophyll do it daily at room temperature. The equation would be as follows:

$$\text{Chlorophyll}: 2H_2O_{(\text{Liquid})} \rightarrow 2H_{2(\text{gas})} + O_{2(\text{gas})} \quad (1)$$

Both melanin and chlorophyll are certain that this is the case [44], but the mechanisms involved are far from understood. But melanin is hundreds of times more efficient than chlorophyll, as chlorophyll only absorbs the ends of visible light, but melanin absorbs the entire electromagnetic spectrum. Moreover, in chlorophyll the dissociation of water is irreversible, and the proof is that the plants expel the toxic oxygen into the atmosphere; but in Melanin, water dissociation is reversible. This is from liquid to gas, and back to liquid, which is possible because melanin supports oxygen toxicity. Then the equation would look as follows:

$$\text{Melanin}: 2H_2O_{(\text{Liquid})} \rightarrow 2H_{2(\text{gas})} + O_{2(\text{gas})} \rightarrow 2H_2O_{(\text{Liquid})} + 4e^- \quad (2)$$

For every two water molecules that are reformed, 4 high-energy electrons are generated. High-energy electrons are easily exchanged, as they travel at near-light speeds are difficult to control, so what is thought to be absorbed quickly, especially by the fibrous parts of the cell, that is, those close to the perinuclear space that is the main location of the melanosomes. On the other hand, molecular hydrogen (H_2) is the main energy hauler in the entire universe, and since it is not combined with water, once it is generated, molecular hydrogen follows the laws of simple diffusion, and targets the areas of highest concentration (where it occurs continuously) to the areas of lower concentration, simply moving through the cytoplasm and reaches even the cell membrane. It is redundant to say that during its path, said molecular hydrogen is captured by the different cellular organelles and chemical reactions that use its precious energy load and its powerful antioxidant effect, being consumed continuously.

Melanin releases energy symmetrically, in all directions, like increasing bubbles of energy. And such spheres also flood the cell nucleus, constituting its source of energy, since it contains no mitochondria, nor ATP.

So is this, that when the generation and distribution of energy from melanin is affected by environmental pollutants, the functions and posteriorly the structures′ cells begin to affect, including genes. Because the functions of the nucleus also depend entirely on the energy coming from melanin. Therefore, nature's insistence on placing melanin in all cells of all living things now has a meaning: energy production.

11. CO_2 levels highest than normal should impoverish melanin's bio-energetic functions

In all lung life forms, mechanisms are in place to accelerate CO_2 expulsion, such as carbon dioxide anhydrase. Elevated CO_2 levels have such a marked effect on the generation and distribution of energy from melanin that they cause death in less than 60 seconds.

That is why we observe in different life forms a rush of nature to expel the carbon dioxide that it continuously generates because of cellular metabolism, which is also continuous, day and night. And the figures are revealing in the air we breathe in, CO_2 makes up 0.04% of the inspired volume, but in the exhaled air, The CO_2 rises to 4%, that is a hundred times.

Conversely, only 5% of inspired oxygen is absorbed as inspired air contains about 21%, and 16% exhaled air. If oxygen were used as intended by biochemistry texts, liters, and liters of oxygen per minute would be needed, which is not the case. In addition, no mechanism has been identified to accelerate the passage of atmospheric oxygen into the body, in any form of life. So, the poor lung absorption of oxygen is due to simple diffusion.

Finally, two of the body's most metabolically active tissues known to date: the cones and rods of the retina and the central portion of the yellow bone marrow, they are completely devoid of blood vessels, which contradicts the dogma that glucose is the universal energy source, because if so, glucose would have to be transported through the blood vessels, and both tissues indicated above, under normal conditions; they completely lack them.

12. Conclusion

Our incidental discovery about the true energy source of the eukaryotic cell, breaks into a thousand pieces the dogma of double glucose paper as a universal precursor to any organic compound of the human body and which, at the same time, serves as an energy source. The discovery of the unsuspected bioenergy role of melanin opens new possibilities in the study, diagnosis, and treatment of disturbances of the functioning of the body that we call acute leukemias.

Aromatic compounds, ionizing radiations, ozone (O_3), Sulfur Dioxide (SO_2), carbon monoxide (CO), nitrogen Oxide (NO_2), Methyl Mercury, PCBs, lead, cadmium, phthalates, brominated flame retardants, heavy metals, per-fluorinated compounds (PFCs), nonylphenol ethoxylates, fungicides, polyvinyl chloride plastic, Arsenic, Aflatoxins, blue-green algae in recreational waters, cyanogenic glycosides in cassava, foxglove, oleander; persistent organic pollutants (POPs),; HCB: hexa-chlorobenzene; HCH: hexachlorocyclohexane; PCBs: polychlorinated biphenyls; DDT: dichlorodiphenyltrichloroethane; PBDEs: polybrominated diphenyl ethers; they are toxic agents whose mechanism of action begins by damaging the distribution and generation of energy from the dissociation of the water molecule by melanin. The effects on bone marrow depend on the dose and whether the poisoning was acute, unique, multiple, chronic, acute over chronic, etc.

It is surprising to find that tissues as metabolically active as cones and rods and the central portion of the yellow bone marrow, which require 10 times more energy than the cerebral cortex in the case of the retina, or the bone marrow that produces about 2.5 million blood cells per second, do not contain any blood vessels under normal conditions.

According to the dogma currently prevalent, they should have numerous blood vessels since glucose is transported that way. But now that we know that the bone marrow gets the energy of light, like any other tissue of the human body, then the focus changes radically and the explanation about the lack of blood vessels is evident.

Since the transformation of sunlight into chemical energy through the dissociation of the water molecule is a grimly accurate process that has not changed in the very way since the beginning of time, we can now unlearn the biochemistry of the usual textbooks and broaden our landscape about diseases, because in reality, such

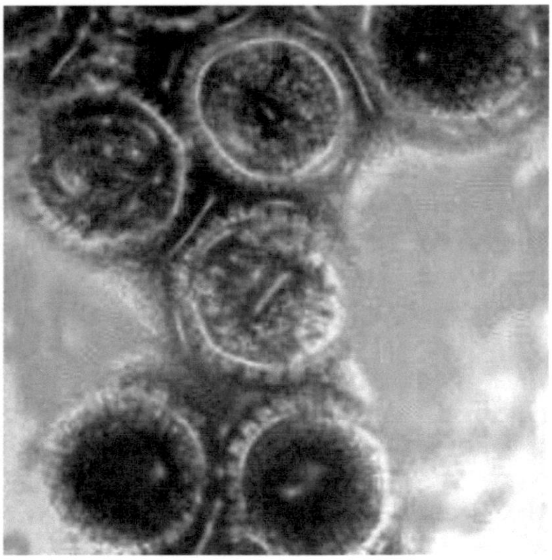

Figure 14.
Melanin is a great electron-acceptor, so in a TEM microphotograph, melanin is seen as a dark area.

diseases do not exist as such as the vast majority are reduced to an imbalance in the generation and distribution of energy from melanin.

The fundamental processes of life, such as energy collection, are astonishingly fast and accurate, so even minor perturbations that we might call transients, for example by the cold, induce a disorganization first of the functioning of the body and then real histochemical alterations that grow and spread rapidly by not being the adequate balance between the mass and energy.

In a few sheets it is not possible to explain all that it involves reordering our thoughts and concepts based on a different form of energy, which we had not even imagined, so it is necessary for the interested reader to deepen and the subject by looking for more information in other articles and books so that concepts about the flow of mass and energy of the body, which we now know is totally different from how it had been considered to date (**Figure 14**), yields fruits that will be reflected in a better quality of life in our patients.

Welcome to a new era in Biology and medicine.

Acknowledgements

This work was made possible thanks to the support of the Center for the Studies of Human Photosynthesis (R) S.C. Aguascalientes 20000, Mexico.

Conflict of interest

There is no conflict of interest to disclose.

Author details

Arturo Solís Herrera[1*], Ruth I. Solís Arias[1] and Luis F. Torres Solís[2]

1 Human Photosynthesis(R) Research Center, Aguascalientes, México

2 Universidad Autónoma de Aguascalientes, Aguascalientes, México

*Address all correspondence to: comagua2000@gmail.com

References

[1] Wasserman, H. P. Lymphocytes, and the transport of melanin. *J. Invest. Derm.* 41: 473, 1963. Pp: 377-385

[2] Pienaar, U. de V.: Haematology of some South African reptiles. Witwatersrand Univ. Press, Johannesburg, 1962.

[3] Sundberg, R. D.: Metastatic malignant melanoma of the bone marrow. *Anat. Rec.*, 124: 368, 1956.

[4] Laidlaw, G. F. and Blackberg, S. N.: Mela- noma studies: Simple technique for dopa reaction. *Amer. J. Path.*, 8: 491, 1932.

[5] Pearse, A. G. E.: Histochemistry—Theoretical and applied. 2nd Edition, London, J. & A. Churchill, 1960

[6] Warter A, George-Diolombi G, Chazal M, Ango A (1990) Melanin in a dentigerous cyst and associated adenomatoid odontogenic tumor. *Cancer* 66, 786-788

[7] Soames JV (1982) A pigmented calcifying odontogenic cyst. *Oral Surg Oral Med Oral Pathol* 53, 395-400.

[8] Buchner A, David R, Carpenter W, Leider A (1996) Pigmented lateral periodontal cyst and other pigmented odontogenic lesions. *Oral Dis* 2, 299-302

[9] Takeda Y, Sato H, Satoh M, Nakamura S, Yamamoto H (2000) Pigmented ameloblastic fibrodentinoma: a novel melanin-pigmented intraosseous odontogenic lesion. *Virchows Arch* 437, 454-458.

[10] Kitano M, Tsuda-Yamada S, Semba I, Mimura T, Nozoe E, Setoyama M (1994) Pigmented ameloblastic fibro-odontoma with melanophages. *Oral Surg Oral Med Oral Pathol* 77, 271-275.

[11] Üzüm N, Akyol G, Asal K, Köybaşioğlu A (2005) Ameloblastic carcinoma containing melanocyte and melanin pigment in the mandible: a case report and review of the literature. *J Oral Pathol Med* 34, 618-620.

[12] Caggiati, A. Rosi, C. Franceschini, M. Innocenzi, D. The Nature of Skin Pigmentations in Chronic Venous Insufficiency: A Preliminary Report. *Eur J Endovasc Surg* 35, 111-118. DOI: 10.1016/j.ejvs.2007.08.007

[13] Farmer, ER. Hood, AF. Pathology of the skin. 2nd ed. New York: McGraw-Hill, Health Professions Division; 2000. pp. 795

[14] Pearse, AGE. Histochemistry. Theoretical and applied. 3rd ed., vol.2. Edinburgh London: Churchill Livingstone; 1972. pp. 1130

[15] Jordan, H. E.: A source of origin of pigmented leucocytes in Amphibia. *Am. Ass. Anat. Abstr*. 20(a) Anat. Rec., 29: 387, 1925

[16] Johnson, Rachelle W. Sowder, Miranda E. Giaccia, Amato J. Hypoxia and Bone Metastatic Disease. *Curr Osteoporos Rep* 2017 August; 15(4): 231-238. Doi: 10.1007/s11914-017-0378-8

[17] Mohyeldin A, Garzon-Muvdi T, Quinones-Hinojosa A. Oxygen in stem cell biology: a critical component of the stem cell niche. *Cell Stem Cell*. 2010; 7(2):150-61. DOI: 10.1016/j.stem. 2010.07.007 [PubMed: 20682444]

[18] Harrison JS, Rameshwar P, Chang V, Bandari P. Oxygen saturation in the bone marrow of healthy vol . Rankin EB, Giaccia AJ, Schipani E. A central role for hypoxic signaling in cartilage, bone, and hematopoiesis. *Current osteoporosis reports*. 2011; 9(2):46-52. DOI: 10.1007/s11914-011-0047-2 [PubMed: 21360287] unteers. *Blood*. 2002; 99(1):394. [PubMed: 11783438

[19] Chow DC, Wenning LA, Miller WM, Papoutsakis ET. Modeling pO2 Distributions in the Bone Marrow Hematopoietic Compartment. I. *Krogh's Model. Biophys J.* 2001; 81(2):675-84. [PubMed: 11463616]

[20] Kraemer, Michael J. Hunter, Robert. Rosse, Cornelius. Smith, Nathan J. Race. Related differences in Peripheral blood and in Bone Marrow Cell Populations of American Black and American White Infants. *JAMA*, Vol. 69, No. 5, 1977.

[21] O Landgren, B I Graubard, J A Katzmann, R A Kyle, I Ahmadizadeh, R Clark, S K Kumar, A Dispenzieri, A J Greenberg, T M Therneau, L J Melton, N Caporaso, N Korde, M Roschewski, R Costello, G M McQuillan, S V Rajkumar. **Racial disparities in the prevalence of monoclonal gammopathies: a population-based study of 12 482 persons from the National Health and Nutritional Examination Survey**. *Leukemia*, 2014; DOI: 10.1038/leu.2014.34

[22] Kassissia, Ibrahim G. Goresky, Carl A. Rose, Colin P. Schwab, Andreas J. Simard, André. Huet, Pierre. Michel. Bach, Glen G. Tracer Oxygen Distribution is Barrier-Limited in the Cerebral Microcirculation. *Circ Res* 1995: 77: 1201-1211. Doi: 10.1161/01.RES.77.6.1201.

[23] Garn SM, Smith NJ, Clark DC: The Magnitude and the implications of apparent race differences in hemoglobin values. *Am J Clin Nutr* 28:563-566, 1975

[24] Caramihai E, Karayalcin G, Aballi AJ, et al: Leukocyte count differences in healthy white and black children. *J Pediatr* 86:252-254, 1975

[25] Wehrhan, Falk. Weber, Manuel. Neukam, Friedrich W. Geppert, Carol-Immanuel. Kesting, Marco. Preidl, Raimund H.M. Fluorescence-guided bone resection: A histological analysis in medication-related osteonecrosis of the jaw. *J Cranio- Maxillofacial Surg.* Volume 47, Issue 10, October 2019, pp. 1600-1607. Doi: 10.1016/j.jcms,2019. 07.012.

[26] Slominski, Radomir M. Zmijewski, Michal A. Slominski, Andrzej T. The role of melanin pigment in melanoma. *Exp Dermatol.* 2015 April ; 24(4): 258-259. doi:10.1111/exd.12618.

[27] Sarna M, Zadlo A, Hermanowicz P, et al. *Exp Dermatol.* 2014; 23:813-818. [PubMed: 25180917]

[28] Slominski A, Zmijewski MA, Pawelek J. *Pigment Cell Melanoma Res.* 2012; 25:14-27. [PubMed: 21834848]

[29] Schallreuter KU, Kothari S, Chavan B, et al. *Exp Dermatol.* 2008; 17:395-404. [PubMed: 18177348]

[30] Albert DM, Jacobiec FA. Svitra PP, Perry H. (1994) Vogt–Koyanagi–Harada (uveomeningitic) syndrome. in *Principles and practice of ophthalmology.* eds Albert DM, Jacobiec FA (Saunders, Philadelphia), pp 481-488

[31] Norose K, Yano A, Aosai F, Segawa K. (1990) Immunologic analysis of cerebrospinal fluid lymphocytes in Vogt–Koyanagi–Harada disease. *Invest Ophthalmol Vis Sci* **31**:1210-1216.

[32] Nakamura S, Nakazawa M, Yoshioka M, *et al.* (1996) Melanin-laden macrophages in cerebrospinal fluid in Vogt–Koyanagi–Harada syndrome. *Arch Ophthalmol* **114**:1184-1188

[33] Takeshita, Takayuki. Nakazawa, Mitsuru. Murakami, Kazuko. Tamai, Makoto, Nakamura Shozo, A patient With long standing melanin laden macrophages in cerebrospinal fluid in Vogt- Koyanagi- Harada syndrome. BJ Ophthalmol. Volume 81, issue 12. dx.doi.org/10.1136/bjo.81.12.1113b

[34] Appelbaum, Frederick R. Acute Leukemias in adults. **Abeloff's Clinical Oncology (Sixth Edition)** 2020,

Pages 1783-1797.e1 /doi.org/10.1016/B978-0-323-47674-4.00095-5

[35] Houlston RS, Sellick G, Yuille M, Matutes E, Catovsky D. Causation of chronic lymphocytic leukemia--insights from familial disease. *Leuk Res* 2003; 27:871-876. [PubMed: 12860003]

[36] Ishibe N, Sgambati MT, Fontaine L, et al. Clinical characteristics of familial B-CLL in the National Cancer Institute Familial Registry. *Leuk Lymphoma* 2001; 42:99-108. [PubMed: 11699227]

[37] Goldin, Lynn R. Landgren, Ola. Marti, Gerald E. Caporaso, Neil E. Familial aspects of chronic lymphocytic leukemia, monoclonal B-cell lymphocytosis (MBL) and related lymphomas. *European J Clin Med Oncol*. 2010 February; 2(1): 119-126

[38] Hillestad LK. Acute promyelocytic leukemia. *Acta Medical Scandinava.* 1957; 159: 189-194. http://dx.doi.org/10.1111/j.0954- 6820. 1957.tb00124.x

[39] Bernard J, Mathe G, Boulay J, Ceoard B, Chome J. Acute promyelocytic leukaemia: a study made on 20 cases. *Schweiz Medical Wochenschrifte.* 1959; 89: 604-608. PMid:13799642

[40] Rand JJ, Moloney WD, Sise HS. Coagulation defects in acute promyelocytic leukemia. *Arch Intern Med.* 1969 Jan;123(1):39-47. http://dx.doi.org/10.1001/archinte.1969.00300110041007 PMid:5248747

[41] McClellan JS, Kohrt HE, Coutre SS, Gotlib JR, Majeti R, Alizadeh AA, Medeiros BC. Treatment advances have not improved the early death rate in acute promyelocytic leukemia. *Haematologica*. 2011 Oct 11

[42] Lengfelder, Eva. Hofmann, Wolf-Karsten. Nolte, Florian. Management of elderly patients with acute promyelocytic leukemia: progress and problems. *Ann Hematol* (2013) 92:1181-1188 DOI 10.1007/s00277-013-1788-z

[43] Silverman, Richard B. Organic Chemistry of Enzyme-Catalized reaction. Chapter 9 – Isomerizations. Elsevier, 2002, pages 359-397. doi.org/10.1016/B978-0-08-051336-2.50014-0

[44] Solís- Herrera, A. Arias- Esparza, MC. Ashraf, Ghulam Md. Zamyatnin Jr, Andrey A. Aliev, Gjumrakch. Beyond mitochondria, what would be the energy source of the cell? CNS Agents Med Chem. 2015, Vol. 15, No. 1; pp. 32-41. **DOI** : 10.2174/1871524915666150203093656 PubMed: 128159

Chapter 6

Self-Renewal Pathways in Acute Myeloid Leukemia Stem Cells

Jonason Yang, Nunki Hassan, Sheng Xiang Franklin Chen, Jayvee Datuin and Jenny Y. Wang

Abstract

Acute myeloid leukemia (AML) is a difficult-to-treat blood cancer. A major challenge in treating patients with AML is relapse, which is caused by the persistence of leukemia stem cells (LSCs). Self-renewal is a defining property of LSCs and its deregulation is crucial for re-initiating a new leukemia after chemotherapy. Emerging therapeutic agents inhibiting aberrant self-renewal pathways, such as anti-RSPO3 monoclonal antibody discovered in our recent study, present significant clinical potential that may extend beyond the scope of leukemogenesis. In this chapter, we provide an overview of normal and malignant hematopoietic stem cells, discuss current treatments and limitations, and review key self-renewal pathways and potential therapeutic opportunities in AML.

Keywords: acute myeloid leukemia, leukemia stem cells, self-renewal, signaling, WNT, β-Catenin, G protein-coupled receptor, GPR84, LGR4, RSPO3, targeted therapy

1. Introduction

AML is a heterogenous clonal disorder characterized by blocked differentiation and increased proliferation of hematopoietic progenitors. The heterogeneity of AML can be attributed to diverse driver mutations that may be present in combination with multiple cells of origin and epigenetic abnormalities [1–3]. The main treatment for AML is chemotherapy, which kills rapidly dividing leukemic blasts but is ineffective against quiescent, self-renewing LSCs leading to relapse and poor clinical outcomes. The discovery of LSCs not only as the origin but also the culprit of therapeutic resistance in AML is a milestone in our understanding of malignancy and thus targeting LSCs is a critical and challenging step in developing anticancer therapy [4]. Recent evidence has shown that aberrant activation of self-renewal pathways, such as WNT/β-catenin and RSPO3-LGR4 pathways, is essential for the initiation and development of LSCs [5, 6], unveiling a potential target for curative therapies in AML.

2. Normal and malignant hematopoietic stem cells

2.1 Hematopoietic stem cells

Normal hematopoiesis is a hierarchically organized process where hematopoietic stem cells (HSCs) can self-renew to produce new copies of themselves via symmetric

IntechOpen

division or differentiate into lineage-committed progenitors via asymmetric division [7], which ultimately give rise to all blood lineage cells (**Figure 1**). A tight balance between self-renewal and differentiation is critical for sustaining the functional integrity of hematopoiesis, which prevents HSC exhaustion or hematologic malignancies such as leukemia. HSCs preferentially reside in a hypoxic microenvironment within the bone marrow in which they are maintained in a quiescent state [8]. Quiescence is important to preserve the genetic integrity of HSCs during adult homeostasis as frequent DNA replication may incur oncogenic mutations. Therefore, dysregulation of key HSC properties is essential for leukemia initiation as they enable the accumulation of genetic lesions and promote malignant transformation.

2.2 Leukemia stem cells

The discovery of the first cancer stem cell in AML two decades ago has led to a paradigm shift in our understanding of cancer cell biology and the way cancer can be treated and cured [9]. Cancer stem cells have been subsequently identified in a variety of tumors. Similar to normal HSCs, LSCs are a subpopulation of leukemic cells, which reside at the apex of a malignant hierarchy and possess the ability to self-renew and to differentiate into non-LSC bulk blasts [10]. LSCs with unlimited self-renewal capacity and chemoresistance are responsible for disease initiation and progression and are believed to be the root cause of cancer relapse. It was initially hypothesized that only HSCs could undergo malignant transformation into LSCs due to their inherent ability to self-renew. However, the study of acute promyeloid leukemia (APML), a subset of AML, showed that committed progenitors might be capable of developing into LSCs. The APML-associated fusion gene PML/retinoic acid receptor-α (RARA), resulting from the t(15, 17) balanced reciprocal translocation, was present in CD34-CD38+ cell population but not in CD34+CD38- cell population [11]. As APML only represents a unique subset of AML, further

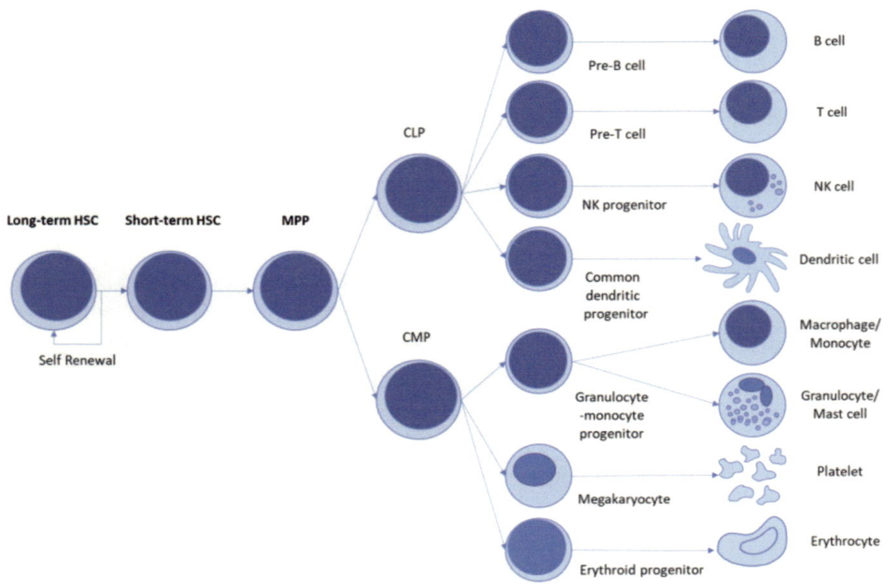

Figure 1.
Hierarchical organization of normal hematopoiesis. HSCs are categorized as long-term HSCs, which are highly self-renewing cells that last a lifespan, and short-term HSCs that self-renew for a limited period and differentiate into multipotent progenitor (MPP). MPP differentiates further into lineage-restricted progenitors including common lymphoid progenitor (CLP) and common myeloid progenitor (CMP) from which all mature blood cells arise. NK, natural killer.

studies looked at mixed-lineage leukemia (MLL) fusion proteins and isolated cell populations of committed progenitors with MLL fusion mutations to examine their leukemogenesis potential. By injecting sublethally irradiated mice with the aforementioned cell population, leukemogenesis was observed and thus the ectopic renewal of genes in committed progenitors associated with self-renewal is a definite possibility [12, 13]. The cancer stem cell model implies that eradication of LSCs is crucial for developing relapse-free therapies and to achieve a long-term remission in AML. However, eradication of LSCs remains a hefty challenge, whose difficulty lies in the therapeutic targeting of key oncogenic pathways driving LSC formation and maintenance without affecting normal adult HSCs and hematopoiesis.

3. Cause of chemotherapy failure: leukemia stem cells

Chemotherapy remains the first line treatment for AML, which has been relatively unchanged since its inception more than four decades ago. The chemotherapy drugs often used for AML treatment are a combination of cytarabine and an anthracycline drug such as daunorubicin. Insufficient inhibition of quiescent LSCs may be the culprit behind the failure of chemotherapy for the treatment of AML. Similar to their normal HSC counterpart, most LSCs remain quiescent or in the G0 phase of the cell cycle [14, 15]. This proves challenging as chemotherapy only interferes with DNA replication via DNA polymerase inhibition (e.g. cytarabine) or with DNA restructuring via topoisomerase II inhibition (e.g. daunorubicin) to induce apoptotic cell death in actively replicating cells [16, 17]. It is noted that LSCs can retain chemoresistant adaptations present in HSCs such as expression of P-glycoprotein, an efflux pump that may export chemotherapeutic agents and is associated with multidrug resistance and poor disease outcomes [18]. Consequently, most chemotherapy-induced cell deaths occur within leukemic blasts rather than in LSCs. Thus, the residual disease within patients is often characterized by the subpopulation of LSCs which are often quiescent and resistant to conventional chemotherapy leading to relapse (**Figure 2A**). This highlights the need for stem cell-targeted therapies so that the subpopulation of LSCs can be eliminated allowing for long-term remission (**Figure 2B**).

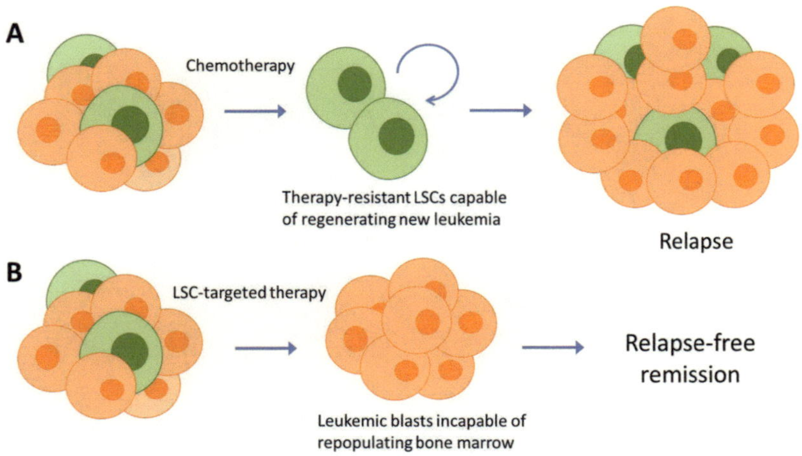

Figure 2.
Conventional chemotherapy versus targeted therapies for AML treatment. (A) Chemotherapy is unable to eradicate LSCs, leading to relapse. (B) Targeted therapy specifically kills LSCs, resulting in relapse-free remission.

4. Self-renewal signaling in leukemia stem cells

Self-renewal is a key property of LSCs and its deregulation is responsible for leukemia initiation and progression, which could be targeted for LSC eradication. Several pathways controlling LSC self-renewal have been identified in AML, such as WNT/β-catenin signaling and G protein-coupled receptors including GPR84 and LGR4 [5, 6, 19, 20].

4.1 WNT/β-catenin signaling pathway

β-catenin was first associated with colon cancer almost thirty years ago via its interaction with adenomatous polyposis coli (APC) [21, 22]. It later became evident that the canonical WNT/β-catenin pathway is dysregulated in various cancers, including AML [23, 24]. We and others have demonstrated that aberrant activation of WNT/β-catenin signaling contributes to the transformation of normal HSCs into LSCs [5, 25]. Our studies show that WNT/β-catenin signaling pathway is required for self-renewal of LSCs derived from either normal HSCs or lineage-committed progenitors in AML [5].

The WNT/β-catenin pathway was initially explored in normal HSCs (**Figure 3**). Constitutive activation of β-catenin results in an increase in the number of HSCs *in vitro* [26]. However, *in vivo* studies challenge the *in vitro* observation, where the conditional deletion of β-catenin in adult HSCs does not cause the self-renewal defect in mice [27].

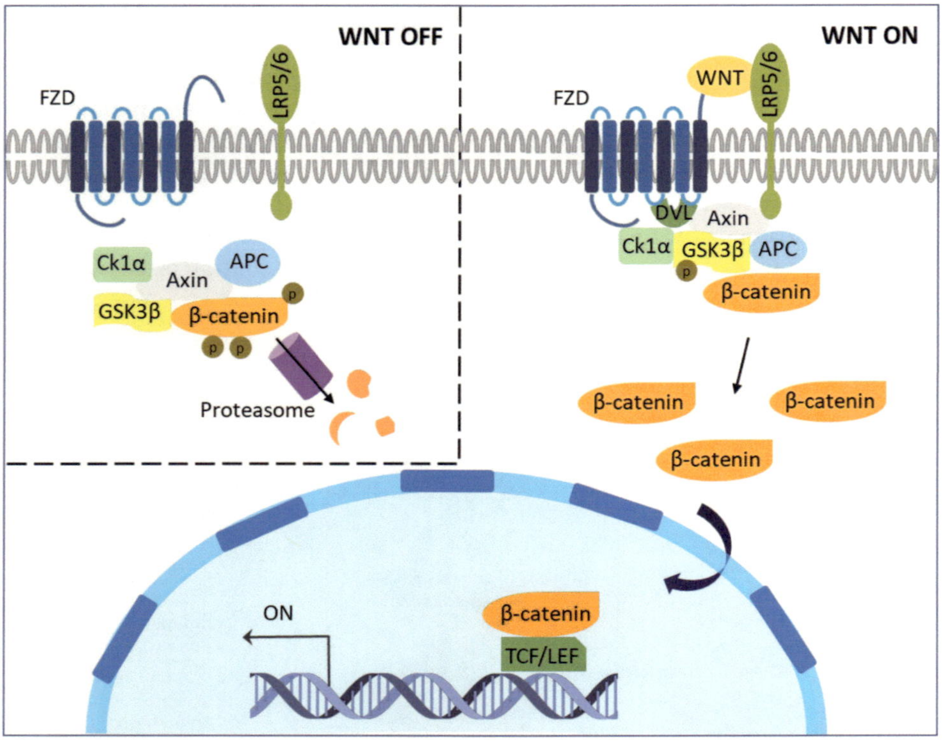

Figure 3.
Schematic diagram of the canonical WNT/β-catenin signaling pathway. In the OFF state, defined by the absence of a WNT ligand, β-catenin is repressed via a destruction complex composed of APC, scaffold protein Axin, glycogen synthase kinase 3 (GSK3) and casein kinase 1 (CK1) that phosphorylates β-catenin leading to its proteasomal degradation [28–30]. In the ON state, a WNT ligand binds to the receptor complex consisting of lipoprotein receptor-related proteins 5 and 6 (LRP5/6) and frizzled receptors (FZD), which recruits the destruction complex, leading to inhibition of β-catenin phosphorylation and therefore ensuring nuclear translocation and the subsequent accumulation of active β-catenin [31].

On the other hand, several lines of evidence including our own have demonstrated the importance of WNT/β-catenin pathway in regulation of LSC self-renewal in AML [5, 25]. Our studies have shown that deletion of β-catenin impairs LSC function and blocks AML progression in mice [5]. β-catenin can promote leukemogenesis through cooperation with homeobox (HOX) oncoproteins in HSCs [5]. Conversely, lack of endogenous β-catenin in lineage-committed progenitors limits the ability of HOX genes to efficiently transform the progenitor cells [5]. Despite the recognized importance, treatments directly targeting WNT/β-catenin pathway have been elusive, mainly due to our limited understanding of precise mechanisms of the pathway and lack of key druggable molecules involved in driving constitutive activation of the pathway.

Of note, while aberrant activation of β-catenin frequently occurs in human LSCs [25, 32] and is associated with poor patient outcomes in AML [33], increased expression of WNT proteins has not been observed. This suggests that aberrant activation of WNT/β-catenin signaling in AML may require other developmental signaling molecules that function as agonists.

4.2 G protein-coupled receptors serving as modulators of WNT/β-catenin signaling

G protein-coupled receptors (GPCRs) are a large superfamily of cell surface signaling proteins that bind extracellular ligands to transduce signals into cells via heterotrimeric G proteins [20]. GPCRs can act as modulators of WNT/β-catenin signaling and have a critical role in embryonic development and stem cell maintenance [20, 34, 35]. Dysregulation of GPCRs have detrimental consequences including malignant transformation and have emerged as crucial players in promoting tumor growth and metastasis [6, 19, 20].

The mechanism of action of GPCRs when stimulated by an appropriate ligand (or agonist) is understood in conjunction with its interaction with the G protein heterotrimer, which contains α, β and γ subunits. Ligands binding to GPCRs stimulate conformational changes within the receptor causing the Gα subunit to exchange bound guanosine diphosphate (GDP) for guanosine-5′-triphosphate (GTP). This step is key to the activation of the G protein as it causes the dissociation between the α subunit and the βγ subunit [36]. Each of the G protein subunits is responsible for several downstream effects. The Gα subunits have been classified into four families: $G\alpha_s$, $G\alpha_q$, $G\alpha_{i/o}$ and $G\alpha_{12/13}$ each with a distinct function. Typically, $G\alpha_s$ and $G\alpha_i$ moderate cyclic AMP (cAMP) levels by stimulating or inhibiting adenylyl cyclase respectively [37]. $G\alpha_{13}$ typically activates the Rho family of GTPases and $G\alpha_q$ stimulates phospholipase Cβ (PLCβ), leading to activation of intracellular Ca^{2+} [20]. The βγ dimer subunits activate downstream signaling partners such as Src, phospholipase C, adenylyl cyclase, phosphodiesterases and ion channels [36]. Aberrant activation of GPCRs has a profound effect on many cellular processes and may ultimately lead to malignant progression.

Although therapeutic targeting of GPCR signaling pathways in non-cancer disease is not a new phenomenon, our limited understanding of the role played by these receptors in tumorigenesis has hindered the development of therapeutic approaches for cancer treatment.

4.2.1 G protein-coupled receptor 84

G protein-coupled receptor 84 (GPR84) is often described as a pro-inflammatory receptor. We have documented a crucial role for GPR84 in sustaining LSC self-renewal through positive regulation of β-catenin signaling in established AML [19]. Overexpression of GPR84 augments activation of β-catenin and its transcriptional co-factors TCF7L2 and c-FOS, and positively modulates a subset of genes associated with WNT activation and *in vivo* dissemination as well as oncogenic potential of AML cells. On the other hand, GPR84 depletion impairs LSC function and inhibits the development of an aggressive and drug-resistant subtype of AML. The GPR84-deficient phenotype is dependent on β-catenin status as the restoration of β-catenin activation is capable of rescuing the functional defeat [19]. In addition, levels of GPR84 expression are significantly upregulated in human and mouse AML LSCs compared with normal HSCs, thus providing a therapeutic window to selectively target LSCs while sparing normal HSCs [19, 38]. These observations demonstrate a strong rationale for inhibiting GPCR/β-catenin signaling as a novel therapeutic strategy to target drug-resistant malignant stem cells in cancer.

GPR84 is also implicated in pro-inflammatory and fibrotic processes due to its action in macrophages, fibroblasts/myofibroblasts, and epithelial cells [39, 40]. Whilst the precise mechanism of action is unclear, GPR84 antagonist GLPG1205 has been developed to treat idiopathic pulmonary fibrosis patients in a phase II clinical trial (NCT03725852). However, the efficacy of GLPG1205 in AML is yet to be investigated.

4.2.2 Leucine-rich repeat-containing G protein-coupled receptor 4

Leucine-rich repeat-containing G protein-coupled receptor 4 (LGR4) is another GPCR that we have recently reported to act as a positive modulator of WNT/β-catenin signaling in AML initiation and progression [6]. The cell of origin determines the dependence of LSCs on LGR4 signaling. LSCs derived from HSCs depend primarily on LGR4 signaling for self-renewal and the establishment of an aggressive phenotype in mice; conversely, LSCs derived from lineage-committed progenitors only reveal a partial dependency on LGR4 signaling [6]. LSCs derived from different cellular origins may utilize distinct endogenous signaling mechanisms driving tumorigenesis, where LGR4 in HSC-derived LSCs relays signals via coupling to $G\alpha_s$ to upregulate WNT/self-renewal target genes but LGR4 in progenitor-derived LSCs signals through $G\alpha_q$ to potentiate WNT/β-catenin activation [6, 41]. The origin-dependent difference in pathway requirements contributes to the heterogeneity of an LSC pool within a tumor.

The mechanism underlying the enhanced aggressive leukemia phenotype associated with elevated LGR4 may involve functional cooperation between LGR4 and HOXA9 in LSCs [6]. High level of HOXA9 expression is a characteristic feature of AML, including cases with MLL rearrangements, and is associated with poor patient outcome [42]. Enforced expression of HOXA9/MEIS1 transforms normal HSC-enriched cells where β-catenin is often active, but cannot fully transform committed progenitors that inherently lack β-catenin activity and self-renewal ability [5]. This indicates an indispensable requirement for β-catenin activation in HOXA9-mediated transformation. Consistent with the role of LGR4 as an essential upstream effector of β-catenin signaling, we uncover that LGR4 cooperates with HOXA9/MEIS1 in HSC-enriched cells contributing to a highly tumorigenic phenotype characteristic of MLL-rearranged AML in mice. Thus, functional cooperation between LGR4 activation and a HOXA9 gene expression program drives LSC self-renewal and leukemogenesis in AML [6].

4.2.3 Therapeutic targeting of LGR4-RSPO3 signaling

The LGR family members (e.g. LGR4) have been identified as receptors for R-spondin (RSPO) proteins [43]. RSPOs function as WNT agonists [44] that synergize with low levels of WNT to potentiate β-catenin activation [45, 46]. An important feature of RSPOs is their coexpression with and dependence on WNT ligands during mouse development where RSPO expression is reduced by the double knockout of WNT1 and WNT3 [47], and the RSPO activity is inhibited by depletion of WNT3

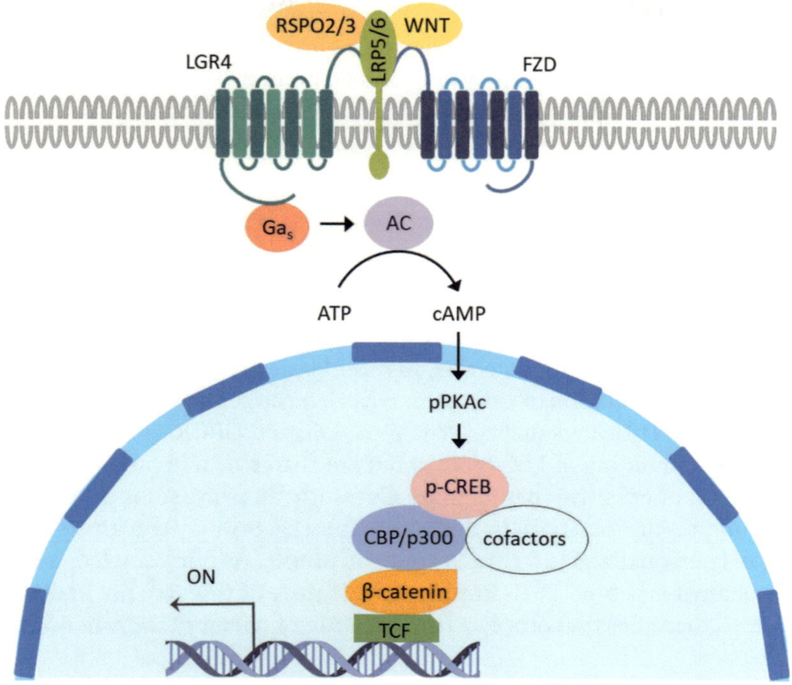

Figure 4.
Schematic diagram describing RSPO2/RSPO3-mediated augmentation of the canonical WNT/β-catenin signaling through an LGR4-dependent mechanism in HOXA9-dependent AML [6].

[46, 48] or WNT antagonists (i.e. DKK1) [49]. Although all four RSPO proteins (RSPO1–4) augment WNT/β-catenin signaling, RSPO2 and RSPO3 appear more effective than RSPO1, and RSPO4 is relatively inactive [50]. RSPO3 is prominently expressed in hematopoietic organs [51]. Our study has demonstrated that RSPO2 and RSPO3 can serve as stem cell growth factors to block differentiation and promote proliferation of primary AML patient blasts, and are capable of potentiating β-catenin activation in AML LSCs via an LGR4-dependent mechanism (**Figure 4**) [6].

The link between RSPO-LGR4 and WNT/β-catenin pathway has opened a new opportunity to specifically target key self-renewal signaling for LSC eradication. We have discovered that RSPO3-LGR4 pathway can be effectively inhibited by a clinical-grade anti-RSPO3 monoclonal antibody (rosmantuzumab), which disrupts the RSPO3-LGR4 interaction and abrogates leukemia-initiating capacity of patient-derived LSCs without affecting the healthy stem cell compartment [6]. Rosmantuzumab has proven to be safe and well tolerated in Phase I clinical trials conducted on patients with advanced solid tumors [52]. While the therapeutic efficacy of anti-RSPO3 antibody will need further preclinical validation in a large number of patient-derived xenograft models with different mutational profiles, these findings indicate differential dependence of normal and malignant stem cells on RSPO-LGR4 signaling and underline a therapeutic opportunity for selective targeting of AML LSCs.

5. Limitations of current studies

As our understanding of cancer continues to grow, we increasingly realize it to be a myriad of heterogenous diseases that defy simple classifications and AML is no exception. As a result, current studies tend to focus on specific tumor markings or specific genes present within tumors. Even within the subgroup of LSCs, there exists multiple unique pathways that may work together to achieve a tumorigenic effect. In this regard, the notion of having a single drug to treat AML is archaic. The development of novel therapeutic agents is therefore necessary in order to treat an array of aberrant pathways. Thus, future research must not only focus on the effectiveness of treatment, but also how they relate to specific patient factors.

6. Conclusion

The discovery of LSCs has resulted in a paradigm shift in our understanding of leukemia biology and the way we treat AML. LSCs play a significant part in the origin, drug resistance and relapse of leukemia. In recent years, researchers have shed light on this elusive subpopulation of cells by uncovering the cellular pathways that drive the action of LSCs. Pathways such as Wnt/β-catenin and GPCR signaling are not only vital in our understanding of LSC biology but are also critical in providing avenues for the development of effective therapeutics. Currently there are some promising agents in clinical and pre-clinical trials. In the future these agents may constitute combination therapies personalized to a patient's genetic profile. As our knowledge of the precise mechanisms behind LSCs improves, the future of research lies in developing novel targeted therapies that obsolete the single use of chemotherapy in AML.

Acknowledgements

The authors acknowledge the financial support from NHMRC (APP1128824) and Tour de Cure Senior Research Grants (RSP-024-2018, RSP-148-18/19, and RSP-187-19/20) as well as grant 1165516 awarded through the 2018 Priority-driven Collaborative Cancer Research Scheme and co-funded by Cancer Australia and Leukemia Foundation of Australia.

Conflict of interest

The authors declare no conflict of interest.

Author details

Jonason Yang, Nunki Hassan, Sheng Xiang Franklin Chen, Jayvee Datuin and Jenny Y. Wang*
Cancer and Stem Cell Biology Group, Children's Cancer Institute, Lowy Cancer Research Centre, University of New South Wales, Sydney, Australia

*Address all correspondence to: jenny.wang@unsw.edu.au

References

[1] Li S, Mason CE, Melnick A. Genetic and epigenetic heterogeneity in acute myeloid leukemia. Current Opinion in Genetics & Development. 2016;36:100-6.

[2] O'Brien E, Prideaux S, Chevassut T. The Epigenetic Landscape of Acute Myeloid Leukemia. Advances in hematology. 2014;2014:103175.

[3] Liersch R, Muller-Tidow C, Berdel WE, Krug U. Prognostic factors for acute myeloid leukaemia in adults--biological significance and clinical use. Br J Haematol. 2014;165(1):17-38.

[4] Ishikawa F, Yoshida S, Saito Y, Hijikata A, Kitamura H, Tanaka S, et al. Chemotherapy-resistant human AML stem cells home to and engraft within the bone-marrow endosteal region. Nat Biotechnol. 2007;25(11):1315-21.

[5] Wang Y, Krivtsov AV, Sinha AU, North TE, Goessling W, Feng Z, et al. The Wnt/beta-catenin pathway is required for the development of leukemia stem cells in AML. Science. 2010;327(5973):1650-3.

[6] Salik B, Yi H, Hassan N, Santiappillai N, Vick B, Connerty P, et al. Targeting RSPO3-LGR4 Signaling for Leukemia Stem Cell Eradication in Acute Myeloid Leukemia. Cancer cell. 2020;38(2):263-78.

[7] Yamamoto R, Morita Y, Ooehara J, Hamanaka S, Onodera M, Rudolph KL, et al. Clonal analysis unveils self-renewing lineage-restricted progenitors generated directly from hematopoietic stem cells. Cell. 2013;154(5):1112-26.

[8] Eliasson P, Jonsson JI. The hematopoietic stem cell niche: low in oxygen but a nice place to be. J Cell Physiol. 2010;222(1):17-22.

[9] Dick JE. Stem cell concepts renew cancer research. Blood. 2008;112(13):4793-807.

[10] Bonnet D, Dick JE. Human acute myeloid leukemia is organized as a hierarchy that originates from a primitive hematopoietic cell. Nat Med. 1997;3(7):730-7.

[11] Turhan A, Lemoine F, Debert C, Bonnet M, Baillou C, Picard F, et al. Highly purified primitive hematopoietic stem cells are PML-RARA negative and generate nonclonal progenitors in acute promyelocytic leukemia. Blood. 1995;85(8):2154-61.

[12] Cozzio A, Passegue E, Ayton PM, Karsunky H, Cleary ML, Weissman IL. Similar MLL-associated leukemias arising from self-renewing stem cells and short-lived myeloid progenitors. Genes & development. 2003;17(24):3029-35.

[13] Krivtsov AV, Twomey D, Feng Z, Stubbs MC, Wang Y, Faber J, et al. Transformation from committed progenitor to leukaemia stem cell initiated by MLL–AF9. Nature. 2006;442(7104):818-22.

[14] Chan WI, Huntly BJ. Leukemia stem cells in acute myeloid leukemia. Semin Oncol. 2008;35(4):326-35.

[15] Saito Y, Uchida N, Tanaka S, Suzuki N, Tomizawa-Murasawa M, Sone A, et al. Induction of cell cycle entry eliminates human leukemia stem cells in a mouse model of AML. Nature biotechnology. 2010;28(3):275-80.

[16] Murry DJ, Blaney SM. Clinical Pharmacology of Encapsulated Sustained-Release Cytarabine. Annals of Pharmacotherapy. 2000;34(10):1173-8.

[17] Murphy T, Yee KWL. Cytarabine and daunorubicin for the treatment

of acute myeloid leukemia. Expert Opinion on Pharmacotherapy. 2017;18(16):1765-80.

[18] Chaudhary PM, Roninson IB. Expression and activity of P-glycoprotein, a multidrug efflux pump, in human hematopoietic stem cells. Cell. 1991;66(1):85-94.

[19] Dietrich PA, Yang C, Leung HH, Lynch JR, Gonzales E, Liu B, et al. GPR84 sustains aberrant beta-catenin signaling in leukemic stem cells for maintenance of MLL leukemogenesis. Blood. 2014;124(22):3284-94.

[20] Lynch JR, Wang JY. G Protein-Coupled Receptor Signaling in Stem Cells and Cancer. Int J Mol Sci. 2016;17(5):707.

[21] Su LK, Vogelstein B, Kinzler KW. Association of the APC tumor suppressor protein with catenins. Science. 1993;262(5140):1734-7.

[22] Rubinfeld B, Souza B, Albert I, Muller O, Chamberlain SH, Masiarz FR, et al. Association of the APC gene product with beta-catenin. Science. 1993;262(5140):1731-4.

[23] Clements WM, Wang J, Sarnaik A, Kim OJ, MacDonald J, Fenoglio-Preiser C, et al. beta-Catenin mutation is a frequent cause of Wnt pathway activation in gastric cancer. Cancer Res. 2002;62(12):3503-6.

[24] Dahmen RP, Koch A, Denkhaus D, Tonn JC, Sorensen N, Berthold F, et al. Deletions of AXIN1, a component of the WNT/wingless pathway, in sporadic medulloblastomas. Cancer Res. 2001;61(19):7039-43.

[25] Yeung J, Esposito MT, Gandillet A, Zeisig BB, Griessinger E, Bonnet D, et al. beta-Catenin mediates the establishment and drug resistance of MLL leukemic stem cells. Cancer Cell. 2010;18(6):606-18.

[26] Reya T, Duncan AW, Ailles L, Domen J, Scherer DC, Willert K, et al. A role for Wnt signalling in self-renewal of haematopoietic stem cells. Nature. 2003;423(6938):409-14.

[27] Cobas M, Wilson A, Ernst B, Mancini SJ, MacDonald HR, Kemler R, et al. Beta-catenin is dispensable for hematopoiesis and lymphopoiesis. The Journal of experimental medicine. 2004;199(2):221-9.

[28] Minde DP, Radli M, Forneris F, Maurice MM, Rüdiger SGD. Large extent of disorder in Adenomatous Polyposis Coli offers a strategy to guard Wnt signalling against point mutations. PloS one. 2013;8(10):e77257-e.

[29] Minde DP, Anvarian Z, Rüdiger SG, Maurice MM. Messing up disorder: how do missense mutations in the tumor suppressor protein APC lead to cancer? Molecular cancer. 2011;10:101-.

[30] Giles RH, van Es JH, Clevers H. Caught up in a Wnt storm: Wnt signaling in cancer. Biochim Biophys Acta. 2003;1653(1):1-24.

[31] Griffin JN, del Viso F, Duncan AR, Robson A, Hwang W, Kulkarni S, et al. RAPGEF5 Regulates Nuclear Translocation of β-Catenin. Developmental Cell. 2018;44(2): 248-60.e4.

[32] Majeti R, Becker MW, Tian Q, Lee TL, Yan X, Liu R, et al. Dysregulated gene expression networks in human acute myelogenous leukemia stem cells. Proc Natl Acad Sci U S A. 2009;106(9):3396-401.

[33] Ysebaert L, Chicanne G, Demur C, De Toni F, Prade-Houdellier N, Ruidavets JB, et al. Expression of beta-catenin by acute myeloid leukemia cells predicts enhanced clonogenic capacities and poor prognosis. Leukemia. 2006;20(7):1211-6.

[34] Papayannopoulou T, Priestley GV, Bonig H, Nakamoto B. The role of G-protein signaling in hematopoietic stem/progenitor cell mobilization. Blood. 2003;101(12):4739-47.

[35] Layden BT, Newman M, Chen F, Fisher A, Lowe WL, Jr. G protein coupled receptors in embryonic stem cells: a role for Gs-alpha signaling. PLoS One. 2010;5(2):e9105.

[36] Bar-Shavit R, Maoz M, Kancharla A, Nag JK, Agranovich D, Grisaru-Granovsky S, et al. G Protein-Coupled Receptors in Cancer. International journal of molecular sciences. 2016;17(8):1320.

[37] Taussig R, Iñiguez-Lluhi JA, Gilman AG. Inhibition of adenylyl cyclase by Gi alpha. Science. 1993;261(5118):218-21.

[38] Saito Y, Kitamura H, Hijikata A, Tomizawa-Murasawa M, Tanaka S, Takagi S, et al. Identification of therapeutic targets for quiescent, chemotherapy-resistant human leukemia stem cells. Sci Transl Med. 2010;2(17):17ra9.

[39] Gagnon L, Leduc M, Thibodeau J-F, Zhang M-Z, Grouix B, Sarra-Bournet F, et al. A Newly Discovered Antifibrotic Pathway Regulated by Two Fatty Acid Receptors: GPR40 and GPR84. The American Journal of Pathology. 2018;188(5):1132-48.

[40] Recio C, Lucy D, Purvis GSD, Iveson P, Zeboudj L, Iqbal AJ, et al. Activation of the Immune-Metabolic Receptor GPR84 Enhances Inflammation and Phagocytosis in Macrophages. Frontiers in immunology. 2018;9:1419-.

[41] Lynch JR, Yi H, Casolari DA, Voli F, Gonzales-Aloy E, Fung TK, et al. Gaq signaling is required for the maintenance of MLL-AF9-induced acute myeloid leukemia. Leukemia. 2016;30(8):1745-8.

[42] Golub TR, Slonim DK, Tamayo P, Huard C, Gaasenbeek M, Mesirov JP, et al. Molecular classification of cancer: class discovery and class prediction by gene expression monitoring. Science. 1999;286(5439):531-7.

[43] Carmon KS, Gong X, Lin Q, Thomas A, Liu Q. R-spondins function as ligands of the orphan receptors LGR4 and LGR5 to regulate Wnt/beta-catenin signaling. Proceedings of the National Academy of Sciences of the United States of America. 2011;108(28):11452-7.

[44] Kazanskaya O, Glinka A, del Barco Barrantes I, Stannek P, Niehrs C, Wu W. R-Spondin2 is a secreted activator of Wnt/beta-catenin signaling and is required for Xenopus myogenesis. Dev Cell. 2004;7(4):525-34.

[45] Hao HX, Xie Y, Zhang Y, Charlat O, Oster E, Avello M, et al. ZNRF3 promotes Wnt receptor turnover in an R-spondin-sensitive manner. Nature. 2012;485(7397):195-200.

[46] Binnerts ME, Kim KA, Bright JM, Patel SM, Tran K, Zhou M, et al. R-Spondin1 regulates Wnt signaling by inhibiting internalization of LRP6. Proc Natl Acad Sci U S A. 2007;104(37):14700-5.

[47] Kamata T, Katsube K, Michikawa M, Yamada M, Takada S, Mizusawa H. R-spondin, a novel gene with thrombospondin type 1 domain, was expressed in the dorsal neural tube and affected in Wnts mutants. Biochim Biophys Acta. 2004;1676(1):51-62.

[48] Nam JS, Turcotte TJ, Smith PF, Choi S, Yoon JK. Mouse cristin/R-spondin family proteins are novel ligands for the Frizzled 8 and LRP6 receptors and activate beta-catenin-dependent gene expression. J Biol Chem. 2006;281(19):13247-57.

[49] Wei Q, Yokota C, Semenov MV, Doble B, Woodgett J, He X. R-spondin1

is a high affinity ligand for LRP6 and induces LRP6 phosphorylation and beta-catenin signaling. J Biol Chem. 2007;282(21):15903-11.

[50] Kim KA, Wagle M, Tran K, Zhan X, Dixon MA, Liu S, et al. R-Spondin family members regulate the Wnt pathway by a common mechanism. Mol Biol Cell. 2008;19(6):2588-96.

[51] Kazanskaya O, Ohkawara B, Heroult M, Wu W, Maltry N, Augustin HG, et al. The Wnt signaling regulator R-spondin 3 promotes angioblast and vascular development. Development. 2008;135(22):3655-64.

[52] Bendell J, Eckhardt GS, Hochster HS, Morris VK, Strickler J, Kapoun AM, et al. Initial results from a phase 1a/b study of OMP-131R10, a first-in-class anti-RSPO3 antibody, in advanced solid tumors and previously treated metastatic colorectal cancer (CRC). European Journal of Cancer. 2016;69:S29-S30.

Chapter 7

MicroRNAs and Their Role in Acute Lymphoblastic Leukemia

Edgardo Becerra Becerra and Guadalupe García-Alcocer

Abstract

Acute lymphoblastic leukemia (ALL) has been established as the most common acute leukemia in children, accounting for 80–85% of cases. ALL occurs mostly in children and it is considered as a high-risk disease in the elderlies. ALL is characterized by a clonal disorder where the normal hematopoiesis is replaced by a malignant clonal expansion of lymphoid progenitors. Although many therapeutic strategies have been established to treat ALL leading to improved survival rates, the short-term and long-term complications derived from treatment toxicity represent a critical risk for patients. The treatment-related toxicity suggests a need for the development of new therapy strategies to effectively treat high-risk and low-risk disease. Nowadays, an important approach is focused on the identification of molecules involved in the mechanisms that lead to leukemia generation and progression to determine potential targets at the transcriptional level. MicroRNAs (miRNAs) are a group of key molecules that regulate signaling pathways related to lymphopoiesis. miRNAs participate in the regulation of hematopoietic differentiation and proliferation, as well as their activity. The present review details the recompilation of evidences about the relation between miRNAs and lymphopoiesis, ALL development and progression in order to propose and explore novel strategies to modulate ALL-related miRNA levels as a therapeutic approach.

Keywords: miRNAs, therapeutics, lymphopoiesis, acute lymphoblastic leukemia, agomiR, antagomiR

1. Acute lymphoblastic leukemia generalities

Acute lymphoblastic leukemia (ALL) has been established as the most common acute leukemia in children representing 80–85% of cases [1]. The global incidence ranges from three to five cases per 100, 000 population and the lowest incidence occurs in the adults older than 65 years old [2]. Even though ALL occurs mostly in children, it represents a devastating disease in the elderlies. ALL is a clonal disorder where the normal hematopoiesis is replaced by a malignant clonal expansion of lymphoid progenitors (blasts) [3]. Such clonal disorder is characterized by genetic abnormalities that lead to a block in B or T cell differentiation leading to abnormal cell proliferation and apoptosis in the bone marrow, peripheral blood and extramedullary sites [4, 5]. The overall survival of patients with ALL has been improved after treatment stratification according to immunophenotype and genotype. This treatment has allowed to incorporate, into therapy protocols, and more effective drug combinations [6]. Although improved survival rates have been obtained, the short-term and long-term complications derived from treatment toxicity represent a critical risk for patients. This suggests a need for the development of new therapy strategies to diminish the treatment-related toxicity and effectively treat high-risk and low-risk disease. An important approach is focused on the mechanisms that lead to leukemia generation and progression by identifying potential targets at the transcriptional level.

The development of B-lymphocytes and T-lymphocytes from a lymphoid progenitor occurs in the bone marrow and thymus, respectively, and the normal lymphopoiesis is regulated at a transcriptional level involving transcription factors acting as regulators of genes expression [7]. Nevertheless, a question arises: does the transcriptional process is sufficient to control the cell fate, lineage and other aspects of cellular functioning? The answer is "no", and there are other key mechanisms involved. MicroRNAs (miRNAs) are a group of key molecules that regulate signaling pathways related to lymphopoiesis. miRNAs regulate hematopoietic differentiation and proliferation, as well as their activity. Besides, a deregulation in miRNAs expression is observed in leukemias having a main role in the pathogenesis of such clonal disorder [7, 8]. The first connection between miRNAs and leukemia indicated that 13q14 deletion in B-cell chronic lymphocytic leukemias induced the loss of miR-16-1 and miR-15a in 70% of chronic lymphocytic leukemias [9]. In addition, recent studies suggested that at least 50% of miRNAs are located in cancer-associated genomic regions and mRNAs are regulated by these miRNAs populations [5]. Moreover, different patterns of miRNAs are observed in normal lymphopoiesis and leukemias. The investigation of the relation between miRNAs and pathological cellular processes represents an interesting approach for the development of new therapeutic strategies.

2. miRNAs biology

miRNAs are endogenous small non-coding RNAs with a length of 19–25 nucleotides (nt) and their genes are transcribed by RNA polymerase II (Pol II) in the nucleus [10, 11]. miRNAs transcripts are first generated as pri-miRNAs structures (up to 1000 nt of length) which contain cap structures and poly-A tails (**Figure 1**). The pri-miRNAs transcript is briefly processed into precursor miRNA (pre-miRNA) transcript of 60–120 nt of length by the microprocessor complex formed by class 2 ribonuclease III enzyme called DROSHA and the DiGeorge Syndrome Critical Region Gene (DGCR8) protein. The pre-miRNA structure bears a hairpin structure with 2-nt overhang at the 3'end [12, 13]. The next step consists in exporting the pre-miRNA from the nucleus to the cytosol. This process is mediated by the exportin-5 (a RanGTP-dependent dsRNA-binding protein) which recognizes the overhang in the pre-miRNA as a target to be transported [14].

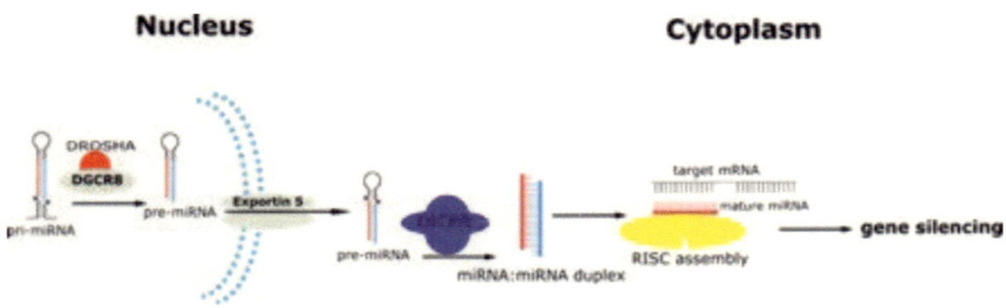

Figure 1.
miRNAs biogenesis and gene silencing mediated by miRNA.

Once in the cytosol, and pre-miRNA is processed by the DICER enzyme (RNAse type III) leading to a mature miRNA duplex (miRNA: miRNA) about 22 nt of length. The miRNA duplex is loaded into the RNA-induced silencing complex (RISC), composed by of the Argonaute2 (Ago2) and the trans-activator RNA (tar)-binding protein (TRBP). Note that the mature single-strand miRNA is retained by the Argo2 protein in the RISC complex to guide the gene silencing by binding to its mRNA target leading to mRNA degradation [10, 13, 15]. Recent evidence indicates that some pri-miRNAs contain open reading fragments about 300 nt and could be transported, without being processed, into the cytosol, and then become translated into micropeptides, having the ability to influence a variety of cellular processes. This is an additional field of opportunity to carry out functional studies with the aim to develop novel therapeutic strategies [16].

3. miRNAs and their implications in lymphopoiesis and ALL development

3.1 Lymphopoiesis regulation by miRNAs

Lymphopoiesis is a process in which hematopoietic stem cells (HSCs) differentiate into an immature form called lymphoid progenitor and finally into mature B- or T-lymphocytes [17]. The miRNAs play a key role in the process of cell differentiation by regulating several signaling pathways. The pattern of miRNAs expression is different according to normal or malignant lymphopoietic process.

The miRNA-150 (miR-150) is expressed in B- and T-cells and the lymphoid progenitors express the miR-150 to promote B-cell maturation and by assisting in the transition of the progenitor B-cells (pro-B) to precursor B-cell (pre-B) stage. When a premature miR-150 expression occurs, the result is a blocked transition from pro-B to pre-B stage [18, 19]. In the thymus, the expression of miR-150 enhances T-cell development and its key pathways (Notch pathway) and prevents an alternative lineage differentiation (B-cell differentiation) in the progenitors. Since C-myb is an essential transcription factor involved in the early lymphoid development, a downregulation eventually leads to an arrest from pro-B to pre-B stage. This event is accompanied by miR-150 overexpression [15, 17].

The miRNA-155 (miR-155) is upregulated in both B- and T-cells in their activated and mature stage. In the case of B-cells differentiation, miR-155 inhibits PU.1 expression leading to Pax5 downregulation and the initiation of the plasma cell differentiation pathway. This event is known as the miR-155-PU.1 axis. The role of miR-155 in T-cells differentiation depends on the level of miR-155 expression. The expression of miR-155 mediates the differentiation of T-cells into T-helper type 1, while its absence leads to T-cells transition into T-helper type [20, 21].

The miRNA-181 (miR-181) is a family of miRNAs and is composed of three clusters located in a different chromosome. Hsa-miR-181a-1 and hsa-miR181b-1 are located on chromosome 1; hsa-miR-181a-2 and hsa-miR181-b-2 are located on chromosome 9 and finally hsa-miR181c-1 and hsa-miR-181c-2 are located on chromosome19 [22]. miR-181 family have been reported to be implicated in lung and breast cancers [23]. miR-181a can act as inhibitor of the normal cellular response to DNA damage by affecting the expression and activity of the stress-sensor kinase ataxia telangiectasia mutated (ATM). In the early stage of B-cells differentiation, the expression of miR-181 is high and decreases subsequently within differentiation [17], and during T-cell development, the miR-181 is highly expressed in double-positive T-cells. The targets for miR-181 are BCL-2, CD89, EGR1 and T-cell receptor [24, 25].

miRNA	Function	Target	miRNA expression in ALL vs. normal samples	References
miR-150	Transition from pro-B to pre-B stage	C-MYB	High	He *et al.*, 2015 [26]
miR-155	Promotes T-cell differentiation into Th type 1 cells	PTEN	High	Seddiki et al., 2014 [21]
miR-181	B-cell differentiation and T-cell development	BCL-2, MYC, CDX2, CD69, GR1, and T-cell receptor	High	Veruci et al., 2015 [24]
miR-17-92	Transition from pro-B to pre-B stage	YLD, HOXA9, BIM, RUNX1, MYC	High	Rao et al., 2015 [27]
miR-126	B-ALL development	MYC and CDX2	High	Fulci et al., 2009 [28]
miR-223	Reduction in cell growth and T-ALL development	IKAROS, PTEN, BIM, PHF6, NF1, and FBXW7	Low	Mavrakis et al., 2011 [29]
miR-19b	T-ALL development	IKAROS, PTEN, BIM, PHF6, NF1, and FBXW7	High	Mavrakis et al., 2011 [29]
miR-20a	T-ALL development	IKAROS, PTEN, BIM, PHF6, NF1, and FBXW7	High	Mavrakis et al., 2011 [29]
miR-92	T-ALL development	IKAROS, PTEN, BIM, PHF6, NF1, and FBXW7	High	Mavrakis et al., 2011 [29]
miR-26a	T-ALL development	KAROS, PTEN, BIM, PHF6, NF1, and FBXW7	High	Mavrakis et al., 2011 [29]
miR-123a	PI3K signaling activation	PTEN	High	Bertacchini et al., 2015 [30]
miR-21	Regulation of PI3K/Akt/ mTOR pathway	PTEN	High	Bertacchini et al., 2015 [30]
miR-99a	Promotes the differentiation of human granulocytes and monocytes cells	mTOR, IGF-1, and MCL1	Low	Li et al., 2012 [31], Li et al., 2013 [32]
miR-100	Promotes the differentiation of human granulocytes and monocytes cells	mTOR, IGF-1, and MCL1	Low	Li et al. 2013 [32]
miR-19	T-ALL development	PTEN, HOXA, CYLD, BIM, and NOTCH1	High	Tsuchida et al., 2011 [33]
miR-29a	T-ALL development	MYC and CDX2	Low	Zaidi et al., 2017 [34]
miR-30a	B-ALL development	NOTCH1, NOTCH2 and MYC	High	Ortega et al., 2015 [35]

Table 1.
Function, targets and expression level of miRNAs related to ALL.

The miR-17-92 cluster is composed of six miRNAs including miR-17, miR-18a, miR-19a, miR19-b-1, miR-20a and miR-92-1 and is highly expressed in both B- and T-lymphoid progenitors and subsequently decreases within maturation [27]. When miR-17-92 cluster is downregulated or absent, occurs B-cell differentiation disorder due to the overexpression of the proapoptotic protein BIM (target of miR-17-92 cluster). On the other hand, when miR-12-92 cluster is overexpressed during lymphopoiesis, promotes lymphoproliferative disorders and severe autoimmunity [36].

The aforementioned miRNAs play a critical role on the lymphopoiesis and the change of their expression pattern leads to blood disorders or malignant lymphopoiesis mechanisms. Such is the reason why miRNAs can be potential targets for treatment, diagnosis and prognosis in ALL.

3.2 The role of miRNAs in ALL development

Besides the involvement of aberrant miRNAs expression in malignant lymphopoiesis, it may be related to drug resistance mechanisms. Focusing on promoting the reversal expression of such miRNA may enhance disease management and improve clinical outcomes. By comparing miRNAs expression in both normal pediatric bone marrow and pediatric ALL, an overexpression of miR-100, miR-196b in ALL and lower expression of let-7e in normal bone marrow were reported [37]. In a study conducted in childhood B-ALL and T-ALL, the miRNA expression profile in the bone marrow was evaluated to discriminate between T-ALL and B-ALL. The results indicated a downregulation of miR-708-5p, miR-497-5p, miR-151a-5p, miR-151b, miR-371b-5p, miR-455-5p, miR-195-5p, miR-1266-5p, miR-574-5p, miR-425-5p and upregulation of miR-450b-5p, miR-450a-5p, miR-542-5p, miR-424-5p, miR-629-5p, miR-29c-5p in T-ALL. Further machine process analyses showed that miR-29c-5p, involved in calcium signaling, is involved in B-cell fate and it is the best discriminator to stablish childhood B-ALL or T-ALL. In addition, clinical samples of T-ALL were studied and reveled that miR-223, miR-19b, miR-20a, miR-92, miR-142-3p, miR-150, miR-93, miR-26a, miR-16, and miR-342., miR-19b,-20a,-26a,-92 and miR-223 target T-ALL tumor suppressors, such as IKAROS, PTEN, BIM, PHF6, NF1 and FBXW7 [37], which means that overexpression of such miRNAs could lead to ALL development and represents a potential therapeutic target.

The identification of miRNAs that target genes of MYC, TFs of CDX2 and IncRNA of XIST could represent an approach to ALL therapeutics, due to that the aforementioned genes may play important role in the development of B-ALL. NOTCH1 is another important target due to mutations of gain of function, which are implicated in T-ALL development as well as NOTCH1 and NOTCH2 that take part in B-malignances [38]. **Table 1** exhibits a list of miRNAs involved in ALL development and pathogenesis considered as potential therapeutic targets.

4. Modulation of miRNAs expression levels in ALL: a therapeutic approach

Children diagnosed with ALL, in most cases follow a standard treatment protocol divided into three phases: induction, consolidation and maintenance, and sometimes a central nervous system-directed therapy. The drugs used in induction and consolidation phases usually include prednisolone (PRED), vincristine (VCR), L-asparaginase (L-ASP) and daunorubicin (DNR), all these drugs presents late effects. The maintenance phase is the most prolongated treatment in childhood ALL, however, it involves a much less intensive regimen than induction and consolidation phases. The maintenance phase has been demonstrated to lower the risk of relapse, but could be a cause for emergence new mutations leading to drug resistance [16]. Even though the great effort in the development of new treatment strategies, drug resistance is the major cause of chemotherapy failure and relapse in pediatric patients. The classification of patients resistant or sensitive to drugs can be carried out based on the expression level of miRNAs.

The multidrug resistance (MDR) represents a problem in the treatment of pediatric ALL. It is considered an ubiquitous and severe clinical problem. MDR is mediated by adenosine triphosphate (ATP)-binding cassette (ABC) transporters. Several chemotherapeutic drugs are actively transported by ABC transporters across the cellular membranes leading to chemotherapy failure. Recent evidence indicates that some miRNAs tend to enhance chemotherapy response by modulating the expression of ABC transporters. In a study, the transfection of miR-326 into HepG2 cells demonstrated enhanced response to chemotherapeutic drugs due to downregulation of ABC transporter ABCC144 [16, 39]. Previous reports indicated that overexpression of ABCA2 and ABCA3 genes increases the risk of MDR and relapse in pediatric ALL patients [40]. Based upon bioinformatics analysis, miR-326 was identified as negative regulator of MDR-related genes, ABCA2 and ABCA3 in particular. Further evaluation of the miR-326 expression levels in pediatric ALL patients resistant to chemotherapy (MDR+) revealed that miR-326 is significantly decreased in MDR+ compared to the MDR- control group, supporting the idea that low level expression of miR-326 impacts directly on chemotherapy treatment response [41, 42].

Glucocorticoids (GC) are a group of drugs clinically used to treat ALL due to their involvement in cell progression, immunoglobulin, lymphokine production and apoptosis in immature lymphoblasts. The MLL rearrangements are common genetic abnormality in ALL. MLL-AF4 is the result of a balanced translocation between MLL and AF4 and it occurs in approximately 50% of ALL cases in infants. MLL-AF4 is an indicative of poor prognosis due to failure in GC-induced apoptosis. miR-128b and miR-221 are downregulated in this type of ALL and leads to overexpression of their targets: CDKN1B, MLL, AF4 and both MLL-AF4 and AF4-MLL fusion genes (involved in AL development). The restoration of miR-128b and miR-221 results in the downregulation of their aforementioned targets and increase the sensitivity to GC therapy [37, 43]. After transiently overexpression of miR-17 in a pre-B cell line (SUP-B15), it was found a reduced dexamethasone (DEX)-induced apoptosis indicating resistance to DEX. Further inhibition of miR-17 by locked nucleic acid inhibitor enhanced the response to DEX. The development of miRNA inhibitors, antagomiRs and agomiRs allows to modulate miRNAs levels in order to obtain a better response in ALL treatment.

AntagomiR is a chemically-modified single-strand miRNA inhibitor used to block miRNA regulation of target gene expression efficiently. AntagomiRs are synthesized to reduce the ability of endogenous miRNAs to silence target mRNA transcripts. They can downregulate the corresponding endogenous miRNAs by either local or systemic injection into the animals. Their structure consists of a single-strand RNA carrying the chemically modifications functioning by blocking a target of miRNA. The strand of the antagomiR has 2 phosphorothionates at the 5'end, 4 phosphorothionates, 1 cholesterol group at the 3'end and full-length nucleotide 2′-methoxy modification. Its stability is significantly higher than miRNA inhibitors. On the other hand, agomiR is a chemically-modified double-strand miRNA mimics which can mimic mature endogenous miRNAs after transfection into cells. They can upregulate the endogenous miRNA activity by utilizing the natural miRNA machinery. The antisense strand of the agomiR has 2 phosphorothionates at the 5'end, 4 phosphorothionates, 1 cholesterol group at the 3'end and full-length nucleotide 2′-methoxy modification. The chemically-modified structure of agomiR increases its stability and activity. Both, agomiRs and antagomiRs are recommended for miRNA functional *in vitro* and *in vivo* studies.

Once a miRNA has been established or identified as a target to be downregulated, or up regulated, agomiRs or antagomiRs can be used to modulate miRNAs levels and further determination of anticancer effects. This is a promising and interesting approach to combine miRNA-based therapy and current chemotherapy to synergistically improve clinical outcomes. The potential therapeutic miRNAs targets described below can be modulated by using agomiR or antagomiR.

The miR-101 has a potential role in drug response to doxorubicin (DOXO) in Jurkat T-ALL. It was shown that miR-101 targets NOTCH1 which is linked to enhanced DOXO sensitivity to myeloma cell lines in mouse. Therefore, miR-101 may enhance DOXO-mediated apoptosis by repressing NOTCH1, while low expression of miR-101 may be related to chemoresistance in T-ALL [44].

For ALL patients with BCR-ABL fusion gene, the treatment with tyrosine-kinase inhibitors (TKI) could be a promising strategy even though the prognosis is suboptimal. BCR-ABL1 and ABL1 are direct targets of miR-203. However, miR-203 is silenced by genetic and epigenetic mechanisms in hematopoietic malignancies as leukemia. It has been reported that the restoration of miR-203 expression reduces BCR-ABL1 and ABL1 levels in cells and leads to arrest in cell proliferation [15, 45]. In addition, the inhibition of the DNMT3A gene, which gives the instructions for making the enzyme DNA methyltransferase alpha involved in DNA methylation and gene silencing, can be assessed by increasing miR-217 or mimics expression. This may prevent drug resistance to TKI in Philadelphia-chromosome-positive ALL patients, being another therapeutic strategy [46]. According to the aforementioned, the demethylation may be a potential therapeutic strategy in ALL. As mentioned before, the miR-143 is epigenetically repressed by promoter hypermethylation in MLL-AF4-positive primary blast, but not in normal bone marrow cells, and neither in MLL-AF4-negative primary blasts. Besides, MLL-AF4 expression is regulated by miR-143, such not being possible in MLL-AF4-positive cells. The restoration of miR-143 levels could induce apoptosis and regulate in a negative way the of the leukemia cells growth [47].

The miR-125b-2 cluster, consisting of miR-125b, miR-99a and let-7c, is increased in ETV6-RUNX1+ leukemia. According to previous reports, the miR-125b-2 cluster expression is not regulated by the ETV6-RUNX1 fusion protein, which indicates that the expression of this cluster may be an independent leukemia event. Further knockdown of miR-125b-2 cluster in the *ETV6-RUNX1*$^{+}$ cell line Reh led to increased cell sensitivity to DOXO and staurosporine treatment. Hence, the overexpression of miR-125b-2 cluster confers to leukemic cells survival advantage through the inhibition of apoptosis and failure in activation of caspase-3 [48]. These findings support the idea that miR-125b-2 cluster is a potential therapeutic target in pediatric ALL.

In pediatric ALL patients, a genome-wide miRNA analysis indicated a reduced miR-335 expression, such being the most significant miRNA abnormality associated with a poor outcome. Furthermore, the overexpression of miR-335 significantly sensitized the ALL cells to PRED. The role of miR-335 in PRED resistance was studied by investigating downstream pathways. The results suggested that low level of miR-335 leads to higher MAPK1-mediated survival. Further treatment with MEK/ERK inhibitor enhanced PRED-induced cell death suggesting that using synthetic miR-335 and overriding MAPK1 activity plus MEK/ERK pathway inhibition may provide a promising therapeutic strategy to overcome PRED resistance [49].

In regards of T-ALL, few studies investigate the role of miRNAs in GC response. GC bind to its receptor (GCR), which acts as a ligand-dependent-transcription factor, inducing cell cycle arrest and apoptosis in cancer cells [50]. The GCR is modulated by miR-142-3p, which represses GCR biosynthesis. The inhibition of miR-142-3p in T-ALL cell lines resulted in increased GC-mediated cell death compared to not inhibited cells. Another protein involved in GC resistance via GCR repression is the FKBP51, which is negatively regulated by miR-100 and miR-99. Both miRNAs are found to be downregulated in the T-ALL as well as the B-ALL. In transfected T-ALL cell lines with mimics of miR-100 and miR-99, the result led to enhanced sensitivity to CG and apoptosis. In addition, previous studies reported that miR-100 and miR-99 act synergistically with miR-125 enhancing resistance to VCR [51, 52]. *In vitro* studies indicate that only the overexpression of the three aforementioned miRNAs led to VCR resistance. Moreover, hypoxia is a crucial microenvironmental factor supporting self-renewal of leukemic stem cells in bone marrow niches. miR-210 is one of the hypoxia-regulated miRNAs most studied in cancer including its role in drug resistance and as a prognostic potential. The miR-210 levels were modified in ETV6-RUNX+ Reh and MLL-AF4 + RS4; 11 pediatric ALL cell lines by introducing antagomiR and agomiR to miR-210. After 24 h of the transfection, both cell lines were treated with the DNR, VCR, DEX and L-ASP, individually or in combinations of the four drugs. In ETV6-RUNX+ Reh cells, the half maximal inhibitory concentrations (IC50s) of DNR, DEX and L-ASP were significantly decreased (in agomiR-transfected cells) or increased (in antagomiR-transfected cells) compared to cells transfected with negative control mimics. At the other extreme, the IC50s of DNR, DEX and VCR were decreased (in agomiR-transfected cells) or increased (in antagomiR-transfected cells) in MLL-AF4 + RS4;11 cells [53]. In regards with these findings, the use of agomiRs and antagomiRs to miRNAs could be an alternative to overcome resistance to chemotherapy. Nevertheless, the great challenge in clinical and nonclinical trials, is the delivery of synthetic miRNAs to leukemia cells effectively.

5. Conclusion and future directions

miRNAs are taking place as therapeutic targets promising in the molecular oncology due to their ability to regulate important cellular processes through multiple targets. Their inherent role in carcinogenesis can be as oncogenes or tumor suppressive genes, and the identification of specific biological functions, type of cancer and targets of miRNAs is a critical aspect in the approach of miRNAs therapeutics. Since miRNAs are differentially expressed in distinct stages of lymphopoiesis and influence ALL development, the aberrant miRNAs signatures observed in ALL may be intensively used to determine biomarkers for diagnosis, classification and prognosis. The changes in the expression level of several miRNAs play a functional role in drug resistance, and the reversal of such expression profiles could improve drug sensitivity to obtain better clinical outcomes. The transfection of agomiRs or antagomiRs to miRNAs allows the increase or decrease of specific miRNA expression levels. However, safety concerns and degradation effects limit their efficacy *in vivo*. There is a need for systemic delivery of miRNA as therapeutic agent in the treatment of ALL. The miRNAs listed before represent a low percentage of the total miRNAs studied as potential therapeutic targets. It is quite difficult to present the entire list, nonetheless, there is an available database considered as a valuable source of information for researchers to understand and investigate miRNAs and their targets with diagnostic and therapeutic potential in ALL. Such database is LeukmiR and can be consulted in this link http://tdb.ccmb.res.in/LeukmiR/

Author details

Edgardo Becerra Becerra and Guadalupe García-Alcocer*
Unidad de Investigación Genética, Posgrado en Ciencias Químico Biológicas, Facultad de Química, Universidad Autónoma de Querétaro, Querétaro, Mexico

*Address all correspondence to: leguga@email.com

References

[1] Noone AM, Howlader N, Krapcho M, Miller D, Brest A, Yu M, Ruhl J, Tatalovich Z, Mariotto A, Lewis DR, Chen HS, Feuer EJ CK. SEER Cancer Statistics Review (CSR) 1975-2015.

[2] Rendón-Macías ME, Reyes-Zepeda NC, Villasís-Keever MÁ, Meneses JS, Núñez AE. Tendencia mundial de la supervivencia en pacientes pediátricos con leucemia linfoblástica aguda. revisión de las últimas cuatro décadas. *Bol Med Hosp Infant Mex*. 2012;69(3):153-163.

[3] Zhao H, Wang D, Du W, Gu D, Yang R. MicroRNA and leukemia: Tiny molecule, great function. *Crit Rev Oncol Hematol*. 2010;74(3):149-155. doi:10.1016/j.critrevonc.2009.05.001

[4] Terwilliger T, Abdul-Hay M. Acute lymphoblastic leukemia: a comprehensive review and 2017 update. *Blood Cancer J*. 2017;7(6):e577-e577. doi:10.1038/bcj.2017.53

[5] Rawoof A, Swaminathan G, Tiwari S, Nair RA, Dinesh Kumar L. LeukmiR: a database for miRNAs and their targets in acute lymphoblastic leukemia. *Database*. 2020;2020. doi:10.1093/database/baz151

[6] Vora A. Childhood leukaemia: an update. *Paediatr Child Health (Oxford)*. 2016;26(2):51-56. doi:10.1016/j.paed.2015.10.007

[7] Johanson TM, Skinner JPJ, Kumar A, Zhan Y, Lew AM, Chong MMW. The role of microRNAs in lymphopoiesis. *Int J Hematol*. 2014;100(3):246-253. doi:10.1007/s12185-014-1606-y

[8] Garzon R, Croce CM. MicroRNAs in normal and malignant hematopoiesis. *Curr Opin Hematol*. 2008;15(4):352-358. doi:10.1097/MOH.0b013e328303e15d

[9] Calin GA, Dumitru CD, Shimizu M, et al. Nonlinear partial differential equations and applications: Frequent deletions and down-regulation of micro- RNA genes miR15 and miR16 at 13q14 in chronic lymphocytic leukemia. *Proc Natl Acad Sci*. 2002;99(24):15524-15529. doi:10.1073/pnas.242606799

[10] Lin S, Gregory RI. MicroRNA biogenesis pathways in cancer. *Nat Rev Cancer*. 2015;15(6):321-333. doi:10.1038/nrc3932

[11] O'Brien J, Hayder H, Zayed Y, Peng C. Overview of MicroRNA Biogenesis, Mechanisms of Actions, and Circulation. *Front Endocrinol (Lausanne)*. 2018;9. doi:10.3389/fendo.2018.00402

[12] Acunzo M, Romano G, Wernicke D, Croce CM. MicroRNA and cancer – A brief overview. *Adv Biol Regul*. 2015;57:1-9. doi:10.1016/j.jbior.2014.09.013

[13] Yeasmin F, Yada T, Akimitsu N. Micropeptides Encoded in Transcripts Previously Identified as Long Noncoding RNAs: A New Chapter in Transcriptomics and Proteomics. *Front Genet*. 2018;9. doi:10.3389/fgene.2018.00144

[14] Zheng L, Tu Q, Meng S, et al. Runx2/DICER/miRNA Pathway in Regulating Osteogenesis. *J Cell Physiol*. 2017;232(1):182-191. doi:10.1002/jcp.25406

[15] Ultimo S, Martelli AM, Zauli G, Vitale M, Calin GA, Neri LM. Roles and clinical implications of microRNAs in acute lymphoblastic leukemia. *J Cell Physiol*. 2018;233(8):5642-5654. doi:10.1002/jcp.26290

[16] Grobbelaar C, Ford AM. The Role of MicroRNA in Paediatric

Acute Lymphoblastic Leukaemia: Challenges for Diagnosis and Therapy. *J Oncol*. 2019;2019:1-14. doi:10.1155/2019/8941471

[17] Chen B, Luan C, Yang Z. The functional role of microRNA in acute lymphoblastic leukemia: relevance for diagnosis, differential diagnosis, prognosis, and therapy. *Onco Targets Ther*. October 2015:2903. doi:10.2147/OTT.S92470

[18] He Y, Jiang X, Chen J. The role of miR-150 in normal and malignant hematopoiesis. *Oncogene*. 2014;33(30):3887-3893. doi:10.1038/onc.2013.346

[19] Lawrie CH, Manterola L, Fernandez-Mercado M, et al. MicroRNAs as B-cell lymphoma biomarkers. *Blood Lymphat Cancer Targets Ther*. February 2015:25. doi:10.2147/BLCTT.S60481

[20] O'Connell RM, Kahn D, Gibson WSJ, et al. MicroRNA-155 Promotes Autoimmune Inflammation by Enhancing Inflammatory T Cell Development. *Immunity*. 2010;33(4):607-619. doi:10.1016/j.immuni.2010.09.009

[21] Seddiki N, Brezar V, Ruffin N, Lévy Y, Swaminathan S. Role of miR-155 in the regulation of lymphocyte immune function and disease. *Immunology*. 2014;142(1):32-38. doi:10.1111/imm.12227

[22] Yang Z, Wan X, Gu Z, et al. Evolution of the mir-181 microRNA family. *Comput Biol Med*. 2014;52:82-87. doi:10.1016/j.compbiomed.2014.06.004

[23] Pop-Bica C, Pintea S, Cojocneanu-Petric R, et al. MiR-181 family-specific behavior in different cancers: a meta-analysis view. *Cancer Metastasis Rev*. 2018;37(1):17-32. doi:10.1007/s10555-017-9714-9

[24] Verduci L, Azzalin G, Gioiosa S, et al. microRNA-181a enhances cell proliferation in acute lymphoblastic leukemia by targeting EGR1. *Leuk Res*. 2015;39(4):479-485. doi:10.1016/j.leukres.2015.01.010

[25] Neilson JR, Zheng GXY, Burge CB, Sharp PA. Dynamic regulation of miRNA expression in ordered stages of cellular development. *Genes Dev*. 2007;21(5):578-589. doi:10.1101/gad.1522907

[26] He Y, Chevillet JR, Liu G, Kim TK, Wang K. The effects of microRNA on the absorption, distribution, metabolism and excretion of drugs. *Br J Pharmacol*. 2015;172(11):2733-2747. doi:10.1111/bph.12968

[27] Rao R, Nagarkatti PS, Nagarkatti M. Δ 9 Tetrahydrocannabinol attenuates Staphylococcal enterotoxin B-induced inflammatory lung injury and prevents mortality in mice by modulation of miR-17-92 cluster and induction of T-regulatory cells. *Br J Pharmacol*. 2015;172(7):1792-1806. doi:10.1111/bph.13026

[28] Fulci V, Colombo T, Chiaretti S, et al. Characterization of B- and T-lineage acute lymphoblastic leukemia by integrated analysis of MicroRNA and mRNA expression profiles. *Genes, Chromosom Cancer*. 2009;48(12):1069-1082. doi:10.1002/gcc.20709

[29] Mavrakis KJ, Van Der Meulen J, Wolfe AL, et al. A cooperative microRNA-tumor suppressor gene network in acute T-cell lymphoblastic leukemia (T-ALL). *Nat Genet*. 2011;43(7):673-678. doi:10.1038/ng.858

[30] Bertacchini J, Heidari N, Mediani L, et al. Targeting PI3K/AKT/mTOR network for treatment of leukemia. *Cell Mol Life Sci*. 2015;72(12):2337-2347. doi:10.1007/s00018-015-1867-5

[31] Li Y, Hu Z, Chen B, et al. Taurine attenuates methamphetamine-induced autophagy and apoptosis in PC12 cells through mTOR signaling pathway. *Toxicol Lett*. 2012;215(1):1-7. doi:10.1016/j.toxlet.2012.09.019

[32] Li X-J, Luo X-Q, Han B-W, Duan F-T, Wei P-P, Chen Y-Q. MicroRNA-100/99a, deregulated in acute lymphoblastic leukaemia, suppress proliferation and promote apoptosis by regulating the FKBP51 and IGF1R/mTOR signalling pathways. *Br J Cancer*. 2013;109(8):2189-2198. doi:10.1038/bjc.2013.562

[33] Tsuchida A, Ohno S, Wu W, et al. miR-92 is a key oncogenic component of the miR-17-92 cluster in colon cancer. *Cancer Sci*. 2011;102(12):2264-2271. doi:10.1111/j.1349-7006.2011.02081.x

[34] Zaidi SK, Perez AW, White ES, Lian JB, Stein JL, Stein GS. An AML1-ETO/miR-29b-1 regulatory circuit modulates phenotypic properties of acute myeloid leukemia cells. *Oncotarget*. 2017;8(25):39994-40005. doi:10.18632/oncotarget.18127

[35] Ortega M, Bhatnagar H, Lin A-P, et al. A microRNA-mediated regulatory loop modulates NOTCH and MYC oncogenic signals in B- and T-cell malignancies. *Leukemia*. 2015;29(4):968-976. doi:10.1038/leu.2014.302

[36] Inaba H, Greaves M, Mullighan CG. Acute lymphoblastic leukaemia. *Lancet*. 2013;381(9881):1943-1955. doi:10.1016/S0140-6736(12)62187-4

[37] Gómez-Gómez Y, Organista-Nava J, Illades-Aguiar B, Antonio Leyva-Vázquez M. miRNAs in Acute Lymphoblastic Leukemia: Diagnosis, Prognosis and Target Therapeutic. In: *Advances in Hematologic Malignancies*. IntechOpen; 2019. doi:10.5772/intechopen.84318

[38] Martínez N, Almaraz C, Vaqué JP, et al. Whole-exome sequencing in splenic marginal zone lymphoma reveals mutations in genes involved in marginal zone differentiation. *Leukemia*. 2014;28(6):1334-1340. doi:10.1038/leu.2013.365

[39] Kibria G, Hatakeyama H, Harashima H. Cancer multidrug resistance: mechanisms involved and strategies for circumvention using a drug delivery system. *Arch Pharm Res*. 2014;37(1):4-15. doi:10.1007/s12272-013-0276-2

[40] Rahgozar S, Moafi A, Abedi M, et al. mRNA expression profile of multidrug-resistant genes in acute lymphoblastic leukemia of children, a prognostic value for ABCA3 and ABCA2. *Cancer Biol Ther*. 2014;15(1):35-41. doi:10.4161/cbt.26603

[41] de Oliveira JC, Brassesco MS, Scrideli CA, Tone LG, Narendran A. MicroRNA expression and activity in pediatric acute lymphoblastic leukemia (ALL). *Pediatr Blood Cancer*. 2012;59(4):599-604. doi:10.1002/pbc.24167

[42] Ghodousi ES, Rahgozar S. MicroRNA-326 and microRNA-200c: Two novel biomarkers for diagnosis and prognosis of pediatric acute lymphoblastic leukemia. *J Cell Biochem*. 2018;119(7):6024-6032. doi:10.1002/jcb.26800

[43] Kotani A, Ha D, Schotte D, Armstrong SA, Lodish HF. A novel mutation in the miR-128b gene reduces miRNA processing and leads to glucocorticoid resistance of MLL-AF4 Acute Lymphocytic Leukemia cells. *Cell Cycle*. 2010;9(6):1037-1042. doi:10.4161/cc.9.6.11011

[44] Qian L, Zhang W, Lei B, et al. MicroRNA-101 regulates T-cell acute lymphoblastic leukemia progression

and chemotherapeutic sensitivity by targeting Notch1. *Oncol Rep*. 2016;36(5):2511-2516. doi:10.3892/or.2016.5117

[45] Faber J, Gregory RI, Armstrong SA. Linking miRNA Regulation to BCR-ABL Expression: The Next Dimension. *Cancer Cell*. 2008;13(6):467-469. doi:10.1016/j.ccr.2008.05.013

[46] Nishioka C, Ikezoe T, Yang J, Nobumoto A, Tsuda M, Yokoyama A. Downregulation of miR-217 correlates with resistance of ph + leukemia cells to ABL tyrosine kinase inhibitors. *Cancer Sci*. 2014;105(3):297-307. doi:10.1111/cas.12339

[47] Dou L, Zheng D, Li J, et al. Methylation-mediated repression of microRNA-143 enhances MLL–AF4 oncogene expression. *Oncogene*. 2012;31(4):507-517. doi:10.1038/onc.2011.248

[48] Gefen N, Binder V, Zaliova M, et al. Hsa-mir-125b-2 is highly expressed in childhood ETV6/RUNX1 (TEL/AML1) leukemias and confers survival advantage to growth inhibitory signals independent of p53. *Leukemia*. 2010;24(1):89-96. doi:10.1038/leu.2009.208

[49] Yan J, Jiang N, Huang G, et al. Deregulated MIR335 that targets MAPK1 is implicated in poor outcome of paediatric acute lymphoblastic leukaemia. *Br J Haematol*. 2013;163(1):93-103. doi:10.1111/bjh.12489

[50] Lv M, Zhang X, Jia H, et al. An oncogenic role of miR-142-3p in human T-cell acute lymphoblastic leukemia (T-ALL) by targeting glucocorticoid receptor-α and cAMP/PKA pathways. *Leukemia*. 2012;26(4):769-777. doi:10.1038/leu.2011.273

[51] Akbari Moqadam F, Lange-Turenhout EAM, Ariës IM, Pieters R, den Boer ML. MiR-125b, miR-100 and miR-99a co-regulate vincristine resistance in childhood acute lymphoblastic leukemia. *Leuk Res*. 2013;37(10):1315-1321. doi:10.1016/j.leukres.2013.06.027

[52] Drobna M, Szarzyńska-Zawadzka B, Dawidowska M. T-cell acute lymphoblastic leukemia from miRNA perspective: Basic concepts, experimental approaches, and potential biomarkers. *Blood Rev*. 2018;32(6). doi:10.1016/j.blre.2018.04.003

[53] Mei Y, Gao C, Wang K, et al. Effect of microRNA-210 on prognosis and response to chemotherapeutic drugs in pediatric acute lymphoblastic leukemia. *Cancer Sci*. 2014;105(4):463-472. doi:10.1111/cas.12370

Section 3

Conventional Treatment of Acute Leukemias

Chapter 8

Acute Lymphoblastic Leukemia in Adolescents and Young Adults

Martha Alvarado-Ibarra, José Antonio De la Peña Celaya, Luara Luz Arana-Luna, Eleazar Hernández-Ruiz, José Luis Alvarez Vera, María Eugenia Espitia Ríos and Juan Manuel Pérez Zúñiga

Abstract

When diagnosed with ALL the age group between 18 and 45 years old (AYA, adolescents and young adults) do not have the good prognosis factors generally observed in children with this diagnosis. For a long time, it was undetermined whether they should be treated with continuous and sustained chemotherapy as children or whether receive sustained chemotherapy, but with longer rest periods like old adults. The medical care of adolescents and young adults with neoplastic diseases, grouped between 15 and 45 years of age, became an emerging research field of treatment in hematological diseases. Outcomes have asses complete response disease-free survival, and overall survival as markers of response, with very poor results reported. Relevant challenges have been identified in the AYA group with ALL that have drawn attention to the need to increase research in this area, particularly in the care of the population under 45 years of age with hematological malignancies.

Keywords: acute lymphoblastic leukemia, remission, relapse, treatment, adult young and adolescents, bone marrow transplant

1. Introduction

Acute lymphoblastic leukemia (ALL) is an oncohematological disease caused by genetic changes that alter the differentiation and proliferation of lymphocytes, distinguished by the infiltration of bone marrow, blood, and other tissues by neoplastic cells of hematopoietic origin [1]. The pathophysiology of these disease include causes for which, certain genes result affected in their function. Patients could present the following symptomatology: fever, lymphadenopathy, coagulation disorders, anemia, hepato-splenomegaly, weight loss, among others.

Another definition of ALL could be a disease caused by an acquired or congenital injury to the hematopoietic cell DNA (the genetic material) developing in the bone marrow, once these cells transform into a leukemic clone multiplies uncontrollably and rapidly in billions of malignant cells called lymphoblasts that prevents the normal cellular production of leukocytes, platelets and red blood cells. As a result, when a patient is diagnosed with acute lymphoblastic leukemia, the number of healthy blood cells (red blood cells, white blood cells, and platelets) could be less than normal, although it is not uncommon to see an exaggerated elevation of white blood cells but all of them lymphoblasts.

It is more frequent in childhood than in adulthood, being the most common type of leukemia in children, with a peak of incidence between the 2 and 4 years old. When it appears in adulthood, it implies a worse prognosis.

2. Diagnosis by flow cytometry

There are a group of important cellular markers to make the diagnosis of B cell lineage, those are: CD19, CD20, CD22, CD24, and CD79a. The principal and earlier markers for lineage B cells are CD19, CD22 (membrane and cytoplasm respective) and CD79a [1, 2]. The presence of either of these two markers, without further differentiation markers, identifies the neoplastic cell as pro-B ALL (EGIL BI subtype). Positivity of the CD10 antigen (CALLA) defines the neoplastic cell as "common ALL" (EGIL B-II subtype). Cases with additional identification of the cytoplasmic heavy Mu chain are classified as the pre-B group (EGIL B-III subtype), while the presence of surface immunoglobulin light chains as mature B-ALL (EGIL B-IV subtype) [3].

In recent years, the direct correlation between ontogenetic classification with immunophenotypic expression by flow cytometry and cytogenetic or molecular alterations in type B acute lymphoblastic leukemia has been described (**Table 1**) [3–6].

T-cell ALL constitutes 25% of adult ALL cases. Characteristic T cell markers are CD1a, CD2, CD3 (membrane and cytoplasm), CD4, CD5, CD7, and CD8. CD2, CD5 and CD7 antigens are markers of immature T cells, but none of them is absolutely lineage-specific, so the unequivocal diagnosis of T-ALL is based on the demonstration of superficial / cytoplasmic CD3. In T-ALL CD10 expression is quite common (25%) but non-specific, CD34 andCD13 and / or CD33 myeloid antigens can also be expressed by these cells. The recognized T-ALL subgroups: pro-T EGIL TI (cCD3 +, CD7 +), pre-T EGIL T-II (cCD3 +, CD7 + and CD5 / CD2 +), cortical T EGIL T-III (cCD3 +, Cd1a +, sCD3 + / -) and mature-T EGIL T-IV (cCD3 +, sCD3 +, CD1a−) [3–7].

PRECURSORS	ONTOGENICS	INMUNOPHENOTYPE	MOLECULAR CYTOGENETIC
	Pro B	CD 10(-), CD 34 (++), CD 20(-), TdT(++)	t(v;11q23.3), rearrangement MLL (KMT2A), t(4;11)
CD 19 (+), CD 22 (+), CD79a(+), HLA-DR(+)	Common	CD10 (+++), CD 34(+), CD20 (-/+), Cadena μ (-), TdT (++)	t(9;22) (q34.1;q11.2)(BCR-ABL1), t(12;21)(p13.2;q22.1) (TEL-AML1/ ETV6-RUNX1); t(5;14)(q31.1;q32.3) (IL3-IGH); hiperdyploid, hipodyploid
	Pre B	CD 10(+), CD34(-), CD20(+), Cadena μ (+), TdT ++	t(5;14)(q31.1;q32.3) (IL3-IGH); hiperdyploid, hipodyploid
	Mature	CD20(+), TdT(-), CD10 (+), CD34(-), k(+) o λ(+)	rearregment of MYC, t(8;14), t(2;8), t(8;22)

Table 1.
Immunogenetic classification of B ALL.

PRECURSOR	ONTOGENICS	INMUNOPHENOTYPE	MOLECULAR/ CYTOGENETIC
	Pro T (T I)	CD2(-), CD5(-), CD8(-), CD4 (-), TdT(++), CD34(+/-)	*NOTCH 1 t (10;14) HIX 11-TCR* t (11;14) LMO/TCR NUP213 ABL1 HOX11
CD7(++), (CD3c(+), CD3m(-/+) débil	Early T	CD5(+) d,CD8(-), CD1a(-), CD2(-), TdT(+)	
	Pre T (T II)	CD2(+) y/o CD5(+) y/o CD8 (+), CD1a(-), mCD3(-)	
	Intermedia or cortical T (T III)	CD1a(+),CD34(-), CD4(+), CD8(+), CD3m(+)	
CD7(++), CD3c(+), CD3m(+)	Mature T	CD3m(+), CD1a(-), TCRαβ(+) o TCRγδ(+)	————

Table 2.
Immunogenetic classification of T cell.

The ontogenetic and immunocytogenetic correlation have particular importance due to prognostic relevance in both B-cell and T-cell lymphoid leukemia. **Table 2** shows the correlation between the different T cell-type leukemia.

3. Cytogenetic diagnosis

The karyotype alterations that could be found in ALL are numerical and structural changes as well, that have profound prognostic significance. Cytogenetics analysis represents an important step in ALL classification. The conventional karyotype can be useful in identifying recurring translocations, as well as in the identification of gain or loss of chromosomal material; However, the biggest limitation of this technique is the requirement of the cell to enter in metaphase, what is necessary for the obtaining of the material for the analysis of chromosomes. In such cases the technique of fluorescence in situ hybridization (FISH) can allow direct detection and visualization of virtually all investigated chromosomal abnormalities in ALL, with a sensitivity near of 99%, finally, comparative genomic hybridization of matrices (matrix-CGH, a-CGH) and matrices of single nucleotide polymorphisms(SNPs) can allow the identification of cryptic and/or submicroscopic changes in the genome [8, 9].

3.1 Cytogenetic/genetic risk groups

The aberrations with a good prognosis are: del(12p), t(12p) / t(12; 21) (p13; q22) t(10; 14) (q24; q11) in ALL of lineage B. These abnormalities are relatively rare in adults compared to childhood with ALL.

Aberrations associated with intermediate risk include the normal diploid subset plus cases of hyperdiploidy and various other recurrent or random chromosomal abnormalities.

Other aberrations such as isolated trisomy 21, trisomy 8, and perhaps del(6q) and t(1; 19) (q23;p13) / E2A-PBX1 may constitute an intermediate-high risk group; Recent evidence suggests that the previously poor prognosis reported for t (1, 19) (q23; p13) / E2A-PBX1 could be outweighed by some current therapeutic approaches [10, 11]. Other newly identified aberrations in the intermediate-high risk group are iAMP21 12 and IGH rearrangements, including CRLF2 [12, 13].

Finally, patients with t(9; 22) (q34; q11) or BCR-ABL1 rearrangement with positive FISH test (Philadelphia + ALL), t (4; 11) (q21; q23) or MLL rearrangements at 11q23, monosomy 7, hypodiploidy (and the closely related near triploid group) fell into the high-risk cytogenetic category, with a disease-free survival (DFS) rate of approximately 25%, or 10% in the specific case of Phi + ALL prior to introduction of tyrosine kinase inhibitors (TKI) [14, 15]. The presence of the Phi + chromosome in ALL can constitute 25–50% of CD10 + or pre-B cases and represent the most frequent alteration in adult and elderly patients, found in more than 50% of cases in the 6th decade of life [16]. Secondary chromosomal abnormalities in addition to t(9; 22) (q34; q11) may worsen the prognosis [17] however this has not yet been proven in the TKI era [18]. Currently the most group with the most unfavorable prognosis among cases with known genetic / molecular aberration is represented by t(4; 11) (q21; q23) with MLL1 rearrangement unless an allogeneic hematopoietic stem cell transplantation is performed [19].

Some other karyotypes alterations are exclusive to specific ALL syndromes. Translocations involving chromosome 8 (MYC gene), as well as t (8; 14) (q24; q32) (90% of cases), t (8; 22) (q24; q11) (10% of cases) and t (2;8) (rarely observed) are practically present in 100% of cases of mature B-ALL with L3 / Burkitt morphology and immunoglobulins in the clonal surface. Typical cytogenetic aberrations are also found in the T lineage, the most frequent involve resection points of 14q11, for example, t (10; 14) (q24; q11), t (11; 14) (p13; q11) and others, the presence of t (8; 14) with resection points at q24; q11 (q24; q32 in line B ALL) in T cell ALL is associated with aggressive lymphomatous presentation [20–22].

An interruption in IKZF1 encoding the Ikaros transcription factor has been frequently observed in ALL with BCR / ABL rearrangement (80% of cases). The IKZF1 mutation predicts poor outcome in the treatment of ALL, Phi+ or not [13, 23–25].

By integrating genome-wide technologies the "BCR / ABL-like" subgroup has been suggested and identified in adult and child populations [26, 27] and represents approximately 15% of ALL ontogeny B cases. This subgroup It is characterized by a gene expression that is similar to that of BCR/ABL + patients, with frequent detection of the IKZF1 mutation and CRLF2 rearrangements but with where abysmal differences in the outcomes. Other mutations and / or rearrangements that activate tyrosine kinases has also been revealed as poor prognosis factor such as rearrangement of IGH-CRLF2, NUP214-ABL1, EBD1-PDGRB, BCR-JAK2 fusions and STRN3 JAK2, which have been associated with a very poor prognosis [28].

Hypodiploid ALL, considered a high risk factor has been extensively evaluated in pediatric ALL [29] Alterations involving tyrosine kinase receptors and RAS gene signaling (i.e., NRAS, KRAS, FLT3, and NF1) can be detected in up to 70% of haploid cases, while hypodiploid cases are characterized by lesions involving members of the Ikaros family, particularly IKZF2 and by TP53 interruptions which can be identified in 91.2% of these. In adult ALL, these cases are characterized by non-random chromosome loss and CDKN2A / B with locus deletion as the only recurrent abnormality; As previously reported, in children these cases often harbor TP53 mutations [30].

The TP53 mutation is detected in 6.4% of all ALL cases and a correlation with a worse result has been demonstrated. In adults, TP53 mutations are identified at diagnosis in 8.2% of cases (11.1% of T-ALL and 6.4% of B-ALL), and are preferably identified without molecular aberrations and are associated with refractoriness to chemotherapy [31, 32].

In T cell-ALL, well-recognized aberrations are: Rearrangement of the T-cell receptor (TCR) gene, chromosomal deletions and focal gene deletions, in addition, chromosomal rearrangements can also lead to fusion genes in the framework of Chimeric proteins with oncogenic properties such as thePICALM-MLLT10, NUP214-ABL1 fusion for medin episomes, EML-ABL1, theSET-NUP214 fusion and MLL-type genetic rearrangements have uncertain significance [33, 34].

Cytogenetic alterations	Gene	Frequency in adults	Frequency in children
Hypodiploidy (>50 chromosomes)	–	7%	25%
Hypodiploidy (<44 chromosomes)	–	2%	15
t(9;22) (q34;q11):Philadelphia chromosome(Ph+)	BCR-ABL1	25%	2-4%
t(12,21) (p13;q22)	ETV6-RUNX1 (TEL-AML1)	2%	22%
t(v;11q23), t(4;11), t(11;19)	KMT2A	10%	8%
t(1;19) (q23;p13)	TCF3-PBX1 (E2A-PBX1)	3%	6%
t(5;14) (q31;q32)	IL3-IGH	< 15	<1%
t(8;14), t(2;8), t(8;22)	c-MYC	4%	2%
t(1;14)	TAL-1	12%	7%
t(10;14) (q24;q11)	HOX11 (TLX1)	8%	15
t(5;14) (q35;q32)	HOX11L2	1%	35
t(11;14) (q11)(p13;q11) (p15;q11)	TCR y TCR	20-25%	10-20%
BCR-abl1-like/Ph-like	Multiple	10-30%	15%
LLA-B con iAMP21	RUNX11	–	2%
ETP	Multiple	2%	25%
Ikaros	IKZF1	25-35%	12-17%

Table 3.
Frequency of Chromosomic and molecular alterations by age group.

A large set of mutations in T cell-line ALL has been identified by sequencing techniques including NOTCH1, FBW7, BCL11B, JAK1, PTPN2, IL7R and PHF6, some of them have recognized prognostic importance, while others require further investigation. In fact, NOTCH1 and / or FBW7 mutations that occur in more than 60% and around 20% of cases, respectively, are generally associated with a favorable outcome. A new prognostic model has been recently proposed defining as low risk those with NOTCH1 and FBW7 mutations and those with lesions involving RAS/PTEN as high-risk. JAK1 mutations, which increase JAK activity and impair

Risk	Cytogenetic alterations
Good	• Hypodiploidy (51-65 chromosomes) • Cases with trisomy 4,10 y 17 more favorable results • t(12;21) (p13;q22):ETV6-EUNX1[a]
Poor	• Hypodiploidy • KMT2A, t(4;11) • t(v;14q32)/IgH • t(8;22)(q34;q11.2):BCR-ABL1 • Complex karyotype (5 o more abnormalities) • Ph-like ALL intrachromosomal amplification 21(iAMP21)

Table 4.
Cytogenetic risk groups.

B-lymphoblastic leukemia/lymphoma
B-lymphoblastic leukemia/lymphoma, NOS
B-lymphoblastic leukemia/lymphoma with recurrent genetic abnormalities
B-lymphoblastic leukemia/lymphoma with t(9;22)(q34.1;q11.2);BCR-ABL1
B-lymphoblastic leukemia/lymphoma with t(v;11q23.3);KMT2A rearranged
B-lymphoblastic leukemia/lymphoma with t(12;21)(p13.2;q22.1);ETV6-RUNX1
B-lymphoblastic leukemia/lymphoma with hyperdiploidy
B-lymphoblastic leukemia/lymphoma with hypodiploidy
B-lymphoblastic leukemia/lymphoma with t(5;14)(q31.1;q32.3) IL3-IGH
B-lymphoblastic leukemia/lymphoma with t(1;19)(q23;p13.3);TCF3-PBX1
Provisional entity: B-lymphoblastic leukemia/lymphoma, BCR-ABL1–like
Provisional entity: B-lymphoblastic leukemia/lymphoma with iAMP21
T-lymphoblastic leukemia/lymphoma
Provisional entity: Early T-cell precursor lymphoblastic leukemia
Provisional entity: Natural killer (NK) cell lymphoblastic leukemia/lymphoma
Modified of D´Angelo, 2006 [37].

Table 5.
WHO classification of lymphoblastic leukemia.

proliferation and survival, have been associated with refractoriness of chemotherapy and should be considered as poor prognosis markers [35, 36].

Recurrent chromosomal and molecular abnormalities characterize ALL subtypes in adults and children (**Table 3**) and often provide prognostic information that can influence risk stratification and treatment decisions (**Table 4**). The frequency of certain subtypes differs between adult and child ALL, what partially explains the difference in clinical outcomes between patient populations [6, 30, 34, 36].

The most recent classification of the World Health Organization (WHO) for acute lymphoblastic leukemia ins shown in **Table 5**.

4. Treatment

The evolution in treatment of patients with ALL has progressed over time, this in order to achieve better survival, relapse-free rates and the quest to achieve cure. We will divide this issue into two large groups: AYA group (adolescents and young adults) and the group of people over 40 years old; and subdivided focusing on status of Philadelphia chromosome (positive and negative).

Chemotherapy treatment is divided into treatment phases with different goals: [38, 39].

Induction: it is the phase that seeks to achieve remission normalizing the parameters of the blood count (Hb >10 gr/dl, Neutrophils >1000 /mm3, platelets >100,000/mm3) as well normalization of the organs affected by diagnosis (liver, kidney, lung).

Consolidation: in this phase, the aim is to keep the patient in remission and achieve a negative minimal residual disease (MRD) that will impact the prognosis.

Maintenance: this phase seeks to avoid relapse of the disease and prepare for an elective suspension [38–40].

5. Treatment of the AYA group

This group is considered as a "superimposed" population since pediatric schemes have improved their degrees of response compared to adult designed schemes. Initially, the treatment regimens in this group of patients were based on regimens for adults, showing complete remissions in a low percentage, a couple of examples are the UKALLXII/ECOG [41] case study that reported complete remission (CR) nearly 51% after 1 chemotherapy cycle with increase to 91% after 2 induction cycles and the CALGB8811 [42] study that reported RC of 62–86% after 1 and 2 cycles of induction to remission respectively; On the other hand, the LALA-94 [43] study reported CR rate of 72% after one treatment cycle up to 84% after 2 treatment cycles, thus we have to mention the Hyper-CVAD scheme with a CR rate in the first cycle reported in 81% with increase after 2 cycles to 92% [44]; the DFCI45 pilot study showed an RC of 82% in the first induction cycle. Due to the above, it's clear that treatment schemes based on adults' schemes are ineffective to achieve CR, for these reasons the AYA Group was separated looking for different treatment schemes which includes two large groups, those based on pediatric schemes with expansion in the group of age and modified pediatric inspiration schemes (**Tables 6** and 7).

By reviewing the pediatric regimens with extension to the age group of treatment was possible to increase the degree of response in this group classified as AYA; in adult regimens, complete remissions ranging from 51% to a maximum of 82% were reported after 1 cycle of treatment, however, in **Table 1** we observe that pediatric regimens in general achieved a higher percentage of complete response or remission after applying 1 cycle of induction, showing with the highest degree of complete response in 98% of the cases for the studies: TOTAL TERAPY IV, 46 PETHEMA ALL 96.47 DCOG, 58 ALL97.59, however, it should be noted that the study with greater robustness in this group that showed the highest CR is the

Studies	Number of cases	Age (rank)	% CR	DFS (years/%)	OS (years/%)	Ref.
CCG 1961	262	16-21	95	5/72	5/78	[38]
DFCI9101/9501	51	15-18	94	5/78	5/81	[40]
UKALL 2003	229	16-24	97	5/72	5/76	[39]
TOTAL TERAPY XV	45	15-81	98	5/86	5/88	[45]
PETHEMA ALL 96	81	15-30	98	6/61	6/69	[46]
HOVON (FRALLE 93)	54	17-40	91	2/66	2/72	[47]
NOPHO 2008	221	18-45	NR	5/74	5/78	[48]
FRALL 2000	186	15-19	96	5/74	5/80	[49]
INTERGROUPC10403	296	17-39	NR	2/66	2/79	[50]
FRALLE93	77	15-20	94	5/67	NR	[51]
DCOG	47	15-18	98	5/69	5/79	[52]
ALL97	61	15-17	98	5/65	NR	[53]
AIEOP	150	14-18	94	5/67	5/67	[54]

CR: Complete Remission, Ref. Reference, DFS: Disease Free Survival, OS: Overall Survival, NR: Not Reported.

Table 6.
No comparative studies of pediatric regimens.

Studies	Number of cases	Age (rank)	% CR	DFS (years/%)	OS (years/%)	Ref.
DFCI 01-175	74	18-50	86	4/58	4/67	[55]
MODIFIED DFCI 91-01	42	18-35	98	3/77	3/83	[56]
GRAALL2003/2005	502	15-35	95	5/59	5/65	[57]
GMALL 07/03	887	15-35	91	5/61	5/65	[58]
MODIFIED TPOG	35	15-39	89	2/47	2/50	[59]
LALIN	20	15-25	90	5/70	NR	[60]
NOPHO-92	144	10-14	99	5/65	NR	[61]

CR: Complete Remission, Ref. Reference, DFS: Disease Free Survival, OS: Overall Survival, NR: Not Reported.

Table 7.
Pediatric inspired schemes.

Studies	Number of cases	Age (rank)	% CR	DFS (years/%)	OS (years/%)	Ref.
Hyper-CVAD	185	>60	91	5/39%	5/10	[62]
SMOG 8419	85	50-84	41	5/32	5/<10	[63]
GIMEMA 0288	778	12-59	82	2/50	9/27	[64]
CALGB	280 350 129	<30 30-59 >60	90 81 57	3/47 3/38 3/18	3/58 3/38 3/18	[65]
PETHEMA ALL96	33	56-67	58	2/39	2/46	[66]
MRC UKALLXII/ECOG2993	100	55-64	70	5/19	5/21	[67]
GMALL	268	55-85	76	NR	5/23	[68]
HOSPITAL EDOUARD HERRIOT, LYON	195 118 66	<35 35-60 >60	84 85 58	3/35 3/31 3/11	3/39 3/34 3/11	[69]
MD ANDERSON, HOUSTON	65 64 31 44	<30 30-49 50-59 >60	98 89 93 79	3/53 3/55 3/34 3/36	5/54 5/42 5/29 5/17	[70]
ALL-07FRAIL	72	57-89	54	6.9 month	7.6 month	[71]

CR: Complete Remission, Ref. Reference, DFS: Disease Free Survival, OS: Overall Survival, NR: Not Reported.

Table 8.
Treatment schemes for ALL in adults.

PETHEMA ALL 96.47 study, which shows a reported follow-up at 5 years with evidence of DFS of 61% OS of 69% at 6 years. On the other hand, it is important to mention that the Intergroup C1040351 study observed a 2-year DFS of 66% and an OS of 79%. In all the groups referred to in **Table 8**, the degree of CR registered was greater than 90%, but with different DFS and OS times, the longest DFS time for the DCOG study, which was 69% at 5 years and OS of 79% at 5 years.

Of the pediatric inspiration schemes, we refer to those registered in **Table 9**, all of them report CR greater than 90%, with the exception of studies DFCI01–17552 and MODIFIED TPOG 56 where the lowest degree of CR of 86 and 89%,

Studies	Number of cases	Age (rank)	% CR	DFS (years/%)	OS (years/%)	Ref.
GMALL (Imatinib)	28	54-79	96	2/19	2/42	[72]
PETHEMA ALLOPH07 (Imatinib)	53	56-88	87	38months	37.3 months	[73]
HyperCVAD + Imatinib	54	17-84	93	5/43	5/35	[74]
GIMEMA LAL0201-B (Imatinib)	29	61-83	100	1/48	1/74	[75]
EWAL-PH-01 (Dasatinib)	71	59-83	96	5/27	5/36	[76]
GIMEMA LAL1205 (Dasatinib)	53	18-77	100	2/51	2/69	[77]
HyperCVAD plus Dasatinib.	72	21-80	96	5/42	5/52	[78]
EWALL-PH-02 Nilotinib	65	55-85	87	NR	NR	[79]
Korean study Nilotinib	90	17-77	91	2/72	2/72	[80]
HyperCVAD + Ponatinib	37	27-55	100	2/81	2/80	[81]
GIMEMA + Ponatinib	42	27-85	91	3/69	3/83	[82]

CR: Complete Remission, Ref. Reference, DFS: Disease Free Survival, OS: Overall Survival, NR: Not Reported.

Table 9.
ALL Phi positive treatment.

respectively, is recorded. Likewise, the DFS reported in the MODIFIED TPOG group is lower, being 47% of the cases at 2 years. In this same table we observe the two studies with the largest number of patients, the GRAALL2003 / 200,554 study with a number of subjects analyzed of 502 cases and for the GAMALL55 study 887 cases, with a similarity in the DFS reported for the GRAALL2003 / 2005 of 59% at 5 years and for GMALL07 / 03 from 61% at 5 years and similar OS in both groups from 65% at 5 years; the aforementioned has generated improvement in responses and survival in the AYA groups, so the current recommendations are aimed at treating pediatric schemes or modified schemes of pediatric-inspired protocols.

Those patients over 40 years old are considered as "adults" an represent totally different group when comparing with the pediatric and AYA groups when talking about prognosis and treatment. The age by itself is a conditioning factor for a lower response rate, lower DFS, and poorer OS compared to the AYA group, this data is summarized in **Table 8**. This group have hematological remission variable and those with lesser degree of Response rate are adults over 65 years, with a percentage of CR ranging from 41 to 60% according to the ALL-07FRAIL72 studies and the SMOG 841964 study. As illustrated in **Table 3**, in the Edouard Herriot Lyon Hospital, the population of 35–60 years old reached a CR of 85% but this was lower in the group over 60 years with CR reported in 58% [69]; as well as the study of the MD Anderson with the HyperCVAD [62] scheme where the age groups of 30 to 49 years, 50 to 59 years and over 60 years reached a CR of 98%, 83%, 79% respectively [70]. In the same way, the DFS and OS for the Hyper CVAD group of the GIMEMA study 028865 was lower in the older groups, 39% at 5 years and an OS with a longer duration of 27% at 9, in general we conclude that the older age could be related to lower rate of CR, DFS and OS.

All those previously described have been mainly in the groups cataloged as Phi negative ALL, as they are not carriers of the BCR / ABL oncogene, however, in the group that is a carrier of these genetic alteration treatment will be describe in

Table 9, where the different percentages of response between these and those Phi negatives are observed.

In the GMALL73 study the benefit of adding a tyrosine kinase inhibitor (TKI) to non-intensive regimens in elderly patients was initially observed. In this study a group was randomized to receive chemotherapy (CT) + TKI vs. CT, and was observed that adding an TKI achieved a CR of 96%, the double from the RC of 50% seeing in patients who were not treated with imatinib. In this patient group it is striking that adding TKI to a conventional chemotherapy scheme offers the benefit of even higher CR than those presented in populations older than 40 years, as reported in the studies of the Italian group (GIMEMA, LAL0201-B and GIMEMA LAL1205) [75, 77]with CR of 100% with 1st and 2nd generation inhibitor of TKI, however, the DFS and OS were brief in both groups, being higher in the group that received dasatinib (2nd generation TKI) as induction therapy and with a younger population that predicts the higher degree of response. It is worth mentioning that the second-generation TKI dasatinib has Central Nervous System (CNS) penetration showing improved response and survival of cases with CNS infiltration compared to imatinib that fails to cross the blood–brain barrier. **Table 4** records the treatment given by the MD Anderson group, which showed that adding a 3rd generation TKI as ponatinib to the HyperCVAD scheme achieved 100% CR in the group aged 27 to 55 with DFS and OS at 2 years of 81 and 80% respectively [81]. It should be mentioned that ponatinib has good CNS penetration as does dasatinib, however ponatinib is indicated in patients with the T315I resistance mutation.

A meta-analysis of 15 studies with a total of 11,040 patients with ALL Phi positive shown that the highest prevalence of Phi positive is seeing in those between 11 and 40 years old (25.8% to 26.2%.) By age subgroup the reported prevalence was: 1–10 years 15.6%, 10–20 years 25.6%, 21–40 years of age 26.2% and in the group over 40 years of age 16.9%. In this meta-analysis, the overall 5-year survival rate was 42.8% (CI 95% CI, 23.9–64.1, I2 93) [83].

6. Prophylaxis to CNS

Intrathecal chemotherapy is pivotal in the treatment of ALL since the CNS is a site of relevance in this pathology. In adult ALL involvement of the CNS at diagnosis is reported in 5–7% of cases, mainly with meningeal involvement. The risk factors related to initial infiltration are elevated Lactic Dehydrogenase (LDH), hyperleukocytosis and ALL B subtype at diagnosis, the latter showing CNS involvement in up to 18% of cases. Other factors that contribute to the initial infiltration are increased blast replication rate, mediastinal mass, and positive Phi [84]. These same factors contribute to the early relapse of the disease, systemically or in isolation to the CNS. For the diagnosis of infiltration, the microscopic examination of cerebrospinal fluid (CSF) obtained from a lumbar puncture continues to be the standard and classified the cases into risk groups according to the number of leukocytes, and the presence of blasts (**Table 10**) and the nature of the lumbar puncture, as well as determination by flow cytometry.

Traumatic Lumbar puncture (TLP) is defined as a result of CSF with erythrocyte count>10 /uL. The Stevenherz/Bleyer algorithm evaluates traumatic puncture if the patient has leukemic cells in peripheral blood and the lumbar puncture is traumatic and contains >5 leukocytes/uL and blasts, the following algorithm should be followed to distinguish between CNS2 disease and CNS3: CSF leukocytes/ erythrocytes >2 x leukocytes in blood/red blood cells [84, 85].

Effective prophylaxis to prevent CNS relapse is an essential part of ALL regimens, the most used modalities are based on CNS irradiation, intrathecal

Classification	Lymphoblasts in CSF	Leucocytes in CSF
SNC 1	None	
SNC 2	Present	<5
SNC 3	Present	≥5
TLP	Present	Variable

CSF, cerebrospinal fluid; CNS, central nervous system; traumatic lumbar puncture (TLP).

Table 10.
Classification of the CNS infiltration according to the CSF characteristics.

chemotherapy with a single drug or with steroid-based triplet plus cytarabine and methotrexate at same time as systemic CT is being administrated. With these measures the relapse rate can be reduced from 10 to 5%. Irradiation as a single dose of 24 Gy is recommended as unique therapy to the skull without involving the neuroaxis to avoid cytopenia associated with concurrent CT [86]. In cases of ALL Phi +, although dasatinib and ponatinib are not part of prophylaxis therapy these have been shown to cross the blood–brain barrier and secondarily reduced the risk of isolated relapse to the CNS [87, 88].

7. Hematopoietic stem cell transplant

Hematopoietic stem cell transplant (HSCT) in patients with Acute Lymphoblastic Leukemia is a therapeutic option in those with high risk disease that have reached complete response (CR) and those who are candidates by the Predictive Models of Risk (Disease Risk Index (DRI), EBMT Risk Score, HCT-Comorbidity Index). the patients could be classified in 3 different risk groups (0 points = low risk, 1–2 points = intermediate risk, ≥ 3 = high risk) and this correlated with two years NRM (non relapse mortality (**Table 11**) [90–93].

The modality of transplant recommended is allogenic after the first complete response (CR1) in high-risk patients (**Table 12**) and in patients with second complete response (CR2) [90].

Autologous HSCT is not recommended for an adult with ALL. It could be possible in high-risk patients with negative minimal residual disease (MRD) that are not considered for allo-HSCT, but there is insufficient data to support this option, including Phi + ALL [91].

7.1 Indication for the different modalities of allo-HSCT

It is preferred a matched sibling donor or an unrelated donor very well matched, these options are considered equivalent in terms of results [91, 92].

Haploidentical transplant is always an option in patients without a matched donor, this type of transplant is nowadays frequently used because it allows almost all patients in need for an allo-SCT to undergo allo-SCT without a matched-donor [96].

7.2 Conditioning

The choice of conditioning is based on the patient's physical status, for those fit without relevant comorbidity the recommended regimens are the combination of fractionated TBI (Total Body Irradiation) 12Gy in 6 fractions, plus

Comorbidity	Points	Comorbidity	Points
Liver disease Liver cirrhosis, bilirubin >1.5xULN, or AST/ALT >2.5xULN	3	Obesity BMI of > 35 for adults	1
Severe pulmonary DLco and/or FEV1 ≤ 65%, dyspnea at rest oroxygen at home	3	Hepatic Mild Chronic hepatitis, bilirubin>ULN to 1.5x ULN, or AST/ALT >ULN to 2.5x ULN	1
Previoussolid malignancy Treated at any time point in thepatient'shistory, excluding nonmelanoma skin cancer	3	Psychiatric disturbance Depression/anxiety requiring psychiatric consult and/or treatment at the time of HCT	1
Heart valve disease Diagnosed (except mitral prolapse)	3	Cerebrovascular Disease Transient ischemic attacks or cerebrovascular accident	1
Moderate pulmonary DLco and/or FEV1 66–80% or minimal stress dyspnea	2	Diabetes Requiring treatment with insulin or oral hypoglycemic	1
Renal Creatinine >2mg/dl, dialysis, or previous kidney transplant	2	Inflammatory bowel disease Crohn's disease or ulcerative colitis	1
Rheumatologic SLE, RA, polymyositis, mixed CTD, and polymyalgia rheumatica	2	Coronary artery disease congestive heart failure, myocardial infarction, or EF of ≤ 50%	1
Peptic ulcer Requiring treatment	2	Arrhytmia Atrial fibrillation or flutter, sick sinus syndrome, or ventricular arrhythmias	1
Previous infection Documented infection or fever of unknown etiology requiring antimicrobial treatment before, during and after the start of conditioning regimen	1	Age ≥ 40	1

EF = ejection fraction; ULN= upper limit of normal, AST = aspartate aminotransferase, ALT = alanine aminotransferase, BMI=body mass index, SLE = systemic lupus erythematosus, RA= rheumatoid arthritis, CTD = connective tissue disease, Dlco = diffusion capacity of carbon monoxide, FEV1=forced expiratory volume in one second.

Table 11.
HCT-Comorbidity Index [89].

Cyclophosphamide (Cy) 120 mg/kg or Etoposide (VP) 60 mg/kg. The regimens with TBI seem to have better anti-leukemic activity than busulfan-based regimens [97].

For elderly patients should be considered reduced conditioning regimens as for patients with contraindications for myeloablative regimens [92].

For patients with an haploidentical donor the used scheme is: Cy 14.5 mg/kg/day IV on days −6 and − 5, fludarabine 30 mg/m^2/day IV on days −6 to −2, and 200 cGy of TBI on day −1, on days +3 and + 4, 50 mg/kg Cy with Mesna [98, 99].

Other regimens for transplant with haploidentical donor recommended by the Acute Leukemia Working Party of EMBT are: 1) Myeloablative regimen TBF (thiotepa 10 mg/kg, fludarabine 150 mg/m2, busulfan 9.6 mg/kg IV. 2) RIC (reduced-intensity chemotherapy) Thiotepa 5 mg/kg and busulfan 6.4 mg/kg. ATG and Cyclophosphamide are used as prophylaxis for Graft versus Host Disease (GVHD) at doses of ATG 10 mg/Kg (total dose), or Cy 50 mg/kg +3 and + 4 [96].

High Risk	
Cytogenetics	Hypodiploidy (< 44 chromosomes) t(9:22) (q34;q11.2):BCR-ABL1 Complex karyotype (5 or more chromosomal abnormalities) t(4;11) (q21;q23) t(8;14) (q24.1q32)
Age	>40 years
High WBC count at diagnosis	>30 x 10^9 in B-ALL >100 x 10^9 in T-ALL
ALL subtypes	T-cell precursor ALL
High-risk genetics	IKZF1 deletion in B precursor ALL, unmutated NOTCH1, Ph-like.
MRD	>1X10^{-4} after two courses of therapy, some groups post-induction.
CNS disease	Central Nervous System involvement
Immunophenotype	Pro-B/early and mature-T
Time to CR	>1 cycle

Table 12.
High Risk Patients [91, 92, 94, 95].

7.3 Maintenance post allo-HSCT

It is recommended for patients with Ph +, maintenance with TKI after allo-HSCT. The optimal treatment duration has not been defined. The described options are continuing the treatment until MRD negativity is confirmed by three consecutive tests or sustained for at least three months, or TKI administration for at least one year of continuous PCR negativity, and if a single positive result, then reset the treatment period [100].

7.4 Status of minimal residual disease before HSCT

It is demonstrated that the presence of MRD positivity at the time of HSCT is a significant risk for relapse after the procedure; this asseveration applies for both B-ALL and T-ALL and suggests that novel therapies are a new option to improve the outcome [101–103].

8. Novel Therapies

8.1 Blinatumomab

It is a bispecific T-cell engager antibody construct that binds simultaneously to CD3-positive cytotoxic T cells and CD19-positive B cells, this reaction allows the patient's endogenous T cells to recognize and eliminate CD19-positive ALL blasts.

It is indicated for the treatment of B- ALL in the first or second complete remission with MRD >/= 0.1% and in B-ALL relapse or refractory in adults and children.

In the TOWER study, eligible patients with pretreated B-ALL were randomly assigned to receive Blinatumomab or Standard Chemotherapy. The overall survival was significantly better in patients treated with Blinatumomab compared with those of the standard group. The median OS was 7.7 months (95% confidence interval [CI], 5.6 to 9.6) in the blinatumomab group versus 4.0 months (95% CI, 2.9

to 5.3) in the chemotherapy group (hazard ratio for death, 0.71; 95% CI, 0.55 to 0.93; p = 0.01 [104].

8.2 Inotuzumab ozogamicin (InO)

It is a humanized anti-CD22 monoclonal antibody conjugated to calicheamicin, a potent cytotoxic antibiotic compound that induces double-strand DNA breaks. It is utilized in patients with relapsed or refractory (R/R) B-ALL [105].

Katarjian H. and cols published a phase 3 trial (INO-VATE ALL) where randomly assigned adults with R/R ALL to receive either inotuzumab ozogamicin or standard intensive chemotherapy. The rate of complete remission was 80.7% in the inotuzumab ozogamicin group than in the standard therapy group, 29.4% $p < 0.001$. In the survival analysis OS of 5.0 months vs. 1.8 months (HR0.45 [97.5% CI, 0.34 to 0.6)]; $p < 0.001$. The veno-occlusive disease occurred more frequently in the InO group [106].

8.3 Tisagenlecleucel

It is a CD19-directed, genetically modified, autologous T-cell immunotherapy. It is prepared from an apheresis collection of the patient's peripheral blood mononuclear cells. The autologous T cells are transduced using a lentiviral vector to express an anti-CD19 chimeric antigen receptor (CAR) [107]. Tisagenlecleucel was the first gene-modified cell therapy approved by the FDA for children and young adults with relapsed or refractory B-cell ALL.

These have proven highly efficient at inducing MRD-negative remissions. A CAR induced remission could offer a window to proceed to allo- HSCT [107, 108].

Maude and cols published this trial of tisagenlecleucel in children with R/R B-ALL, the overall remission rate was 81%. All patients with complete remission were negative for MRD. The rate of relapse-free survival in patients with a response to treatment was 80% at 6 months and 59% at 12 months. Neurologic events occurred in 40% [108].

9. Minimal residual disease (MRD)

In the last decade, the measurement of minimal residual disease has become a necessary tool in the follow-up of patients since its impact on progression-free survival and overall survival has been demonstrated in multiple studies, that leads it to be currently an indicator of treatment for patients with acute leukemia.

There are several ways of measurement of MRD and each one presents different sensitivity as describe: New Generation Sequencing (NGS) present a sensitivity of 10^6; Flow cytometry with a 10^4 sensitivity for cytometers of 6 colors and 10^6 for cytometers of 8 colors or more; PCR for specific genes 10^5 of sensitivity. However, to achieve these sensitivity results, it is necessary to perform them on bone marrow samples considered in morphological remission [89, 109].

We have already discussed the prognostic value of having a negative MRD. The GRAALL group demonstrated that the presence of negative MRD at the end of induction was a better prognostic marker than the conventional ones, like the achievement of CR at first line therapy a transplantation in patients with pediatric schemes [109, 110].

In a meta-analysis published in 2017, including 13,637 patients in total, the progression-free survival for the pediatric group was 77% at 10 years in patients with negative MRD, and 64% for adults, while progression free survival for patients with positive MRD were 32% and 21% respectively [111].

Author details

Martha Alvarado-Ibarra*, José Antonio De la Peña Celaya, Luara Luz Arana-Luna, Eleazar Hernández-Ruiz, José Luis Alvarez Vera, María Eugenia Espitia Ríos and Juan Manuel Pérez Zúñiga
Servicio de Hematología Centro Médico Nacional 20 de Noviembre, ISSSTE Ciudad de México, Mexico

*Address all correspondence to: normoblasto@gmail.com

References

[1] Coustan-Smith E, Behm FG, Sánchez J, Boyett J, Hancock M, Raimondi S. Immunological detection of minimal residual disease in children with acute lymphoblastic leukemia. Lancet.1998; 351:550–554.

[2] Janossy G, Coustan-Smith E, Campana D. The reliability of citoplasmic CD3+ and CD22+ antigen expression in the immunodiagnosis of acute leukemia: a study of 500 cases. Leukemia. 1989; 3:170–181.

[3] Mirji G, Bhat J, Kode J, Benavalli S, Sangar M." Genetic and clinical characterization of KMT2A fusion partner genes in 13 cases of pediatric leukemia with complexo r cryptic karyotypes." Leu Res.2016;45:33–39

[4] Moorman, Anthony V. "New and emerging prognostic and predictive genetic biomerkers in B-cell presursor acute lymphoblastic leukemia. Leu Res. 2016; 45:407–416

[5] Aber D, Orazi A, Hasserjian R et al. The 2016 revision of the World Health Organization classification of myeloid neoplasms and acute leukemia. Blood 2016;127: 2391–2405.

[6] NCCN Clinical Practice Guidelines in Oncology (NCCN Guidelines®) Acute Lymphoblastic Leukemia Version 1.20 NCCN.org.

[7] Weinberg, O. K., and Arber, D. B. "Mixed-phenotype acute leukemia: Historical overview and a new definition." Leukemia 24.11 (2010): 1844–1851

[8] Pui CH, Crist WM, A T Look. Biology and clinical significance of cytogenetic abnormalities in childhood acute lymphoblastic leukemia. Blood.1990;76: 1449–1463.

[9] Kolomietz E, Al-Maghrabi J, Brennan S, et al. Primary chromosomal rearrangements of leukemia are frequently accompanied by extensive submicroscopic deletions and may lead to altered prognosis. Blood. 2001; 97: 3581–3588. doi: 10.1182 / Blood. V97.11.3581.

[10] Felice MS, Gallego MS, Alonso CN, et al.Prognostic impact of t(1;19)/ TCF3-PBX1 in childhood acute lymphoblastic leukemia in the context of Berlin-Frankfurt-Münster-based protocols. Leukemia Lymphoma. 2011; 52:1215–1221.

[11] Burmeister T, Gökbuget N, Schwartz S, Fischer L, Hubert D, Sindram A, Hoelzer D, Thiel E. Clinical features and prognostic implications of TCF3-PBX1 and ETV6-RUNX1 in adult acute lymphoblastic leukemia. Haematologica. 2010;95:241–246.

[12] Harrison CJ, Moorman AV, Schwab C, y col. An international study of intrachromosomal amplification of chromosome 21 (iAMP21): cytogenetic characterization and outcome. Leukemia. 2014;28 :1015–1021.

[13] Moorman AV, Schwab C, Ensor HM, et al. IGH@ translocations, CRLF2 deregulation, and microdeletions in adolescents and adults with acute lymphoblastic leukemia. J Clin Oncol. 2012;30:3100–3108.

[14] Schardt C, Ottmann OG, Hoelzer D, Ganser A. Acute lymphoblastic leukemia with the (4;11) translocation: combined cytogenetic, immunological and molecular genetic analyses . Leukemia. 1992;6:370–374

[15] Gleissner B, Gökbuget N, Bartram CR, et al. Leading prognostic relevance of the BCR-ABL translocation in adult acute B- lineage lymphoblastic leukemia: a prospective study of the German Multicenter Trial Group and

confirmed polymerase chain reaction analysis. Blood. 2002;99:1536–1543.

[16] Chiaretti S, Vitale A, Cazzaniga G, et al.Clinico-biological features of 5202 patients with acute lymphoblastic leukemia enrolled in the Italian AIEOP and GIMEMA protocols and stratified in age cohorts. Haematologica. 2013; 98: 1702–1710.

[17] Rieder H, Ludwig WD, Gassmann W, et al. Prognostic significance of additional chromosome abnormalities in adult patients with Philadelphia chromosome positive acute lymphoblastic leukaemia. BrJ Haematol. 1996;95: 678–691.

[18] Ravandi F, Jorgensen JL, Thomas DA, et al. Detection of MRD may predict the outcome of patients with Philadelphia chromosome-positive ALL treated with tyrosine kinase inhibitors plus chemotherapy. Blood. 2013; 122 : 1214–1221.

[19] Marks DI, Moorman AV, Chilton L, et al.The clinical characteristics, therapy and outcome of 85 adults with acute lymphoblastic leukemia and t(4;11)(q21;q23)/MLL-AFF1 prospectively treated in the UKALLXII/ECOG2993 trial. Hematologica. 2013; 98: 945–952.

[20] Schneider NR, Carroll AJ, Shuster JJ, y col. New recurring cytogenetic abnormalities and association of blast cell karyotypes with prognosis in childhood T-cell acute lymphoblastic leukemia: a pediatric oncology group report of 343 cases. Blood. 2000; 96: 2543–2549.

[21] Lange BJ, Raimondi SC, Heerema N, et al. Pediatric leukemia/lymphoma with t(8;14)(q24;q11). Leukemia. 1992; 6:613–618.

[22] Parolini M, Mecucci C, Matteucci C, y col. Highly aggressive T-cell acute lymphoblastic leukemia with t(8;14)(q24;q11):extensive genetic characterization and achievement of early molecular remission and long-term survival in an adult patient. Blood Cancer J. 2014;4: e176.

[23] Martinelli G, Iacobucci I, Storlazzi CT, et al. IKZF1 (Ikaros) deletions in BCR-ABL1-positive acute lymphoblastic leukemia are associated with short disease-free survival and high rate of cumulative incidence of relapse:a GIMEMA AL WP report. J Clin Oncol. 2009; 27: 5202–5207.

[24] Van der Veer A, Zaliova M, Mottadelli F, et al. IKZF1 status as a prognostic feature in BCR-ABL1-positive childhood ALL. Blood.2014;123: 1691–8.

[25] Kuiper RP, Waanders E, van der Velden VH, y col.IKZF1 deletions predict relapse in uniformly treated pediatric precursor B- ALL. Leukemia. 2010; 24:1258–1264.

[26] Haferlach T, Kohlmann A, Schnittger S, et al. Global approach to the diagnosis of leukemia using gene expression profiling. Blood. 2005;106: 1189–1198.

[27] Chiaretti S, Li X, Gentleman R, et al. Gene expression profiles of B-lineage adult acute lymphocytic leukemia reveal genetic patterns that identify lineage derivation and distinct mechanisms of transformation. Clin Cancer Res. 2005; 11:7209–7219.

[28] Roberts KG, Morin RD, Zhang J, et al. Genetic alterations activating kinase and cytokine receptor signaling in high-risk acute lymphoblastic leukemia. Cancer Cell.2012;22:153–166.

[29] Holmfeldt L, Wei L, Díaz-Flores E, et al. The genomic landscape of hypodiploid acute lymphoblastic leukemia. Nat Genet. 2013; 45:242–252.

[30] Muhlbacher V, Zenger M, Schnittger S, et al. Acute Lymphoblastic

leukemia with low hypodiploid/near triploid karyitipe is a specific clinical entity and exhibits a very high TP53 mutation frequency of 93%. Genes Chromosomes and Cancer. 2014; 53: 524–536.

[31] Hof J, Krentz S, Van Schewick, et al. Mutations and deletions of the TP53 gene predict non response to trearment and poor aoutcome in first relapse of clidhood acute lymphoblastic leukemia.J Clin oncol.2011;29: 3185–23.

[32] Stencil A, Schnittger S, Weissmann S, et al. TP 53 mutations occur in 15.7% of ALL and are associated with MYC-rearrangement, low hypodiploidy, and a poor prognosis Blood. 2014;124: 251–258.

[33] Barber KE, Marttineau M, harewood L et al. Amplification ofthe ABL gene in T cell acute lymphoblastic leukemia Leukemia. 2004;18:1153–1156.

[34] Asnafi v, Buzyn A, Le Noir s, et al. NOTCH1/FBXW7 mutation identifies a large subgroup with favorable outcome in adult T- cell acute lymphoblastic leukemia (T ALL): a Group for Research on Adult acute Lymphoblastic Leukemia (GRAALL) study. Blood. 2009;113: 3918–3924.

[35] Flex E, Petrangeli V, Stella L, et al. Somatically acquired JAK1 mutations in adult acute lymphoblastic leukemia. J Exp Med. 2008;205 : 751–758.

[36] Asnafi V, Le Noir S, Lhermitte L, et al. JAK1 mutations are not frequent events in adult T-ALL: a GRAALL study. Fr. J Haematol. 2010;148 :178–179.

[37] Daniel D'Angelo, M.D. Personal Communication May 2006.

[38] Nachman JB, La MK, Hunger SP, Heerema NA, Gaynon PS, Hast- ings C, et al. Young adults with acute lymphoblastic leukemia have an excellent outcome with chemotherapy alone and benefit from intensive postinduction treatment: a report from the chil-dren's oncology group. J Clin Oncol. 2009;27(31):5189–94.

[39] Hough R, Rowntree C, Goulden N, Mitchell C, Moorman A, Wade R, et al. Efficacy and toxicity of a paediatric protocol in teenagers and young adults with Philadelphia chromosome negative acute 2018 lymphoblastic leukaemia : results from UKALL 2003 . Br J Hae-matol. 2016;172(3):439–51.

[40] Barry E, DeAngelo DJ, Neuberg D, Stevenson K, Loh ML, Asse- lin BL, et al. Favorable outcome for adolescents with acute lymph- oblastic leukemia treated on Dana-Farber Cancer Institute Acute Lymphoblastic Leukemia Consortium Protocols. J Clin Oncol. 2007;25(7): 813–9.

[41] Rowe JM, Buck G, Burnett AK, et al. Induction therapy for adults with acute lymphoblastic leukemia: Results of more than 1500 patients from the international ALL trial: MRC UKALL XII/ECOG E 2993. Blood. 2005;106: 3760–3767

[42] Larson RA, Dodge RK, Burns CP, et al. A five-drug remis- sion induction regimen with intensive consolidation for adults with acute lymphoblastic leukemia: Cancer and Leukemia Group B Study 8811. Blood. 1995;85:2025–2037.

[43] Thomas X, Boiron J-M, Huguet F, et al. Outcome of treatment in adults with acute lymphoblastic leukemia: analysis of the LALA-94 trial. J Clin Oncol. 2004; 22:4075–4086.

[44] Kantarjian H, Thomas D, O'Brien S, et al. Long-term follow- up results of hyperfractionated cyclophosphamide, vincristine, doxorubicin, and dexamethasone (Hyper- CVAD), a dose-intensive regimen, in adult acute lymphocytic leukemia. Cancer. 2004; 101:2788–2801.

[45] Pui CH, Pei D, Campana D, Bowman WP, Sandlund JT, Kaste SC, et

al. Improved prognosis for older adolescents with acute lymphoblastic leukemia. J Clin Oncol. 2011;29(4): 386–91.

[46] Ribera JM, Oriol A, Sanz MA, Tormo M, Fernandez-Abellan P, del Potro E, et al. Comparison of the results of the treatment of adolescents and young adults with standard-risk acute lympho- blastic leukemia with the Programa Espanol de Tratamiento en Hematologia pediatric-based protocol ALL-96. J Clin Oncol. 2008;26(11): 1843–9.

[47] Rijneveld AW, van der Holt B, Daenen SM, Biemond BJ, de Weerdt O, Muus P, et al. Intensified chemotherapy inspired by a pediatric regimen combined with allogeneic transplantation in adult patients with acute lymphoblastic leukemia up to the age of 40. Leukemia. 2011;25(11): 1697–703.

[48] Toft N, Birgens H, Abrahamsson J, Griskevicius L, Hallbook H, Heyman M, et al. Results of NOPHO ALL2008 treatment for patients aged 1–45 years with acute lymphoblastic leukemia. Leu- kemia. 2018;32(3):606–15.

[49] Stock W, Luger SM, Advani AS, Geyer S, Harvey RC, Mul- lighan CG, et al. Favorable outcomes for older adolescents and young adults (AYA) with acute lymphoblastic leukemia (ALL): early results of US intergroup trial C10403 [abstract]. Blood. 2014;124 (21):Abstract 796.

[50] Gökbuget N, Beck J, Brandt K, Brüggemann M, Burmeister T, Diedrich H, et al. Significant improvement of outcome in ado- lescents and young adults (AYAs) aged 15–35 years with acute lymphoblastic leukemia (ALL) with a pediatric derived adult ALL protocol: results of 1529 AYAs in 2 consecutive trials of the German Multicenter Study Group for Adult ALL (GMALL) [abstract]. Blood. 2013;122 (21):Abstract 839.

[51] Boissel N, Auclerc M-F, Lheritier V, et al. Should adolescents with acute lymphoblastic leukemia be treated as old children or young adults? Comparison of the French FRALLE-93 and LALA-94 trials. J Clin Oncol. 2003; 21:774–780.

[52] deBont JM, van der Holt B, Dekker AW, van der Does-van den Berg A, Sonneveld P, Pieters R. Significant difference in outcome for adolescents with acute lymphoblastic leukemia treated on pediatric vs adult protocols in the Netherlands. Leukemia. 2004;18: 2032–2035.

[53] Ramanujachar R, Richards S, Hann I, Webb D. Adolescents with acute lymphoblastic leukaemia:emerging from the shadow of paediatric and adult treatment protocols. *Pediatr Blood Cancer*. 2006;47(6):748–756.

[54] Testi AM, Valsecchi MG, Conter V, et al. Difference in outcome of adolescents with acute lymphoblastic leukemia (ALL) enrolled in pediatric (AIEOP) and adult (GIMEMA) protocols. Blood. 2004;104:1954.

[55] DeAngelo DJ, Stevenson KE, Dahlberg SE, Silverman LB, Cou- ban S, Supko JG, et al. Long-term outcome of a pediatric-inspired regimen used for adults aged 18–50 years with newly diagnosed acute lymphoblastic leukemia. Leukemia. 2015;29(3):526–34.

[56] Storring JM, Minden MD, Kao S, Gupta V, Schuh AC, Schim- mer AD, et al. Treatment of adults with BCR-ABL negative acute lymphoblastic leukaemia with a modified paediatric regimen. Br J Haematol. 2009;146(1):76–85.

[57] Dombret H, Cluzeau T, Huguet F, Boissel N. Pediatric-like therapy for adults with ALL. Curr Hematol Malig Rep. 2014;9(2):158–64.

[58] Cluzeau T, Dhedin N, Huguet F, Raffoux E, Maury S, Mannone L, et al. Dose- intensity impacts on survival of adolescents and young adults with acute lymphoblastic leukemia treated in adult departments by a pediatric protocol (FRALLE 2000BT) [abstract]. Blood. 2012;120(21):Abstract 3561.

[59] Ting-Chi Yeh, Der-Cherng Liang, et al Treatment of childhood acute lymphoblastic leukemia with delayed first intrathecal therapy and omission of prophylactic cranial irradiation: Results of the TPOG-ALL-2002 study. *Cancer*. 2018;124(23):4538–4547.

[60] López-Hernández MA, Alvarado-Ibarra M, Jiménez-Alvarado RM, et al. Adolescentes con leucemia aguda linfoblástica de novo: eficacia y seguridad de un protocolo pediátrico versus uno de adultos. Gac Med Mex. 2008;144(6):485–490.

[61] Schmiegelow K, Forestier E, Hellebostad M, et al. Long-term results of NOPHO ALL-92 and ALL-2000 studies of childhood acute lymphoblastic leukemia [published correction appears in Leukemia. 2010 Mar;24(3):670]. *Leukemia*. 2010;24(2): 345–354.

[62] Kantarjian HM, O'Brien S, Smith TL *et al.* Results of treatment with hyper-CVAD, a dose-intensive regimen, in adult acute lymphocytic leukemia. *J. Clin. Oncol.* 18(3), 547–561 (2000).

[63] Petersdorf SH, Kopecky KJ, Head DR *et al.* Comparison of the L10M consolidation regimen to an alternative regimen including escalating methotrexate/L-asparaginase for adult acute lymphoblastic leukemia: a Southwest Oncology Group Study. *Leukemia* 15(2), 208–216 (2001).

[64] Annino L, Vegna ML, Camera A *et al.* Treatment of adult acute lymphoblastic leukemia (ALL): long-term follow-up of the GIMEMA ALL 0288 randomized study. *Blood* 99(3), 863–871 (2002).

[65] Richard A. Larson, Acute Lymphoblastic Leukemia: Older Patients and Newer Drugs Hematology 2005.

[66] Sancho JM, Ribera JM, Xicoy B *et al.* Results of the PETHEMA ALL-96 trial in elderly patients with Philadelphia chromosome-negative acute lymphoblastic leukemia. *Eur. J. Haematol.* 78(2), 102–110 (2007).

[67] Sive JI, Buck G, Fielding A *et al.* Outcomes in older adults with acute lymphoblastic leukaemia (ALL): results from the international MRC UKALL XII/ECOG2993 trial. *Br. J. Haematol.* 157 (4), 463–471 (2012).

[68] Goekbuget N, Beck J, Brueggemann M *et al.* Moderate intensive chemotherapy including CNS-prophylaxis with liposomal cytarabine is feasible and effective in older patients with Ph-negative acute lymphoblastic leukemia (ALL): results of a prospective trial from the German multicenter study group for adult ALL (GMALL). *Blood* 120(21), 1493 (2012).

[69] Thomas X, Olteanu N, Charrin C, et al. Acute lymphoblastic leukemia in the elderly: the Edouard Herriot Hospital experience. Am J Hematol. 2001;67: 73–83.

[70] Kantarjian HM, O'Brien S, Smith TL, et al. Results of treatment with hyper-CVAD, a dose-intensive regimen, for adult acute lymphoblastic leukemia. J Clin Oncol. 2000;18:547–561.

[71] Ribera, Josep-Maria et al. Treatment of Frail Older Adults and Elderly Patients With Philadelphia Chromosome-negative Acute Lymphoblastic Leukemia: Results of a Prospective Trial With Minimal Chemotherapy. Clin Lymphoma Mye loma Leuk ; 2020 Apr 05.

[72] Ottmann OG, Wassmann B, Pfeifer H, et al: Imatinib compared with chemotherapy as front-line treatment of elderly patients with Philadelphia chromosome- positive acute lymphoblastic leukemia (Ph1ALL). *Cancer*. 2007;109(10):2068–2076.

[73] Ribera JM, Garćıa O, Oriol A, et al: Feasibility and results of subtype-oriented protocols in older adults and fit elderly patients with acute lymphoblastic leukemia: Results of three prospective parallel trials from the PETHEMA group. Leuk Res 41:12–20, 2016

[74] Daver N, Thomas D, Ravandi F, et al: Final report of a phase II study of imatinib mesylate with hyper-CVAD for the front-line treatment of adult patients with Philadelphia chromosome-positive acute lymphoblastic leukemia. Haematologica 100:653–661, 2015

[75] Vignetti M, Fazi P, Cimino G, et al: Imatinib plus steroids induces complete remissions and prolonged survival in elderly Philadelphia chromosome-positive patients with acute lymphoblastic leukemia without additional chemotherapy: Results of the Gruppo Italiano Malattie Ematologiche dell'Adulto (GIMEMA) LAL0201-B protocol. Blood 109:3676–3678, 2007

[76] Rousselot P, Coudé MM, Gokbuget N, et al: Dasatinib and low-intensity chemotherapy in elderly patients with Philadelphia chromosome-positive ALL. Blood 128:774–782, 2016

[77] Foà R, Vitale A, Vignetti M, et al: Dasatinib as first-line treatment for adult patients with Philadelphia chromosome-positive acute lymphoblastic leukemia. Blood 118: 6521–6528, 2011

[78] Ravandi F, O'Brien SM, Cortes JE, et al: Long-term follow-up of a phase 2 study of chemotherapy plus dasatinib for the initial treatment of patients with Philadelphia chromosome-positive acute lymphoblastic leukemia. Cancer 121:4158–4164, 2015

[79] Ottmann OG, Pfeifer H, Cayuela J-M, et al: Nilotinib (Tasigna®) and chemotherapy for first-line treatment in elderly patients with de novo Philadelphia chromosome/BCR-ABL1 positive acute lymphoblastic leukemia: A trial of the European Working Group for Adult ALL (EWALL-PH-02). Blood 124, 2014 (abstr 798)

[80] Kim DY, Joo YD, Lim SN, et al: Nilotinib combined with multiagent chemotherapy for newly diagnosed Philadelphia-positive acute lymphoblastic leukemia. Blood 126:746–756, 2015

[81] Jabbour E, Kantarjian H, Ravandi F, et al: Combination of hyper-CVAD with ponatinib as first-line therapy for patients with Philadelphia chromosome-positive acute lymphoblastic leukaemia: A single-centre, phase 2 study. Lancet Oncol 16:1547–1555, 2015

[82] Martinelli G, Piciocchi A, Papayannidis C, et al: First report of the GIMEMA LAL1811 phase II prospective study of the combination of steroids with ponatinib as frontline therapy of elderly or unfit patients with Philadelphia chromosome-positive acute lymphoblastic leukemia. Blood 130:99, 2017

[83] Weerapat Owattnapanich, Pongrueth Rujirachun, et al: Prevalence and Clinical Outcome of Philadelphia-Like Acute Lymphoblastic Leukemia: Systematic Review and Meta-analysis. Clinical Lymphoma, Myeloma & Leukemia January 20.

[84] Elias Jabbour, Debora Thomas, et al: Central Nervous System Prophylaxis in Adults With Acute Lymphoblastic Leukemia. Cancer May 15, 2010

[85] Liron Frishman-Levy, et al: Advances in understanding the

pathogenesis of CNS acute lymphoblastic leukaemia and potential for therapy. British Journal of Haematology, 2017, 176, 157–167

[86] Lazarus HM, Richards SM, Chopra R et al. Central nervous system involvement in adult acute lymphoblastic leukemia at diagnosis: results from the international ALL trial MRC UKALL XII/ECOG E2993. Blood 2006; 108: 465–472.

[87] Kimmo Porka, Perttu Koskenvesa, et al: Dasatinib Crosses the Blood-Brain Barrier and Is an Efficient Therapy for Central Nervous System Philadelphia Chromosome-Positive Leukemia. Blood-2008-02-140665.

[88] Jia-Bao He, Xin Zhang, t al: Ponatinib Therapy in Recurrent Philadelphia Chromosome-Positive Central Nervous System Leukemia With T315I Mutation After Allo-HSCT. International Journal of Cancer 2020; 147: 911–1236.

[89] Sorror ML, Giralt S, Sandmaier BM, et al. Hematopoietic cell transplantation specific comorbidity index as an outcome predictor for patients with acute myeloid leukemia in first remission: combined FHCRC and MDACC experiences. Blood. 2007;110: 4606–13.

[90] Majhail N., et al. Indications for Autologous and Allogeneic Hematopoietic Cell Transplantation: Guidelines from the American Society for Blood and Marrow Transplantation. Biol Blood Marrow Transplant 2015.1863e1869.

[91] Hoelzer D., et al. Acute lymphoblastic leukaemia in adult patients: ESMO Clinical Practice Guidelines for diagnosis, treatment and follow-up. Annals of Oncology 27 (Supplement 5): v69–v82, 2016

[92] Terwilliger T., Abdul-Hay M. Acute lymphoblastic leukemia: a comprehensive review and 2017 update. Blood Cancer Journal.2017; 7:e577.

[93] Marks D., Forman S., et al.A Comparison of Cyclophosphamide and Total Body Irradiation with Etoposide and Total Body Irradiation as Conditioning Regimens for Patients Undergoing Sibling Allografting for Acute Lymphoblastic Leukemia in First or Second Complete Remission . Biology of Blood and Marrow Transplantation .2006;12:438–453.

[94] NCCN Guidelines Version 1.2020 Acute Lymphoblastic Leukemia.

[95] Carreras E., et al. The EBMT Handbook. Hematopoietic Stem Cell Transplantation and Cellular Therapies. Springer Open 2019. P 531–538.

[96] Giebel S., et al.Use of Tyrosine Kinase Inhibitors to Prevent Relapse After Allogeneic Hematopoietic Stem Cell Transplantation for Patients With Philadelphia Chromosome–Positive Acute Lymphoblastic Leukemia:A Position Statement of the Acute Leukemia Working Party of the European Society for Blood and Marrow Transplantation. Cancer 2016;122: 2941–51.

[97] Fuchs E., et al. HLA-Haploidentical Bone Marrow Transplantation for Hematologic Malignancies Using Nonmyeloablative Conditioning and High-Dose, Post transplantation Cyclophosphamide. *Biol Blood Marrow Transplant*. 2008;14(6): 641–650

[98] Bolaños-Meade J., et al. HLA-haploidentical bone marrow transplantation with posttransplant Cyclophosphamide expands the donor pool for patients with sickle cell disease. *Blood*. 2012;120(22):4285–4291.

[99] Santoro N., et al., Unmanipulated haploidentical stem cell transplantation in adults with acute lymphoblastic leukemia:a study on behalf of the Acute

Leukemia Working Party of the EBMT. Journal of Hematology & Oncology.2017;10:113

[100] Brammer JE., et al. Multi-center analysis of the effect of T-cell acute lymphoblastic leukemia subtype and minimal residual disease on allogeneic stem cell transplantation outcomes. Bone Marrow Transplantation.2017; 52, 20–27.

[101] Zhou Yi, et al. The Effect of Peritransplant Minimal Residual Disease in Adults With Acute Lymphoblastic Leukemia Undergoing Allogeneic Hematopoietic Stem Cell Transplantation. Clinical Lymphoma, Myeloma & Leukemia 2014;(14), ISSUE 4, P319–326.

[102] Bar M., et al. Impact of Minimal Residual Disease, Detected by Flow Cytometry, on Outcome of Myeloablative Hematopoietic Cell Transplantation for Acute Lymphoblastic Leukemia.Leukemia Research and Treatment 2014; Article ID 421723.

[103] Kantarjian H., et al. Blinatumomab versus Chemotherapy for Advanced Acute Lymphoblastic Leukemia.N Engl J Med 2017;376:836–47.

[104] Jabbour E., et al., Monoclonal antibodies in acute lymphoblastic leukemia. Blood. 2015;125(26):4010–4016.

[105] Katarjian H., et al., Inotuzumab Ozogamicin versus Standard Therapy for Acute Lymphoblastic Leukemia. N Engl J Med 2016;375:740–53.

[106] O'Leary M. et al, FDA Approval Summary: Tisagenlecleucel for Treatment of Patients with Relapsed or Refractory B-cell Precursor Acute Lymphoblastic Leukemia. Clin Cancer Res; 2019;25(4):1141–1146

[107] Pehlivan K. et al. CAR-T Cell Therapy for Acute Lymphoblastic Leukemia: Transforming the Treatment of Relapsed and Refractory Disease. Current Hematologic Malignancy Reports. https://doi.org/10.1007/s11899-018-0470-x.

[108] Maude S.L., et al. Tisagenlecleucel in Children and Young Adults with B-Cell Lymphoblastic Leukemia.N Engl J Med 2018;378:439–48.

[109] Short N, Jabbour E. Minimal Residual Disease in Acute Lymphoblastic Leukemia:How to Recognize and Treat It. Curr Oncol Rep.2017;19:6–13

[110] Nathalie Dhedin, Anne Huynh, Sebastien Maury, Reza Tabrizi, Kheira Beldjord, Vahid Asnafi, Xavier Thomas, Patrice Chevallier. Role of allogeneic stem cell transplantation in adult patients with Ph-negative acute lymphoblastic leukemia. Blood. 2015,125 (16):2486–2496

[111] Donald A.Berry, Shouhao Zhou, Howard Higley, Lata Mukundan, Shuangshuang Fu, Gregory H. Reaman, Brent L. Wood, Gary J. Kelloff, J. Milburn Jessup, Jerald P. Radich. Association of Minimal Residual Disease With Clinical Outcome in Pediatric and Adult Acute Lymphoblastic Leukemia. A Meta-analysis. JAMA Oncol. doi: 10.1001/jamaoncol.2017.0580 Published online May 11, 2017

Chapter 9

What Is the Best Choice and Dose of Anthracycline for Induction Chemotherapy in Acute Myeloid Leukemia?

Sravanti Rangaraju and Omer Jamy

Abstract

Treatment of patients with acute myeloid leukemia, medically fit to receive intensive chemotherapy, has been standardized over the past four decades and consists of an anthracycline administered along with continuous cytarabine. This combination is traditionally administered as seven days of cytarabine and three days of anthracycline, known as 7 + 3. Selecting the appropriate choice and dose of anthracycline for induction chemotherapy continues to be debated. Daunorubicin, used in three doses of either 45 mg/m^2, 60 mg/m^2 or 90 mg/m^2, and idarubicin 12 mg/m^2 are the two commonly used anthracyclines in clinical practice. Other anthracyclines including mitoxantrone and liposomal daunorubicin are incorporated in the treatment algorithm as well. Our understanding of the underlying biology of acute myeloid leukemia has significantly increased in the past decade, helping us formulate individualized treatment plans. In this chapter, we will discuss pivotal studies comparing the safety and efficacy of different types and doses of anthracyclines, focusing predominantly on daunorubicin and idarubicin. The details of the study design as well as subgroup analysis will be presented to determine which subset of patients with AML may benefit from a particular anthracycline.

Keywords: AML, induction chemotherapy, anthracycline, daunorubicin, Idarubicin

1. Introduction

Acute Myeloid Leukemia (AML) is a heterogenous clonal stem cell disorder, resulting in proliferation of immature hematopoietic cells in the bone marrow, peripheral blood and occasionally in other tissues. Consequentially, normal hematopoiesis is inhibited, resulting in neutropenia, anemia and thrombocytopenia. Patients usually present with signs and symptoms of underlying bone marrow failure including fatigue, lethargy, shortness of breath, bruising, bleeding and infections [1–3].

The incidence rate of AML increases progressively with advancing age. It is primarily a disease of the elderly with the median age at diagnosis being 68 years and accounts for 80–90% of all acute leukemias in adults. There are approximately 20,000 new cases of AML diagnosed every year in the United States, accompanied by nearly 10,000 deaths [1, 3, 4].

IntechOpen

Our understanding of the molecular pathogenesis of AML has increased significantly in the last decade. Unfortunately, this understanding has not been matched in terms of therapeutic advances, though this has slowly changed since 2017. Age, cytogenetics and molecular aberrations play a significant role in determining prognosis as well as choice of treatment in patients with AML [2, 5, 6].

Treatment of AML can broadly be divided into intensive and non-intensive chemotherapy. Currently, in addition to age, performance status and medical fitness influence intensity of treatment. Traditionally, young and medically fit patients are treated with an intensive chemotherapy regimen. An arbitrary cutoff of 55 to 65 years has commonly been used to define 'older' and 'younger' patients. Medical fitness can be determined relatively accurately by assessing variables including performance status, organ function and frailty. A combination of age and medical fitness routinely form the basis for the assignment to the intensity of treatment [7–12].

Intensive chemotherapy generally involves a remission induction phase, to achieve complete remission, followed by a post-remission or consolidation phase, to stay in remission and prevent relapse. A combination of an anthracycline and cytarabine is almost always used as upfront intensive therapy for patients with AML. Nearly four decades ago, 7 days of cytarabine and 3 days of daunorubicin was established as the standard of care for patients with AML. Even today, this regimen, commonly known as 7 + 3, serves as the backbone in the treatment algorithm for AML. Since the 1970s, many trials have attempted to improve upon this combination either by using different doses of anthracyclines, different types of anthracyclines or adding a third agent. With very few exceptions, 7 + 3 remains standard of care outside of clinical trials [13, 14].

To this day, it is not entirely clear which type and dose of anthracycline is ideal when used during induction chemotherapy. Daunorubicin and idarubicin have been compared extensively in randomized studies. Mitoxantrone is also considered at times. CPX-351 (liposomal daunorubicin:cytarabine) is FDA approved, as induction therapy, in a subset of patients with AML.

In this chapter, we will present the data comparing the different types and doses of anthracyclines used in induction chemotherapy. Whereas details on all agents will be provided, the main focus will revolve around daunorubicin (45 mg/m^2, 60 mg/m^2 and 90 mg/m^2) and idarubicin (mainly 12 mg/m^2) since they are the most commonly used anthracyclines. Furthermore, randomized studies where induction chemotherapy was not given in a 7 + 3 manner have also been discussed.

2. Daunorubicin

Daunorubicin, a topoisomerase II inhibitor, inhibits both DNA and RNA synthesis by intercalating between DNA base pairs, inhibiting transcription by inhibiting DNA-dependent RNA polymerase as well as steric obstruction. It was discovered as an antitumor antibiotic in the 1960s and has since been used as part of the treatment algorithm for AML [15]. In 1973, Yates et al. shared their findings of using 7 days of continuous cytarabine infusion and 3 days of daunorubicin in patients with AML. They reported a complete remission rate of 63% in 8 untreated patients with AML. The superiority of this regimen was confirmed by CALGB 7421, a trial comparing 7 + 3 to 5 days of continuous cytarabine infusion and 2 days of anthracycline (5 + 2) [13, 14]. Thus, 7 + 3 became the backbone of AML treatment for the next four decades and remains the standard to which other therapies are compared to even today.

The dose of daunorubicin used by Yates et al. as well as CALGB 7421 was 45 mg/m^2 and this dose was used as standard going forward after confirmatory results of CALGB 7721. Since then, several attempts have been made to modify the dose of daunorubicin, as part of standard induction therapy, to further improve outcomes of patients with AML [6, 16–19].

2.1 Daunorubicin 45 mg/m^2 vs. 90 mg/m^2

2.1.1 Older adults

A HOVON-SAKK-AMLSG collaboration investigated escalated daunorubicin dose (90 mg/m^2) vs. standard daunorubicin dose (45 mg/m^2) with 200 mg/m^2 of cytarabine continuous infusion (7 + 3) in older adults with AML [20]. The study enrolled 813 patients with a median follow-up of 40 months. The median age of the study population was 67 years (range 60–83). Around 60% of the study population had intermediate-risk cytogenetics. All patients received a second cycle of cytarabine at a dose of 1000 mg/m^2, every 12 hours, for 6 days.

The escalated dose was associated with higher rates of complete remission when compared to standard dose (64% vs. 54%, $p = 0.002$) as well as higher rates of complete remission after first cycle of induction (52% vs. 35%, $p < 0.001$). There were no significant differences in terms of toxicities and early mortality between the 2 doses. For the overall population, there was no difference in overall survival, event-free survival and disease-free survival between the 2 doses. In a subset analysis of patients between the ages of 60 and 65, the escalated dose was associated with higher rates of complete remission, event-free survival (29% vs. 14%) and overall survival (38% vs. 23%). Within the limitations of the small numbers, older patients with core-binding factors abnormalities also seemed to derive survival benefit with the escalated dose.

2.1.2 Younger adults

In ECOG 1900, Fernandez et al. investigated 3 days of high dose daunorubicin at 90 mg/m^2 vs. standard dose daunorubicin at 45 mg/m^2, in combination with 100 mg/m^2 of cytarabine as continuous infusion (7 + 3), in young patients with AML [21]. The study enrolled 657 patients with a median age of 48 years (range 17–60). A second round of induction was given to patients with residual disease on day 14 bone marrow biopsy. The regimen was 7 + 3 with a daunorubicin dose of 45 mg/m^2. Approximately 41% of the patients had intermediate-risk cytogenetics and 14% and 19% had favorable and unfavorable-risk cytogenetics, respectively.

The rates of complete remission were higher with high dose daunorubicin compared to standard dose (70.6% vs. 57.3%, $p < 0.001$). The rates of complete remission after first induction were also higher in the high dose arm (83.3% vs. 72%). There was no difference in early mortality between the 2 doses. High dose daunorubicin was associated with a higher 4-year overall survival (39% vs. 31%, $p = 0.001$), median overall survival (25.4 m vs. 16.6 m, $p = 0.001$) and event-free survival (28% vs. 20%, $p < 0.001$). Subgroup analysis demonstrated that patients younger than 50 years benefit significantly with high dose daunorubicin with higher complete remission rates (74.3% vs. 59.4%) and improved survival (median overall survival: 34.3 m vs. 19.0 m, HR 0.65, $p = 0.004$). The benefit of high dose daunorubicin did not extend to patients ≥50 years.

Survival with high dose daunorubicin was numerically longer, but statistically insignificant, in patients with favorable-risk cytogenetics, when compared to standard dose. Patients with intermediate-risk cytogenetics benefitted from high dose daunorubicin, compared to standard dose, with a median overall survival of 32.3 m vs. 17.8 m (HR 0.67, p = 0.02). There was no difference in survival between the 2 doses for patients with unfavorable cytogenetics as well as those with FLT3-ITD or MLL-PTD mutations.

An updated report of ECOG 1900 was presented in 2016 with a longer follow-up time period (median 80.1 months amongst survivors) [22]. The update confirmed the benefit of high dose daunorubicin in patients younger than 50 years of age (44.7 m vs. 20.7 m, 9 = 0.002). Older patients did not gain survival advantage with the high dose.

The benefit of high dose daunorubicin, compared to standard dose, was shown in patients with both favorable (NR vs. 39.4 m, HR 0.51, p = 0.03) and intermediate-risk cytogenetics (33.5 m vs. 20.1 m, HR 0.68, p = 0.01). After controlling for confounding variables, a benefit for patients with unfavorable-risk cytogenetics was also seen with the high dose (HR 0.66, p = 0.04).

Subset analysis based on molecular subgroups revealed that FLT3-ITD, DNMT3A and NPM1 mutant-AML derived benefit from high dose daunorubicin. Patients with FLT3-ITD mutated AML had a 4-year overall survival of 28% with high dose daunorubicin compared to 17% with standard dose. The data suggests that an additional 10% of patients with FLT3-ITD mutated AML can be cured with the higher dose. Further analysis demonstrated that both younger and older patients with FLT3-ITD mutant AML derived benefit from high dose daunorubicin. Patients with DNMT3A mutant AML had longer median overall survival with high dose daunorubicin, compared to standard dose (16.5 m vs. 14.1 m). However, the benefit of high dose daunorubicin, in DNMT3A mutant AML, was limited to patients younger than 50 years of age. Both younger and older patients with NPM1 mutant AML derived benefit with high dose daunorubicin. The median overall survival with high dose daunorubicin was 75.9 months, compared to 16.9 months with standard dose. The 4-year overall survival increased with high dose daunorubicin to 52% from 29% with standard dose.

Another phase III study compared high dose daunorubicin at 90 mg/m^2 for 3 days with standard dose daunorubicin at 45 mg/m^2 for 3 days, in addition to cytarabine 200 mg/m^2 as continuous infusion, in adults ≤60 years of age with AML [23]. The study enrolled 383 patients. A second round of abbreviated induction was given to patients with residual disease on day 14 bone marrow biopsy. Approximately 62% of the patients had intermediate-risk cytogenetics and 21% and 15% had favorable and unfavorable-risk cytogenetics, respectively.

The rates of complete remission were higher with daunorubicin 90 mg/m^2 when compared to 45 mg/m^2 (82.5% vs. 72.0%, p = 0.014). After a median follow-up of 52.6 months, high dose daunorubicin, compared to standard dose, was associated with improved overall survival (46.8% vs. 34.6%, p = 0.03) and event-free survival (40.8% vs. 28.4%, p = 0.03). There was no difference in the toxicity profile in both arms. In multivariable analysis, high dose daunorubicin was associated with higher complete remission rate (HR, 1.802, P = 0.024), improved overall survival (HR, 0.739, P = 0.032) and event-free survival (HR, 0.774, P = 0.04). Based on cytogenetic risk group, the benefit was of high dose daunorubicin was mainly seen in patients with intermediate risk disease. Molecular subgroup analysis was not available.

2.2 Daunorubicin 45 mg/m^2 vs. 60 mg/m^2

There is no randomized data comparing daunorubicin 60 mg/m^2 to daunorubicin 45 mg/m^2. One retrospective study evaluated 56 patients and reported complete remission rates of 88% with daunorubicin 60 mg/m^2 and 67% with daunorubicin 45 mg/m^2 ($p = 0.05$). Details on disease-free and overall survival were not available [24].

2.3 Daunorubicin 60 mg/m² vs. 90 mg/m²

The UK NCRI AML17 trial compared daunorubicin 60 mg/m^2 to 90 mg/m^2 in AML induction [25]. The induction chemotherapy regimen was not administered as standard 7 + 3 and used a modified strategy of giving the anthracycline on days 1, 3 and 5, in combination with cytarabine 100 mg/m^2, every 12 hours, on days 1 to 10. Furthermore, a second round of induction was given to all patients in morphological remission after the first induction and consisted of daunorubicin 50 mg/m^2 on days 1, 3 and 5 and cytarabine 100 mg/m^2, every 12 hours, on days 1–8. Hence the cumulative dose of daunorubicin in the 90 mg/m^2 and 60 mg/m^2 arms was 420 mg/m^2 and 330 mg/m^2, respectively. The cumulative dose for both doses, if used in a 7 + 3 regimen, would have been 270 mg/m^2 and 180 mg/m^2, respectively.

The study enrolled 1206 patients with a median age of 53 years (range 16–72 years). Nearly three fourths of the patients in the study had intermediate risk cytogenetics. After a median follow-up of 14.8 months, the study was terminated prematurely due to higher risk of mortality by day 60 in the daunorubicin 90 mg/m^2 arm, with an intention-to-treat analysis showing no benefit of the higher dose. There was no difference in the rate of complete remission between the 2 arms (D60 75% vs. D90 73%, $p = 0.6$). There was no difference in 30-day mortality between the 2 arms, but 60-day mortality was higher with daunorubicin 90 mg/m^2, compared to 60 mg/m^2 (10% vs. 5%, $p = 0.001$). Furthermore, there was no statistical difference between the 2 arms in terms of overall survival (D60 60% vs. D90 59%, $p = 0.15$), relapse-free survival (D60 48% vs., D90 51%, $p = 0.7$) and 2-year overall survival censored at stem cell transplant (D60 60% vs. D90 60%). An exploratory analysis did not identify any subgroup that benefited with the higher dose of daunorubicin.

An updated intention-to-treat analysis, after a median follow-up of 28 months, revealed no differences in terms of rates of complete remission, overall survival, and relapse-free survival [26]. However, subgroup analysis indicated that the higher dose of daunorubicin may benefit patients with FLT3-ITD mutant AML, (Cumulative incidence of relapse: 44% vs. 60%; HR, 0.58; $p = .01$; RFS: 45% vs. 33%; HR, 0.63; $p = .02$; OS: 54% vs. 34%; HR, 0.65; $p = .03$). The survival benefit seemed to be independent of the allelic burden of the mutation as well as coexisting NPM1 mutations.

Data from the DaunoDouble trial were recently presented at the European Hematology Association in the form on an abstract [27]. The trial compared daunorubicin 60 mg/m^2 to daunorubicin 90 mg/m^2 when given as 7 + 3. Daunorubicin was given on days 3 to 5. The study enrolled 262 patients and the median age of the population was 52 years. Per the European Leukemia Network 2017 classification, there were 39% patients with favorable, 40% with intermediate and 21% with adverse risk disease. Response assessment was based on a day 15 bone marrow and patients with <5% blasts were further randomized to either receive a second induction with 7 + 3 or to no further induction. The results of the second randomization are not yet available. The rate of remission with a maximum of two rounds of induction was 67% with daunorubicin 60 mg/m^2 and 61% with daunorubicin 90 mg/m^2 ($p = 0.32$). With a median follow-up of 40 months, there was no difference in cumulative incidence of relapse ($p = 0.343$) and treatment related mortality ($p = 0.994$). There was no difference in 4-year overall survival ($p = 0.108$), event-free survival ($p = 0.207$) and relapse-free survival (0.394) between the 2 groups and

Study	Patients (n)	Age (median, range)	Anthracycline comparison	Induction schedule	Cumulative anthracycline dose (mg/m^2)	Complete remission	Overall survival	Subset analysis
HOVON-SAKK-AMLSG	813	67 (60–83)	D90 vs. D45	7 + 3	D90 270 D45 130	Favors D90	No significant difference	60–65 years: CR, EFS and OS improved with D90
ECOG 1900	657	48 (17–60)	D90 vs. D45	7 + 3	D90 270 D45 130	Favors D90	Favors D90	Cytogenetics: All risk groups had improved OS with D90 FLT3: Improved OS with D90 NPM1 Improved OS with D90 DNMT3A & <50 years: Improved OS with D90
Lee et al.	383	N/A (15–60)	D90 vs. D45	7 + 3	D90 270 D45 130	Favors D90	Favors D90	Cytogenetics: Intermediate risk had improved OS with D90
UK NCRI AML17	1206	53 (16–72)	D90 vs. D60	10 + 3	D90 420 D60 330	No significant difference	No significant difference	FLT3: May benefit from D90
Daunodouble	262	52 (N/A)	D90 vs. D60	7 + 3	D90 270 D60 180	No significant difference	No significant difference	Complete data not available

D90: daunorubicin 90 mg/m^2, D60: daunorubicin 60 mg/m^2, D45: daunorubicin 45 mg/m^2, 7 + 3: 7 days of cytarabine and 3 days of anthracycline, CR: complete remission, EFS: event-free survival, OS: overall survival.

Table 1.
Summary of trials comparing different doses of daunorubicin.

there was no difference in outcomes based on daunorubicin dose on multivariable analysis. Although these results support the use of daunorubicin 60 mg/m^2, results from the second randomization in the study will facilitate with data interpretation.

A summary of the trials comparing different doses of daunorubicin is presented in **Table 1.**

2.4 FLT3-mutant AML

A randomized study compared the addition of midostaurin, a multitarget kinase inhibitor, or placebo to 7 + 3 in FLT3 mutated AML. The dose of daunorubicin was 60 mg/m^2 and patients were < 60 years of age. Compared to placebo, the addition of midostaurin prolonged overall and event-free survival in this population [18]. Whether using daunorubicin 90 mg/m^2 or idarubicin would have yielded even better results remain unknow. There is data (discussed below) that daunorubicin 90 mg/m^2 may be the optimal choice to use in FLT3 mutated AML.

3. Idarubicin

3.1 Idarubicin 12 mg/m^2 vs. daunorubicin 45 mg/m^2

Idarubicin was introduced into the treatment of AML, as a newer anthracycline, in the 1990s. Four trials during that time compared idarubicin 12–13 mg/m^2 for 3 days to daunorubicin 45–50 mg/m^2 for 3 days, given with cytarabine as induction chemotherapy for AML. Three of those studies found idarubicin to be superior to daunorubicin and there was a signal of rapid response to idarubicin, compared to daunorubicin, in the fourth study [28–31]. Another study compared daunorubicin 50 mg/m^2 for 3 days to idarubicin 8 mg/m^2 for 5 days, given with seven days of cytarabine, and found idarubicin to be more effective than daunorubicin in AML patients between 55 and 75 years of age [32]. In summary, idarubicin at an average dose of 12 mg/m^2 is most likely superior to daunorubicin 45 mg/m^2, when administered with cytarabine as induction chemotherapy.

3.2 Idarubicin vs. high dose daunorubicin

3.2.1 Idarubicin 12 mg/m^2 vs. daunorubicin 90 mg/m^2

Since idarubicin was found to be superior to standard dose daunorubicin (45 mg/m^2), the next obvious comparison was between idarubicin and high dose daunorubicin. Studies that compare idarubicin to dose intensified daunorubicin delivered as either higher daily doses or prolonged administration of the standard dose have been conducted. In general, regimens with dose intensified daunorubicin have targeted to achieve a cumulative dose of 240–280 mg/m^2 during induction. Key prospective randomized studies comparing these strategies are summarized here.

A Phase III randomized, noninferiority study conducted in South Korea was reported in 2017 [33]. There were 299 patients with a median age of 49 years (range 15–65). They were randomized to receive infusional cytarabine 200 mg/m^2 for 7 days with either idarubicin 12 mg/m^2 or daunorubicin 90 mg/m^2 for 3 days. If Day 14 bone marrow assessment revealed persistent disease, patients received an additional round of induction with infusional cytarabine for 5 days plus idarubicin 8 mg/m^2 or daunorubicin 45 mg/m^2. Patients received consolidation therapy followed by transplantation (either allogeneic or autologous) in first remission based on their cytogenetic risk stratification and donor availability. There was a higher proportion of secondary (4.7% vs. 11.3%), poor risk (14.5% vs. 27.5%) and good risk (18.6% vs. 23.5%) disease in the daunorubicin arm, while more intermediate risk disease (66.9% vs. 49%) was present in the idarubicin arm. These differences did not have significant impact on outcomes. Other baseline characteristics as well as post remission therapies received were similar between the two treatment arms.

In this study, rates of complete remission (80.5% v 74.7%; P = .224), 4-year overall survival (51.1% vs. 54.7%, p = 0.756), cumulative incidence of relapse (35.2% v 25.1%; P = .194) and event-free survival (45.5% v 50.8%; p = 0.772) did not differ between the idarubicin and daunorubicin arms, respectively. However, in the subgroup analysis of FLT3-ITD-mutant AML (n = 44; idarubicin n = 27; daunorubicin n = 17) the median overall survival (not reached vs. 15.2 m, p = 0.03) and event-free survival (not reached vs. 11.9 m, p = 0.03) favored the daunorubicin arm, while remission rates were similar (88.2% vs. 74.1%) in both groups. No differences were noted in the non FLT3-ITD-mutant subgroup. Adverse events were similar between both groups.

In summary, this study showed noninferiority of high dose daunorubicin compared to standard dose idarubicin. There is a suggestion that high dose daunorubicin improved survival, but not remission rate, in FLT3-ITD-mutant AML. However, the study was not powered adequately to draw definitive conclusions in this subgroup analysis.

3.2.2 Idarubicin 12 mg/m^2 vs. daunorubicin 50 mg/m^2 (over 5 days)

The JASLG AML 201 phase III randomized, noninferiority study compared standard dose idarubicin to high dose daunorubicin defined as 50 mg/m^2 over 5 days (as opposed to 90 mg/m^2 over 3 days) [34]. This study had a second phase of randomization for consolidation therapy after complete remission was attained. There were 1057 patients, with a median age of 47 years (range 14–65), randomized in the first phase to receive infusional cytarabine 100 mg/m^2 for 7 days plus idarubicin or daunorubicin at the above-mentioned doses. Baseline characteristics were well balanced between the two groups. In this study, overall complete remission rate was 77.9% and did not differ between the idarubicin (78.2%) and daunorubicin (77.5%) arms, establishing non-inferiority of high dose daunorubicin. Furthermore, 64.1% vs. 61.1% of patients achieved a CR after the first round of induction in the idarubicin and daunorubicin arms, respectively. There was no difference in overall and relapse-free survival between the 2 arms.

3.2.3 Idarubicin 12 mg/m^2 vs. daunorubicin 80 mg/m^2

ALFA 9801, a randomized study, compared daunorubicin 80 mg/m^2 for 3 days to standard dose idarubicin 12 mg/m^2 (IDA3) in patients aged 50–70 years. A third arm of idarubicin 12 mg/m^2 for 4 days (IDA4) was also added [35]. Patients who had residual disease on a day 20 bone marrow assessment could receive additional induction with a pre-specified mitoxantrone based regimen. Those who achieved complete remission then received 2 cycles of consolidation with intermediate dose cytarabine + anthracycline based on their randomization group. This study had a second phase of randomization which investigated the role of recombinant IL-2 in maintenance therapy, which will not be discussed in this chapter. Four hundred and seventy-eight patients underwent the first phase of randomization and baseline characteristics were well balanced in the three arms. Overall complete remission rate was found to be lower in the daunorubicin arm (70%) compared to the IDA3 (83%) or IDA4 (78%) arms and this difference was statistically significant. However, there was no difference in remission rates after the first induction therapy.

No significant difference was noted in the secondary outcomes of event-free survival, overall survival, and cumulative incidence of relapse between the three arms. Induction related deaths, cytopenias and duration of hospitalization was also similar between the groups. Thus, in this older population of AML patients, while the overall complete remission rates appear to be higher in the idarubicin group, no differences were noted in remission after first induction, overall survival or event-free survival.

3.2.4 Idarubicin 8 mg/m^2 (5 days) vs. daunorubicin 60 mg/m^2

Another trial comparing idarubicin to high dose daunorubicin based induction was the phase III GOELAMS LAM-2001 trial, which included patients between the ages of 17–60 years [36]. The study was primarily designed to compare single vs. tandem autologous hematopoietic stem cell transplant strategies as post remission therapy, however the initial phase randomized 832 patients to receive either idarubicin or daunorubicin based induction. The induction regimen used here was infusional cytarabine 200 mg/m^2 for 7 days plus either idarubicin 8 mg/m^2 for 5 days (cumulative dose of 40 mg/m^2 during induction) or daunorubicin 60 mg/m^2 for 3 days. This study revealed similar complete remission rates between the two groups (83% vs. 81%). Seven-year long term follow up of the patients randomized in the first phase of the study was reported in 2013, looking at a variety of cox proportional models to account for interactions with the second randomization arm. Patients in the idarubicin arm had an improved 7-year OS, compared to daunorubicin, unless they had unfavorable cytogenetics. A subset analysis of patients with intermediate risk cytogenetics (n = 393) demonstrated improved 7-year overall survival (p = 0.005) as well as event-free survival (p = 0.025) with idarubicin [37].

3.2.5 Idarubicin 9 mg/m^2 (4 days) vs. daunorubicin 45 mg/m^2 (4 days)

ALFA 9803 was designed to compare two different post-remission strategies but included a first phase of randomization comparing idarubicin to daunorubicin. There were 416 patients aged 65 years or older, randomized to receive infusional cytarabine for 7 days, with either daunorubicin 45 mg/m^2 for 4 days (cumulative dose 180 mg/m^2) or idarubicin 9 mg/m^2 for 4 days (36 mg/m^2). There was no difference in complete remission rates or toxicity profiles between the two induction strategies [38].

Finally, combined long term outcomes of patients enrolled in the ALFA 9801 and 9803 studies have been reported to identify factors associated with improved long-term survival. This report interestingly revealed randomization to idarubicin to be associated with an improved cure rate (16.6% vs. 9.8%), although standard survival analysis in the independent trials did not reveal any differences between idarubicin and daunorubicin based induction [39].

3.2.6 Idarubicin 12 mg/m^2 vs. daunorubicin 60 mg/m^2

There is no randomized or retrospective data comparing idarubicin 12 mg/m^2 to daunorubicin 60 mg/m^2, when administered with continuous cytarabine as 7 + 3. Both these doses are frequently used interchangeably in clinical trials but whether their efficacy is equivalent is not well defined.

Two meta-analysis compared the efficacy of idarubicin to daunorubicin. One focused on high dose daunorubicin only and found that idarubicin was associated with higher rates of complete remission and lower rates of refractory disease compared to daunorubicin. There was no difference in early mortality, febrile

Study	Patients (n)	Age (range)	Anthracycline comparison	Induction schedule	Cumulative anthracycline dose (mg/m2)	Complete remission	Overall survival	Subset analysis
NCT01145846	299	49 (15–65)	D90 vs. Ida12	7 + 3	D90 270 Ida 36	No significant difference	No significant difference	FLT3: Improved OS and EFS with D90
JASLG AML 201	1057	47 (14–65)	D50 vs. Ida12	7 + 3 (Ida) 7 + 5 (D50)	D50 250 Ida 36	No significant difference	No significant difference	—
ALFA 9801	468	60 (50–70)	D80 vs. Ida12	7 + 3	D80 240 Ida 36	Favors Ida	No significant difference	—
GOELAMS LAM-2001	832	48 (17–60)	D60 vs. Ida8	7 + 3 (D60) 7 + 5 (Ida)	D60 180 Ida 40	No significant difference	Favors Ida	Cytogenetics: Intermediate risk had improved OS and EFS with Ida
ALFA 9803	416	72 (65–85)	D45 vs. Ida9	7 + 4	D45 180 Ida 36	No significant difference	No significant difference	—

D90: daunorubicin 90 mg/m^2, D80: daunorubicin 80 mg/m^2, D60: daunorubicin 60 mg/m^2, D50: daunorubicin 50 mg/m^2, D45: daunorubicin 45 mg/m^2, Ida12: idarubicin 12 mg/m^2, Ida8: idarubicin 8 mg/m^2, Ida9: idarubicin 9 mg/m^2, 7 + 3: 7 days of cytarabine and 3 days of anthracycline, CR: complete remission, EFS: event-free survival, OS: overall survival.

Table 2.
Summary of trials comparing idarubicin and daunorubicin.

neutropenia, cardiotoxicity and overall survival between the 2 drugs. The second study also showed that idarubicin was associated with improved rates of complete remission as well as overall survival, compared to daunorubicin [16, 40].

A summary of the trials comparing idarubicin and high dose daunorubicin is presented in **Table 2.**

4. Mitoxantrone

Mitoxantrone, an anthraquinone derivative, has been extensively used with cytarabine as part of induction chemotherapy in patients with AML. It has been shown to be equally effective, if not better, when compared to daunorubicin. Nonetheless, it has not been adapted readily into the clinical practice of upfront induction chemotherapy and is often incorporated into the treatment algorithm in the relapse and refractory setting. There are 2 randomized trials comparing mitoxantrone, idarubicin and daunorubicin which will be discussed in the subsequent section.

The AML-10 study was a randomized phase III study comparing daunorubicin, idarubicin and mitoxantrone in 2157 patients, ≤60 years of age, with AML [41]. Remission induction was not given in the traditional 7 + 3 manner and consisted of cytarabine 100 mg/m^2 on days 1–10, etoposide 100 mg/m^2 on days 1–5 and either daunorubicin 50 mg/m^2, idarubicin 10 mg/m^2 or mitoxantrone 12 mg/m^2 on days 1, 3 and 5. A second round of the same regimen was given to those with a partial remission to the first round.

There was no difference in the rate of complete remission between the 3 anthracyclines. Nearly a quarter of patients, in each arm, proceeded to allogeneic stem cell transplant. After a median follow-up of 5.6 years, there was no difference in median and 5-year overall survival between the 3 arms. Even after adjusting for other variables, the results remained the same. For patients without a donor, the disease-free survival and survival from complete remission were longer in the idarubicin and mitoxantrone arm than in the daunorubicin arm. There was no difference for patients with a donor.

An ECOG phase III compared daunorubicin 45 mg/m^2, idarubicin 12 mg/m^2 and mitoxantrone 12 mg/m^2, given with continuous cytarabine, as 7 + 3 in older adults with AML [42]. The study enrolled 362 patients with a median age of 67 years. A second round of the same induction was given to patients with residual disease (>5% blasts) on day 14 bone marrow biopsy. There was no statistically significant difference for the rates of complete remission between the 3 arms. Furthermore, there was no difference observed in terms of toxicity profile, disease-free survival and overall survival between the 3 induction regimens.

5. CPX-351 (Vyxeos)

CPX-351 is a liposomal encapsulation of cytarabine and daunorubicin at a fixed synergistic molar ratio of 5:1. Using ratio-metric dosing, instead of the traditionally used maximum tolerated dose (MTD), potentially enhances the efficacy of drugs by maintaining the fixed drug ratio for a longer time in the blood. In the conventional form (MTD), the blood concentration or ratio of the drug(s), after infusion, may change immediately depending on the individual agent's pharmacokinetics, raising concern for inferior efficacy. A liposomal encapsulation, by evading first pass metabolism, may overcome this concern and lead to greater uptake by leukemia cells. Through this mechanism, an increased cytotoxic effect of the drugs is observed, leading to prolonged myelosuppression, in addition to apoptosis of leukemia cells [43, 44].

The liposome of daunorubin:cytarabine 44 mg/m^2:100 mg/m^2 is FDA approved for the treatment of adults with therapy related AML or AML with myelodysplasia-related changes. A phase III study compared cytarabine + liposomal daunorubicin (CPX-351, Vyxeos) to 7 + 3 (daunorubicin 60 mg/m^2), in older patients (60–75 years) with secondary AML. The study enrolled 309 patients. CPX-351 was associated with a higher remission rate (47.7% vs. 33.3%, $p = 0.016$) as well as improved median overall survival (9.6 m vs. 5.9 m, HR 0.69, $p = 0.003$) compared to 7 + 3. There was no difference in early mortality between the two treatments. Prolonged neutropenia and thrombocytopenia were observed with CPX-351 [19].

Although the study above was limited to older patients, the FDA approved CPX-351 for all adults. The reason being that therapy related AML or AML with myelodysplasia-related changes are thought to be biologically aggressive subtypes, regardless of age. Whether CPX-351 is superior, in patients <60 years old, to 7 + 3 using either daunorubicin 90 mg/m^2 or idarubicin is not known. The results of ongoing studies in younger patients as well as planned clinical trials using CPX-351 in combination with targeted therapy or immunotherapy should help identify additional subsets of patients that may derive benefit from this drug.

6. Conclusion

AML is a heterogenous disease and the treatment plan for every patient is different. Both patient and disease related variables help determine the appropriate treatment option for each case. It is challenging to state the outright superiority of one anthracycline over another, but some useful conclusions can be drawn from the evidence presented above.

When choosing between 45 mg/m^2, 60 mg/m^2 and 90 mg/m^2 of daunorubicin, it is reasonable to look at patient age and cytogenetic and molecular abnormalities (if available in a timely manner), before picking one. Daunorubicin 45 mg/m^2 should be used for older patients >65 years of age based on the available evidence. It is probably safe and effective to use daunorubicin 60 mg/m^2 in this age group, but unfortunately there is lack of randomized data to support one dose over the other. For patients younger than 65 years of age, daunorubicin 90 mg/m^2 is superior to daunorubicin 45 mg/m^2. All cytogenetic risk categories and FLT3, NPM1 and DNMT3A-mutant AML seem to derive benefit from daunorubicin 90 mg/m^2. However, data is emerging to suggest that daunorubicin 60 mg/m^2 can effectively replace daunorubicin 90 mg/m^2.

Idarubicin is superior to daunorubicin 45 mg/m^2, when used as 7 + 3, in younger patients. It also appears to be as safe and effective as daunorubicin 90 mg/m^2, except for FLT3-mutant AML where daunorubicin 90 mg/m^2 may have a slight advantage. One caveat to the idarubicin vs. high dose daunorubicin studies is the small representation of older patients (>65 years). For older patients fit for intensive therapy, daunorubicin 45 mg/m^2, may still be the first choice.

Mitoxantrone is comparable to both idarubicin and daunorubicin. It's use in upfront therapy is still not as common as the other 2 available agents. CPX-351 should be the first choice in patients with secondary AML.

Whereas novel drug regimens are emerging in the treatment of AML, intensive chemotherapy still plays a significant role. Anthracyclines will serve as the backbone of AML treatment in fit patients and therefore it is important to know which type and dose to select in the appropriate setting.

Conflict of interest

The authors declare no conflict of interest.

Author details

Sravanti Rangaraju and Omer Jamy*
Division of Hematology/Oncology, Department of Medicine, University of Alabama at Birmingham, Birmingham, AL, USA

*Address all correspondence to: omerjamy@gmail.com

References

[1] Hahn AW et al. *How center volumes affect early outcomes in acute myeloid leukemia*. Clinical Lymphoma, Myeloma & Leukemia. 2015;**15**(11):646-654

[2] Döhner H et al. *Diagnosis and management of AML in adults: 2017 ELN recommendations from an international expert panel*. Blood. 2017;**129**(4):424-447

[3] Song X et al. *Incidence, survival, and risk factors for adults with acute myeloid leukemia not otherwise specified and acute myeloid leukemia with recurrent genetic abnormalities: Analysis of the surveillance, epidemiology, and end results (SEER) database, 2001-2013*. Acta Haematologica. 2018;**139**(2):115-127

[4] Jamy O et al. *Observation versus immediate Reinduction for acute myeloid leukemia patients with indeterminate day 14 bone marrow results*. Clinical Lymphoma, Myeloma & Leukemia. 2020;**20**(1):31-38

[5] Patel JP et al. *Prognostic relevance of integrated genetic profiling in acute myeloid leukemia*. New England Journal of Medicine. 2012;**366**(12):1079-1089

[6] Jamy O et al. *Outcomes of fludarabine, high dose cytarabine and granulocyte-colony stimulating factor (FLAG) as re-induction for residual acute myeloid leukemia on day 14 bone marrow*. Leukemia Research. 2018;**74**:64-67

[7] Etienne A et al. *Comorbidity is an independent predictor of complete remission in elderly patients receiving induction chemotherapy for acute myeloid leukemia*. Cancer. 2007;**109**(7):1376-1383

[8] Malfuson JV et al. *Risk factors and decision criteria for intensive chemotherapy in older patients with acute myeloid leukemia*. Haematologica. 2008;**93**(12):1806-1813

[9] Dombret H, Itzykson R. *How and when to decide between epigenetic therapy and chemotherapy in patients with AML*. Hematology. American Society of Hematology. Education Program. **2017**;**2017**(1):45-53

[10] Sorror ML et al. *Development and validation of a novel acute myeloid leukemia-composite model to estimate risks of mortality*. JAMA Oncology. 2017;**3**(12):1675-1682

[11] Vey, N., Low-intensity regimens versus standard-intensity induction strategies in acute myeloid leukemia. Ther Adv Hematol, 2020. 11: p. 2040620720913010.

[12] DiNardo CD et al. *Azacitidine and venetoclax in previously untreated acute myeloid leukemia*. The New England Journal of Medicine. 2020;**383**(7):617-629

[13] Rai KR et al. *Treatment of acute myelocytic leukemia: A study by cancer and leukemia group B*. Blood. 1981;**58**(6):1203-1212

[14] Yates J et al. *Cytosine arabinoside with daunorubicin or adriamycin for therapy of acute myelocytic leukemia: A CALGB study*. Blood. 1982;**60**(2):454-462

[15] Pophali P, Litzow M. *What is the best daunorubicin dose and schedule for acute myeloid leukemia induction?* Current Treatment Options in Oncology. 2017;**18**(1):3

[16] Wang J et al. *Meta-analysis of randomised clinical trials comparing idarubicin + cytarabine with daunorubicin + cytarabine as the induction chemotherapy in patients with newly diagnosed acute myeloid leukaemia*. PLoS One. 2013;**8**(4):e60699

[17] Wiedower E, Jamy O, Martin MG. *Induction of acute myeloid leukemia with*

Idarubicin. Cytarabine and Cladribine. Anticancer Res. 2015;**35**(11):6287-6290

[18] Stone RM et al. *Midostaurin plus chemotherapy for acute myeloid leukemia with a FLT3 mutation*. The New England Journal of Medicine. 2017;**377**(5):454-464

[19] Lancet JE et al. *CPX-351 (cytarabine and daunorubicin) liposome for injection versus conventional cytarabine plus daunorubicin in older patients with newly diagnosed secondary acute myeloid leukemia*. Journal of Clinical Oncology. 2018;**36**(26):2684-2692

[20] Löwenberg B et al. *High-dose daunorubicin in older patients with acute myeloid leukemia*. The New England Journal of Medicine. 2009;**361**(13):1235-1248

[21] Fernandez HF et al. *Anthracycline dose intensification in acute myeloid leukemia*. The New England Journal of Medicine. 2009;**361**(13):1249-1259

[22] Luskin MR et al. *Benefit of high-dose daunorubicin in AML induction extends across cytogenetic and molecular groups*. Blood. 2016;**127**(12):1551-1558

[23] Lee JH et al. *A randomized trial comparing standard versus high-dose daunorubicin induction in patients with acute myeloid leukemia*. Blood. 2011;**118**(14):3832-3841

[24] Khattry N et al. *Comparison of 2 doses of daunorubicin (45mg/m2 vs 60mg/m2) in induction therapy of patients of de novo acute myeloid leukemia*. Journal of Clinical Oncology. 2006;**24**(18_suppl):6581-6581

[25] Burnett AK et al. *A randomized comparison of daunorubicin 90 mg/m2 vs 60 mg/m2 in AML induction: Results from the UK NCRI AML17 trial in 1206 patients*. Blood. 2015;**125**(25):3878-3885

[26] Burnett AK, Russell NH, Hills RK. *Higher daunorubicin exposure benefits FLT3 mutated acute myeloid leukemia*. Blood. 2016;**128**(3):449-452

[27] Christoph Röllig, B.S., Christoph Schliemann, Nael Alakel, Regina Herbst, Alwin Krämer, et al., *REMISSION AND SURVIVAL AFTER 90 MG VERSUS 60 MG DAUNORUBICIN IN 7+3 STANDARD INDUCTION FOR NEWLY DIAGNOSED ACUTE MYELOID LEUKEMIA: RESULTS FROM THE RANDOMIZED CONTROLLED SAL-DAUNODOUBLE TRIAL.* European Hematology Association 2020.

[28] Berman E et al. *Results of a randomized trial comparing idarubicin and cytosine arabinoside with daunorubicin and cytosine arabinoside in adult patients with newly diagnosed acute myelogenous leukemia*. Blood. 1991;**77**(8):1666-1674

[29] Mandelli F et al. *A randomised clinical trial comparing idarubicin and cytarabine to daunorubicin and cytarabine in the treatment of acute non-lymphoid leukaemia. A multicentric study from the Italian Co-operative Group GIMEMA*. Eur J Cancer. 1991;**27**(6):750-755

[30] Vogler WR et al. *A phase III trial comparing idarubicin and daunorubicin in combination with cytarabine in acute myelogenous leukemia: A southeastern cancer study group study*. Journal of Clinical Oncology. 1992;**10**(7):1103-1111

[31] Wiernik PH et al. *Cytarabine plus idarubicin or daunorubicin as induction and consolidation therapy for previously untreated adult patients with acute myeloid leukemia*. Blood. 1992;**79**(2):313-319

[32] Reiffers J et al. *A prospective randomized trial of idarubicin vs daunorubicin in combination chemotherapy for acute myelogenous leukemia of the age group 55 to 75*. Leukemia. 1996;**10**(3):389-395

[33] Lee JH et al. *Prospective randomized comparison of Idarubicin and high-dose daunorubicin in induction chemotherapy for newly diagnosed acute myeloid leukemia*. Journal of Clinical Oncology. 2017;**35**(24):2754-2763

[34] Ohtake S et al. *Randomized study of induction therapy comparing standard-dose idarubicin with high-dose daunorubicin in adult patients with previously untreated acute myeloid leukemia: The JALSG AML201 study*. Blood. 2011;**117**(8):2358-2365

[35] Pautas C et al. *Randomized study of intensified anthracycline doses for induction and recombinant interleukin-2 for maintenance in patients with acute myeloid leukemia age 50 to 70 years: Results of the ALFA-9801 study*. Journal of Clinical Oncology. 2010;**28**(5):808-814

[36] Chevallier P et al. *Tandem versus single autologous peripheral blood stem cell transplantation as post-remission therapy in adult acute myeloid leukemia patients under 60 in first complete remission: Results of the multicenter prospective phase III GOELAMS LAM-2001 trial*. Leukemia. 2010;**24**(7):1380-1385

[37] Récher C et al. *Long-term results of a randomized phase 3 trial comparing idarubicin and daunorubicin in younger patients with acute myeloid leukaemia*. Leukemia. 2014;**28**(2):440-443

[38] Gardin C et al. *Postremission treatment of elderly patients with acute myeloid leukemia in first complete remission after intensive induction chemotherapy: Results of the multicenter randomized acute leukemia French association (ALFA) 9803 trial*. Blood. 2007;**109**(12):5129-5135

[39] Gardin C et al. *Superior long-term outcome with idarubicin compared with high-dose daunorubicin in patients with acute myeloid leukemia age 50 years and older*. Journal of Clinical Oncology. 2013;**31**(3):321-327

[40] Owattanapanich W et al. *Efficacy and toxicity of Idarubicin versus high-dose daunorubicin for induction chemotherapy in adult acute myeloid leukemia: A systematic review and meta-analysis*. Clinical Lymphoma, Myeloma & Leukemia. 2018;**18**(12):814-821.e3

[41] Mandelli F et al. *Daunorubicin versus mitoxantrone versus idarubicin as induction and consolidation chemotherapy for adults with acute myeloid leukemia: The EORTC and GIMEMA groups study AML-10*. Journal of Clinical Oncology. 2009;**27**(32):5397-5403

[42] Rowe JM et al. *A phase 3 study of three induction regimens and of priming with GM-CSF in older adults with acute myeloid leukemia: A trial by the eastern cooperative oncology group*. Blood. 2004;**103**(2):479-485

[43] Alfayez M et al. *CPX-351 (vyxeos) in AML*. Leukemia & Lymphoma. 2020;**61**(2):288-297

[44] Tzogani K et al. *EMA review of daunorubicin and cytarabine encapsulated in liposomes (Vyxeos, CPX-351) for the treatment of adults with newly diagnosed, therapy-related acute myeloid leukemia or acute myeloid leukemia with Myelodysplasia-related changes*. The Oncologist. 2020;**25**(9):e1414-e1420

Chapter 10

Treatment of AML in Older Patients

Jacobien Hilberink and Gerwin Huls

Abstract

Acute myeloid leukaemia (AML) is a disease mostly diagnosed in older adults. Treatment of older patients with AML remains challenging with higher rates of intrinsic chemotherapeutic resistance and decreased treatment tolerance. Indeed AML in older patients has different clinical and biologic characteristics compared to younger patients. Several treatment options are available for treatment of AML in older patients, namely conventional intensive chemotherapy ('3 + 7'), low-dose cytarabine, and hypomethylating agents. Combinations with new drugs have been recently approved or are in advanced stages of clinical testing, namely venetoclax, midostaurin, glasdegib. Clinical decision making should take into account disease characteristics (e.g. cytogenetic and molecular abnormalities, white blood cell count), patient characteristics (e.g. performance, comorbidities, geriatric assessment) and patients' preference when considering which treatment option is most suitable for the older patient. Allogeneic haematopoietic cell transplantation (HCT) as post-remission strategy should also be considered for older patients with AML. Allogeneic HCT following reduced-intensity conditioning or non-myeloablative conditioning has made this treatment option more suitable for older patients with a reduction in treatment-related mortality.

Keywords: AML, older patients, hypomethylating agents, venetoclax, transplantation

1. Acute myeloid leukaemia: a disease of older individuals

Acute myeloid leukaemia (AML) is a heterogeneous group of malignant haematological diseases. It is predominantly a disease of older adults, with a median age at diagnosis of 68 years [1]. Indeed, 75% of the AML patients are older than 60 years (**Figure 1**). Besides a higher incidence of AML at older age, AML in older adults differs biologically and clinically from AML in younger adults [2]. AML in older adults is characterised by a markedly reduced long-term survival resulting from the combination of poor chemotherapeutic tolerance and inherent chemotherapy resistance compared with younger AML patients [3]. AML in older adults has a lower frequency of favourable core-binding chromosomal abnormalities and a higher incidence of complex aberrant karyotypes [4, 5]. These differences in clinical and cellular behaviour of AML in older adults suggest activation of different target genes by oncogenic events in aged stem or progenitor cells compared with younger stem or progenitor cells. Indeed a distinct gene-expression profile noted for older compared to younger adults with AML supports a molecular basis for disparities in outcome related to age [2, 5, 6]. In addition, more frequent comorbid conditions,

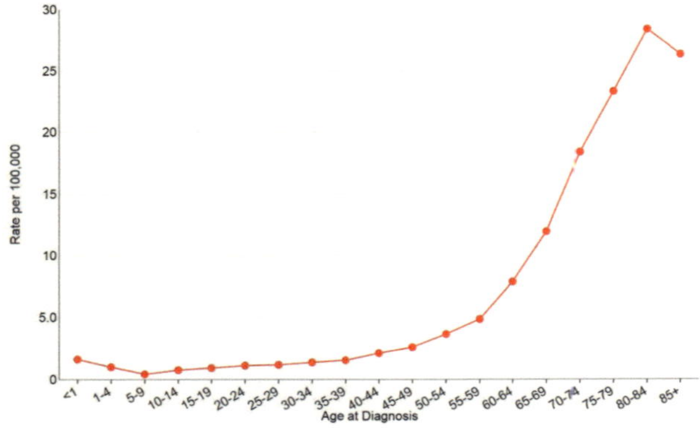

Figure 1.
AML incidence rates by age at diagnosis (2013–2017). Reproduced from: SEER Cancer Stat Facts: Acute Myeloid Leukaemia. National Cancer Institute. Bethesda, MD, https://seer.cancer.gov/statfacts/html/amyl.html

the decreased immune competence of older patients and psychosocial factors influence treatment outcome of AML in older adults. The effects of age on both disease- and patient-related factors result in a lower rate of disease remission, a higher incidence of early death during chemotherapy, and a reduced probability of long-term survival [2, 3]. In light of this, population based studies report a treatment percentage of only 30% in AML patients aged 65 and older [7, 8]. Indeed, regardless of treatment, outcomes for older AML patients are unsatisfactory, with median overall survival (OS) of 5–10 months and 5-year survival of about 10% [9–11]. In contrast with the progress made for younger adults with AML, the treatment in older adults has not improved significantly in recent decades, despite numerous efforts to find effective and tolerable treatments [12].

2. Treatment options in older adults with AML

The optimal treatment of older adults with AML in daily clinical practice remains challenging, and is dependent on patient characteristics (age, performance, comorbidities), disease characteristics (cytogenetic and molecular abnormalities, white blood cell count) and the preference of the patient [3]. Regular treatment options include: best supportive care (BSC), low-dose chemotherapy (e.g. low dose cytarabine (LDAC)), hypomethylating agents (HMA), and intensive chemotherapy (IC) (**Table 1**).

Population data from the Swedish Acute Leukaemia Registry suggest the majority of older patients should be considered candidate for antileukemic therapy [13]. However, only few prospective randomised studies in older AML patients are available to guide treatment decisions. A pivotal clinical trial, although with a limited number of patients (n = 60), showed that standard IC decreases early death rates and improves long-term survival compared with BSC [14]. Also LDAC and gemtuzumab ozogamicin (GO) have been reported to result in superior survival compared with BSC; although neither had an effect in patients with adverse cytogenetics [15, 16].

In addition to IC and LDAC, the armamentarium for the treatment of AML has been expanded in recent years with two cytosine analogues with DNA hypomethylating properties: azacitidine and decitabine. The hypomethylating agents (HMAs) azacitidine and decitabine have relatively mild side effects and are particularly feasible for the treatment of AML in older patients and patients with comorbidities.

	Response: CR/CRi (%)	Median OS (months)	2-year OS (%)	5-year OS (%)
Intensive chemotherapy [9, 14, 30]	41–70	10–20	12–42	10–30
+ **Gemtuzumab ozogamicin** [31, 32, 35, 36]	36–78	7–34	53	36
Low dose chemotherapy [15]	18	4	—	—
Hypomethylating agents [17, 18, 40, 41, 44]	15–47	8–13 (25)	20–50	Not curative, unless consolidated with HCT
New agents	—	—	—	—
A. Venetoclax	—	—	—	
+ HMA [19]	66	14.7	—	
+ LDAC [60]	48	8.4	—	
B. IDH inhibitors [61, 62]	30–40	11–13	—	
	—	—		
C. FLT3-inhibitors + IC [33]	78		45.6	
D. Glasdegib				
+ IC [65]	40	14.7		
+ LDAC [66]	17	8.8		
D. CPX-513 (68,67)	53–67	15		

Table 1.
Treatment options and outcomes for older AML patients.

Importantly, both azacitidine and decitabine have proven efficacy in patients with adverse cytogenetic abnormalities. Although not in their primary analyses, recent phase III trials have shown the superiority of azacitidine and decitabine treatment compared with conventional care for older AML patients [17, 18].

New combinations of HMAs with targeted drugs are being explored. Recently, the results of a phase 3 study of azacitidine in combination with venetoclax versus azacitidine alone in treatment-naïve adults with AML, who were ineligible for standard induction therapy, have been reported (VIALE-A trial; NCT02993523). This study confirmed the additive value of venetoclax to azacitidine treatment by an increase in remission rate from 28–66% and an increase in median OS from 9.6 months to 14.7 months [19]. The high remission rate which was achieved by adding venetoclax to azacitidine treatment is striking. Studies are ongoing to explore the added value of IDH1 or IDH2 inhibitors (ivosidenib or enasidenib) in combination with azacitidine and azacitidine plus venetoclax, for those older AML patients with mutated *IDH1* or *IDH2*.

2.1 Treatment selection: who is fit and who is not fit?

Optimal treatment selection for older patients also requires consideration of treatment tolerance and life expectancy, derived from the evaluation of comorbidities, physical function and cognition [2]. Charlson comorbidity index >1 and haematopoietic cell transplantation comorbidity index (HCT-CI) >2 have been reported to be associated with lower remission rates, increased early mortality and decreased survival in patients treated with IC [20–22]. In a study on 177 patients aged ≥65 years who received IC the early death rates were 3% if the HCT-CI score was 0, 11% if the HCT-CI score was 1 to 2, and 29% if the HCT-CI score was ≥3 [20].

In addition, performance status, scored according to ECOG or WHO guidelines, has shown to be associated with survival in several studies [10, 23, 24].

To adequately assess fitness in older patients, beyond performance status and comorbidities, geriatric assessment (GA) is attracting more attention. GA is an approach to the evaluation of multiple patient characteristics (i.e. physical function, comorbid disease(s), cognitive function, psychological state, social support, polypharmacy, nutritional status) to help characterise individual patient complexity and discriminate among fit, vulnerable and frail patients. GA in older AML patients has been associated with treatment outcomes. In a single-institution prospective study conducted with AML patients ≥60 years of age treated with IC, geriatric assessment performed at diagnosis was associated with survival. In this study (n = 74, median age 68 years), impaired physical performance (measured as short physical performance battery (SPPB) score < 9) and impaired cognition (measured as modified mini-mental state (3MS) exam score < 77) were independently associated with OS, after accounting for other disease and patient characteristics [25]. In a study of 107 non-intensively treated AML patients, the scores for independence in activities of daily living and the Karnofsky score for performance status were associated with survival in multivariate analysis [21]. Although randomised data of comprehensive assessment of older AML patients are lacking, the above mentioned studies support the use of pre-treatment performance and comorbidity assessment in the setting of AML therapy.

2.2 Treatment selection: predicting outcome with algorithms.

Various studies have been undertaken with the aim to create prediction models for treatment effectiveness and to provide support for an educated treatment choice in the setting of AML. These algorithms include patient-specific factors (e.g. performance, comorbidity, body temperature, age) and disease-specific factors (e.g. cytogenetics, white blood cell counts, blast counts, primary or secondary leukaemia, haemoglobin level, platelet count, fibrinogen level, serum concentration of lactate dehydrogenase (LDH)) [23, 24, 26, 27]. However, most prediction models have not been successfully validated in independent cohorts of older patients. In addition, the data used to create most of these algorithms come from a patient population selected to receive intensive chemotherapy and therefore likely do not reflect the real world of older patients with AML. Although prediction models might be useful in identifying patients who are 'fit' for intensive chemotherapy, this does not automatically imply for AML patients with specific disease characteristics (or combinations) associated with poor outcome. This includes the high-risk AML subtypes with mutant *TP53*, complex cytogenetic abnormalities (in particular monosomal karyotype), mutations in *ASXL1* or *RUNX1* and high allelic burden *FLT3*-ITDs. An inclusive and validated prediction model for older AML patients has yet to be published.

3. Treatment of patients considered to be fit

The combination of anthracycline and cytarabine ('3 + 7') has been the standard of care for patients with AML for the last four decades [28]. However, the use of this regimen in older patients with AML does not yield similar results to those reported for younger patients, even in carefully selected patients. Although 50–60% of patients will attain a complete remission (CR), this does not translate into a similar survival benefit as for younger patients, with a 2-year survival of only 15–20% [3, 29]. To improve the outcome for older AML patients receiving intensive chemotherapy (IC) many studies have evaluated modifications of the traditional '3 + 7' combination. Strategies have included dose attenuation [9, 30], addition of gemtuzumab ozogamicin (GO) [31, 32], addition of midostaurin [33], addition of lenalidomide [34], and other attempts (e.g. growth factors, modulation of multidrug resistance).

The HOVON43 study assessed the effect of an escalated daunorubicin dose (90 mg/m^2 vs. 45 mg/m^2) in older AML patients (> 60 years) receiving conventional '3 + 7' chemotherapy [9]. Median age was 67 years and 24% of patients had an unfavourable or very unfavourable cytogenetic risk. Although the CR rate was higher in the escalated-treatment group (64% vs. 54% [P = 0.002]), this did not translate into a survival benefit (2-year OS 31% vs. 26% [P = 0.16]). However, an unplanned post-hoc analysis showed that patients in the escalated-treatment group who were 60 to 65 years of age had higher CR rates and increased survival compared to patients aged 60 to 65 years in the conventional dose group (CR rates 73% vs. 51% and 2-year OS 38% vs. 23%, respectively). These data suggest the survival benefit of an escalated dose of daunorubicin was limited to the younger part of older patients. The MRC-AML-14 study randomised patients four times to a higher (50 mg/m2) or lower (35 mg/m^2) dose of daunorubin, a higher (400 mg/m^2) or lower (200 mg/m^2) dose of cytarabine, allocation to receive the multidrug resistance modulator PSC-833 or not, and to receive three or four courses of treatment [30]. The CR rate was 54% and 5-year OS 12% for all patients, and no benefits were observed in either dose escalation groups, or from a fourth course of treatment.

Several studies investigated the addition of GO to standard chemotherapy to improve outcome in older AML patients. The MRC-AML-16-I study (addition of 3 mg/m^2 GO on day 1 of course 1) found 3-year relapse incidence and survival was significantly better in the GO arm (relapse 68% vs. 76%; survival 25% vs. 20%), although there was no difference in CR rate between both arms [31]. There was no difference in 30- or 60-day mortality and no major increase in toxicity with GO. The French ALFA-0701 trial investigated addition of fractionated doses of GO (3 mg/m^2 on day 1, 4, and 7) to standard chemotherapy and found similar results in patients aged 50–70 years. The CR rate did not differ between both arms (81% in GO-arm vs. 75% in no GO-arm), but survival was increased in the GO-arm (median 34 vs. 19 months; 2-year OS 53.2% vs. 41.9%) [35]. However, in the EORTC-GIMEMA-AML17 trial, randomising patients to a course of GO (6 mg/m^2 on day 1 and 15) followed by IC or IC alone, a trend for inferior survival in the GO-arm was observed (median OS 7.1 vs. 10 months) [32]. Patients aged ≥70 years did significantly worse with GO due to the combined effect of increased induction mortality and poorer OS among those not achieving CR. This study incorporated a higher dose of GO (6 mg/m^2 vs. 3 mg/m^2). GO, especially in higher doses, has been associated with increased toxicity and after initial FDA approval in 2000 was voluntarily withdrawn in 2010 after safety concerns. Since then fractionated doses have been proved safe and efficacious in a large meta-analysis of five randomised controlled trials, leading to re-approval in 2017 [36].

There is ongoing discussion whether older AML patients benefit from treatment with intensive chemotherapy. Retrospective analysis of the outcomes 446 older AML patients (≥70 years) treated with intensive chemotherapy between 1990 and 2008 showed that despite a reasonable CR rate of 45%, the median OS was only 4.6 months and 1-year survival 28% [37]. The surprisingly low median OS was due to high 4-week and 8-week mortality rates of 26% and 36%, and the authors concluded that intensive chemotherapy may not be beneficial to most older patients with AML, although some subgroups (e.g. CBF AML and good risk status) might benefit. In response to this, a Swedish group published updated outcomes of 998 unselected older AML patients, of who 55% received intensive chemotherapy between 1997 and 2006 and concluded that older patients do benefit from intensive treatment with a median OS in *de novo* AML of over 1 year [13]. This highlights that choosing the optimal treatment for older patients with AML remains challenging.

4. Treatment of patients considered unfit for intensive chemotherapy: hypomethylating agents

For patients not eligible for intensive chemotherapy treatment a choice can be made between best supportive care (BSC), low dose chemotherapy (LDAC) or hypomethylating agents (HMAs). Several studies have shown the efficacy of the HMAs azacitidine and decitabine. In addition, HMAs are well-tolerated and have low extra-medullary toxicity. Therefore HMAs are very suitable for the treatment of older patients with AML.

Azacitidine was first studied in the context of high-risk myelodysplastic syndromes (MDS). A phase III trial conducted in intermediate-2 and high-risk MDS patients included a subset of patients with 20–30% blasts, who were reclassified to AML according to redefined WHO criteria [38, 39]. The relative efficacy and safety of azacitidine versus conventional care regimens (CCR; comprising prespecified allocation to BSC, LDAC, or IC) was thus compared in this subgroup of patients (n = 113) and showed an increased median OS (24.5 vs. 16.0 months, P = 0.005) and increased 2-year survival (50% vs. 16%, P = 0.001) for azacitidine-treated patients compared with CCR patients [40]. In addition, a phase III study on the efficacy of azacitidine versus CCR (standard IC, LDAC or BSC) in newly diagnosed AML patients with >30% blasts was conducted [17]. The median OS was longer in the azacitidine group compared to the CCR group (10.4 vs. 6.5 months), although in multivariate analysis significance was lost (HR 0.85 [95% CI 0.69–1.03], P = 0.101). However, in a pre-planned sensitivity analysis censoring for subsequent AML therapy, the median OS was 12.1 months versus 6.9 months in the azacitidine-arm and CCR-arm respectively, with a stratified HR 0.76 (95% CI 0.60–0.96, P = 0.019). Azacitidine was well tolerated as more than half of the patients received six or more treatment cycles. The difference in median OS between the two reported studies (24.5 months vs. 12.1 months) could be explained by the lower blast count in the first study and thereby selection of more indolent disease. Unfortunately both studies were not powered to detect direct differences between azacitidine treatment and intensive chemotherapy.

Decitabine is another hypomethylating agent registered for treatment of AML. Two decitabine schedules are currently in use in clinical practice: the 5-day schedule and the 10-day schedule. A randomised phase III trial compared the efficacy and safety of 5-day decitabine (20 mg/m^2) (n = 242) with treatment choice of BSC (n = 28) or LDAC (n = 215) in older patients ($\geq$ 65 years) with newly diagnosed AML and poor- or intermediate-risk cytogenetics [18]. The CR rate in the decitabine group was 15.7%. Although the planned primary analysis after 396 deaths did not show a significant improvement of OS with decitabine versus treatment choice (median OS 7.7 months vs. 5.0 months), an unplanned analysis after 446 deaths showed a significant benefit for decitabine (HR 0.82 [95% CI 0.68–0.99], P = 0.037). A small but pivotal phase II trial in 53 patients evaluated the effect of a longer 10-day decitabine schedule and found an increased CR rate of 47% and overall response of 64% with a median OS of 13 months [41]. The beneficial effects of the 10-day decitabine schedule were confirmed in two large single-centre retrospective studies that found response rates and median OS of 40% and 11 months, and 35% and 11 months, respectively [42, 43]. Recently, the result of a phase II trial directly comparing 5-day versus 10-day decitabine treatment was reported. The researchers concluded both schedules have similar efficacy (CR rates 29% vs. 30% [P = 0.88], median OS 5.5 vs. 6.0 months [P = 0.47]), although there was an uncorrected imbalance in disease characteristics favouring the 5-day schedule and the randomisation allocation was skewed towards the 10-day schedule [44]. Therefore caution has to be taken when interpreting the results. However, these data show that decitabine, both in 5-day and 10-day schedules, is efficient and suggest that decitabine as a single agent might provide a framework upon which to build future combination studies to improve outcomes for older AML patients.

Guadecitabine is a next generation HMA given subcutaneously which provides prolonged in vivo exposure to its active metabolite decitabine, thus offering potential clinical advantages over current HMAs. In a large randomised trial 815 untreated AML patients not eligible for IC were randomised to either guadecitabine (5 days 60 mg/m^2 every 4 weeks) or a preselected treatment of azacitidine, decitabine, or LDAC (ASTRAL-1 trial, NCT02920008). Although this trial showed that guadecitabine is an effective drug, the trial did not achieve its primary endpoints of statistically significant superiority of guadecitabine vs. preselected treatment for CR or OS [45].

ASTX727 is a next generation HMA with a unique fixed-dose combination of the hypomethylating agent decitabine and the novel cytidine deaminase inhibitor, E7727 (cedazuridine). ASTX727 was designed to deliver decitabine by oral administration. By inhibiting cytidine deaminase, cedazuridine inhibits the major mechanism by which decitabine is degraded in the gastrointestinal tract and liver, and the combination therefore permits the efficient delivery of decitabine orally. It has shown promising effects in a phase II trial conducted in intermediate- and high-risk myelodysplastic syndromes and chronic myelomonocytic leukaemia patients [46]. This trial is now expanding to include AML patients (NCT04093570).

An important question is whether intensive chemotherapy is superior to hypomethylating agents in older AML patients. The results of the above reported clinical trials cannot be directly compared due to differences in patient population studied. The MD Anderson Cancer Center reported the results of a retrospective cohort study of 671 patients, including 114 patients treated with HMAs (either azacitidine or decitabine) and 557 patients treated with IC [47]. Both groups were balanced according to cytogenetics and performance status and were older than 65 years. Patients who had received IC had a higher CR rate compared to patients who had received HMAs (42% vs. 28% [P = 0.001], respectively). However, the median OS was comparable in the 2 groups (6.7 vs. 6.5 months, P = 0.41). Multivariate analysis confirmed that type of AML therapy (IC or HMAs) was not an independent prognostic factor for survival. Interestingly, this study revealed that decitabine was associated with improved median OS compared with azacitidine (8.8 vs. 5.5 months, respectively, P = .03), also in multivariate analysis. No published prospective randomised trials have compared the efficacy of azacitidine with decitabine nor the efficacy of intensive chemotherapy ('3 + 7') with hypomethylating agents. The results of the EORTC-1301 phase III trial, comparing upfront treatment with intensive chemotherapy or decitabine, are eagerly awaited (NCT02172872).

5. Treatment of patients considered not to be fit: LDAC

Low-dose cytarabine (LDAC) (20 mg twice daily for 10 days) has been used in the treatment of AML for several years. Treatment with LDAC has low toxicity and a higher CR rate than best supportive care (18% vs. 1%) [15]. Although the OS for the LDAC-treated group has been demonstrated to be statistically significantly better, it is worth noting that in absolute terms, the therapeutic advantage is marginal, with a prolongation of OS of only a few months. Additionally, the benefit is restricted to the small fraction of patients who achieve a response (median survival 19 months vs. 2 months in responders vs. non-responders respectively) [15]. Patients with adverse cytogenetics do not seem to benefit from LDAC. Combinations of LDAC with other agents have been tested in clinical trials and although some additions resulted in higher CR rates survival was not improved [48–53]. Thus, the OS in patients receiving LDAC is still highly unsatisfactory (median 5 months) [3]. Recently, the results of the VIALE-C trial have been reported, demonstrating an increased efficacy by adding venetoclax to LDAC (see 7.1).

6. New developments

Since 2017 the FDA has approved 8 new drugs for the treatment of AML [54]. New developments to treat AML, especially in older patients, include 1) drugs targeting specific signalling pathways (like the hedgehog pathway or apoptosis); 2) drugs specifically targeting mutations in AML (e.g. targeting the epigenetic modifiers IDH1/IDH2 and mutated cytokine receptor FLT3) and 3) an alternative formulation of classic chemotherapeutic drugs (CPX-315).

6.1 Venetoclax

Venetoclax (ABT-199/GDC-0199), an orally available inhibitor of the anti-apoptotic molecule Bcl-2, has shown great efficacy in chronic lymphocytic leukaemia [55–57]. After observing single-agent activity in AML cell lines [58], venetoclax has been tested as monotherapy in relapsed and refractory AML patients showing activity with a CR/CRi rate of 19% [59]. Promising results have been reported for combinatorial studies with venetoclax in AML. In the randomised phase 3 trial VIALE-C (LDAC +/− venetoclax) 211 patients were randomised 2:1 to venetoclax (n = 143) or placebo (n = 68) in 28-day cycles, plus LDAC on days 1 to 10 [60]. The primary analysis showed a 25% reduction in risk of death with venetoclax plus LDAC vs. LDAC alone, although not statistically significant (hazard ratio [HR], 0.75; P = .11), and a median OS of 7.2 vs. 4.1 months, respectively. An unplanned analysis with additional 6-month follow-up did demonstrate a significant benefit with a median OS of 8.4 months for venetoclax added to LDAC (HR, 0.70; P = .04).

In addition, the results of a phase 3 study of venetoclax in combination with azacitidine versus azacitidine alone in treatment-naïve older AML patients, who were ineligible for standard induction therapy, have recently been reported (VIALE-A trial; NCT02993523). This study confirms the additive value of venetoclax to azacitidine by a significant increase in CR/CRi rate from 28–66% and an increase in median OS from 9.6 months to 14.7 months [19]. The high remission rate which can be achieved by adding venetoclax to azacitidine treatment is striking. The impressive results of this study will likely make the combination of an hypomethylating agent with venetoclax the new standard for the treatment of older unfit AML patients.

6.2 IDH inhibitors

IDH mutations are present in approximately 20% of AML patients and are more frequent in older patients. Mutations in *IDH* lead to the production of the oncometabolite 2-hydroxyglutarate and result in DNA hypermethylation and arrest of myeloid differentiation [54]. Inhibition of these mutant metabolic enzymes by ivosidenib (IDH1) and enasidenib (IDH2) induces myeloid differentiation of leukaemic blasts. In a subgroup analysis of 34 newly diagnosed AML patients unfit for standard chemotherapy harbouring IDH1 mutations, monotherapy with ivosidenib resulted in a remission rate of 42.4% and median OS of 12.6 months [61]. In a phase I/II trial of older untreated AML patients, enasidenib induced a response in 30.8% of patients of whom 18% had a complete remission and a median OS of 11.3 months [62]. In addition to the proven efficacy and tolerability, ivosidenib and enasidenib are orally available, making them attractive for treatment of older AML patients. Both inhibitors are under investigation in combination with other AML treatments, including intensive chemotherapy ("3 + 7") and hypomethylating agents.

6.3 FLT3 inhibitors: midostaurin and gilteritinib

The *FLT3* mutations (mainly *FLT3* internal tandem duplications (*FLT3*-ITD), but also tyrosine kinase mutations (*FLT3*-TKD)) occur in about 20–30% of adult AML patients, although its prevalence decreases in older patients. The RATIFY study proved the favourable impact of adding midostaurin to intensive chemotherapy for AML patients with mutated *FLT3* under 60 years of age [63]. In older patients with *FLT3*-ITD the CR rate and 2-year OS was 77.9% and 45.6% respectively with the addition of midostaurin to conventional chemotherapy [33]. In comparison to historical controls, addition of midostaurin resulted in significant risk reduction for an event (refractory disease, relapse, death) with an HR of 0.42. Based on the results of this study the treatment label of midostaurin was expanded to include older patients with mutated *FLT3*. New FLT3 inhibitors, like gilteritinib, have shown to be potent inhibitors of mutated *FLT3* in relapsed/refractory AML patients, though limited data is available on the safety and efficacy of gilteritinib when combined with intensive chemotherapy or hypomethylating agents.

6.4 Glasdegib

Glasdegib is small molecule inhibitor of the hedgehog receptor smoothened. The hedgehog pathway is important during embryogenesis but repressed after birth. However, aberrant hedgehog signalling has been identified in AML, particularly in leukaemic stem cells, and has been associated with chemoresistance [64]. Inhibition of hedgehog signalling with glasdegib has shown promising results. A phase II study evaluating the combination of glasdegib and intensive chemotherapy in patients over 55 years of age with newly diagnosed AML reported a CR rate of 40% and median OS of 14.7 months [65]. Glasdegib was also evaluated in combination with LDAC in older patients unfit for intensive chemotherapy. Patients receiving glasdegib + LDAC had increased CR rates, 17.0% vs. 2.3%, and improved median OS 8.8 vs. 4.9 months, compared to patients receiving LDAC alone [66]. Based on these results, the FDA has approved glasdegib in combination with LDAC for AML patients ≥75 years or patients ineligible for intensive chemotherapy. In addition, glasdegib is being evaluated in combination with hypomethylating agents and a phase III trial of glasdegib in combination with intensive chemotherapy is ongoing (BRIGHT AML1019, NCT03416179).

6.5 CPX-315

CPX-315 is a liposomal formulation that delivers a 5:1 fixed-molar ratio of cytarabine and daunorubicine. With the liposomal encapsulation both drugs can be delivered in a fixed ratio with the highest proportion of synergy to enhance treatment efficacy [67]. CPX-351 preferentially targets leukaemic cells to a greater degree than non-leukaemic cells in the bone marrow, leading to decreased cytotoxicity against normal haematopoietic cells [68]. A small study of CPX-351 as first-line therapy in 30 newly-diagnosed AML patients ≥65 years showed a promising remission rate of 53.2% with a median OS 14.5 months [68]. In a randomised phase II trial in older adults with untreated AML comparing CPX-351 and conventional '3 + 7' treatment a trend towards increased response rates was observed in the CPX-351 group, 66.7% vs. 51.2%. Survival was comparable between both treatment groups (14.7 vs. 12.9 for the CPX-351 and '3 + 7' group respectively). However, CPX-351 treatment was superior in the subset of secondary AML patients with a median OS of 12.1 months vs. 6.1 months in the '3 + 7' group [67]. Superiority of CPX-351 to conventional '3 + 7' chemotherapy in secondary AML, also including AML with MDS related changes, was confirmed in a phase III trial including 309 older AML patients. The observed remission rates were 47.7% vs. 33.3% and median OS was 9.6 vs. 6.0 months in favour of CPX-351 [69]. The safety profile of CPX-351 was similar to that of conventional chemotherapy.

7. Allogeneic haematopoietic cell transplantation in older patients

Allogeneic haematopoietic cell transplantation (HCT), as post-remission treatment, offers the highest potential for long-term survival and cure for patients with AML. For younger patients, the choice for consolidation with an allogeneic transplant is nuanced, as particular younger patients with high-risk disease, entailing high-risk mutations and presence of measurable residual disease after treatment, benefit post-remission treatment with an allogeneic HCT. As older patients generally have low chance for long-term survival, also if they have "good-risk" cytogenetic abnormalities, allogeneic HCT should be considered in older (fit) AML patients [10, 70, 71]. Nevertheless, only a minority of older patients actually receives an allogeneic HCT [72, 73]. Allogeneic HCT in older patients is limited by concerns related to treatment-related mortality (TRM) (e.g. TRM is >40% in patients with a HCT-comorbidity score ≥ 3) [74]. However, the development of less toxic conditioning regimens (reduced intensity conditioning (RIC) and non-myeloablative (NMA)), has been an important conceptual change that has created the opportunity for older patients with AML to receive an allogeneic HCT. These conditioning regimen are less dependent on cytotoxic effects of the conditioning regimen and more dependent on the graft-versus-leukaemia effect.

Several studies evaluating allogeneic HCT after RIC in older AML patients have shown promising results. A phase II study of 114 older patients receiving an allogeneic HCT after RIC with fludarabine and busalfan reported a 2-year OS of 48% with a non-relapse mortality (NRM) of 15%. However, cumulative incidence of relapse was 44% at 2 years [75]. A large retrospective study analysing the outcomes of 1080 AML patients who underwent allogeneic HCT after RIC found a 2-year OS of 36% in patients age ≥ 65 years, a NRM of 34%, and 2-year relapse probability of 33% [76]. This analysis included several age groups ranging from 40 to above 65 years and found no significant impact of age on NRM, relapse, disease-free survival, or OS. In addition, studies comparing allogeneic HCT after RIC to conventional post-remission treatments have reported favourable outcomes with allogeneic HCT after RIC. A study comparing allogeneic HCT after RIC (n = 97), chemotherapy (n = 44), autologous transplantation (n = 23), and no further treatment (n = 336) as post-remission therapy reported a 5-year OS of 35% for patients receiving allogeneic HCT after RIC compared to 26% and 21% for chemotherapy/autologous transplantation and no treatment, respectively [77]. Multivariate analysis confirmed the beneficial effect allogeneic HCT after RIC on 5-year survival. A comparison between allogeneic HCT after RIC and chemotherapy in patients age 60–70 years showed that allogeneic HCT after RIC was associated with a lower risk of relapse at 3 years (32 vs. 81%) although NRM was increased (36% vs. 4%), leading to an OS of 37% vs. 25% at 3 years [78]. These studies underscore the delicate balance between sufficient antileukemic effect and treatment toxicity, which is challenging in post-remission treatment of older AML patients.

The efficacy and safety of NMA conditioning consisting of low-dose total body irradiation alone or combine with fludarabine (90 mg/m^2) in older patients was evaluated in a prospective cohort of 372 patients aged 60 to 75 years. The OS at 5 years post-transplantation was 35% with an NRM of 27%. Relapse rate was 41% at 5 years indicating the need for further improvement [73]. Nevertheless, these data compare very favourably with historical data on long-term survival of about 10% after treatment of older AML patients with intensive chemotherapy without post-remission treatment with allogeneic HCT.

8. Refractory/relapsed AML

Treatment of relapsed or refractory (R/R) AML, in general, has presented challenges for haematologists for decades. Despite numerous clinical studies, outcomes are consistently disappointing with 5-year OS rates of ~10%. Allogeneic HCT at the time of second complete remission remains the only reliable option with curative potential. For older patients, treatment of R/R AML is even more difficult and outcomes poorer. However, the availability of new drugs, like venetoclax, gilteritinib, ivosidenib and enasidenib offer reasonable chances of temporally disease control with acceptable side effects. This implies the importance of detailed molecular analysis, also in the R/R setting, as the R/R disease might contain different (targetable) mutations. Phase 1 studies are generally an option for those patients with a strong wish to receive treatment. Finally, only best supportive care with antibiotics and transfusions can be a preferable option.

Author details

Jacobien Hilberink and Gerwin Huls*
Universitair Medisch Centrum Groningen, University of Groningen, The Netherlands

*Address all correspondence to: g.huls@umcg.nl

References

[1] Juliusson G, Antunovic P, Derolf A, Lehmann S, Mollgard L, Stockelberg D, et al. Age and acute myeloid leukemia: real world data on decision to treat and outcomes from the Swedish Acute Leukemia Registry. Blood. 2009;113(18):4179-87.

[2] Klepin HD, Rao AV, Pardee TS. Acute myeloid leukemia and myelodysplastic syndromes in older adults. J Clin Oncol. 2014;32(24):2541-52.

[3] Ossenkoppele G, Lowenberg B. How I treat the older patient with acute myeloid leukemia. Blood. 2015;125(5):767-74.

[4] Grimwade D, Walker H, Harrison G, Oliver F, Chatters S, Harrison CJ, et al. The predictive value of hierarchical cytogenetic classification in older adults with acute myeloid leukemia (AML): analysis of 1065 patients entered into the United Kingdom Medical Research Council AML11 trial. Blood. 2001;98(5):1312-20.

[5] de Jonge HJ, de Bont ES, Valk PJ, Schuringa JJ, Kies M, Woolthuis CM, et al. AML at older age: age-related gene expression profiles reveal a paradoxical down-regulation of p16INK4A mRNA with prognostic significance. Blood. 2009;114(14):2869-77.

[6] Pollyea DA, Kohrt HE, Medeiros BC. Acute myeloid leukaemia in the elderly: a review. Br J Haematol. 2011;152(5):524-42.

[7] Oran B, Weisdorf DJ. Survival for older patients with acute myeloid leukemia: a population-based study. Haematologica. 2012;97(12):1916-24.

[8] Menzin J, Lang K, Earle CC, Kerney D, Mallick R. The outcomes and costs of acute myeloid leukemia among the elderly. Arch Intern Med. 2002;162(14):1597-603.

[9] Lowenberg B, Ossenkoppele GJ, van Putten W, Schouten HC, Graux C, Ferrant A, et al. High-dose daunorubicin in older patients with acute myeloid leukemia. N Engl J Med. 2009;361(13):1235-48.

[10] Appelbaum FR, Gundacker H, Head DR, Slovak ML, Willman CL, Godwin JE, et al. Age and acute myeloid leukemia. Blood. 2006;107(9):3481-5.

[11] Dohner H, Weisdorf DJ, Bloomfield CD. Acute Myeloid Leukemia. N Engl J Med. 2015;373(12):1136-52.

[12] Burnett A, Wetzler M, Lowenberg B. Therapeutic advances in acute myeloid leukemia. J Clin Oncol. 2011;29(5):487-94.

[13] Juliusson G, Swedish AMLG. Most 70- to 79-year-old patients with acute myeloid leukemia do benefit from intensive treatment. Blood. 2011;117(12):3473-4.

[14] Lowenberg B, Zittoun R, Kerkhofs H, Jehn U, Abels J, Debusscher L, et al. On the value of intensive remission-induction chemotherapy in elderly patients of 65+ years with acute myeloid leukemia: a randomized phase III study of the European Organization for Research and Treatment of Cancer Leukemia Group. J Clin Oncol. 1989;7(9):1268-74.

[15] Burnett AK, Milligan D, Prentice AG, Goldstone AH, McMullin MF, Hills RK, et al. A comparison of low-dose cytarabine and hydroxyurea with or without all-trans retinoic acid for acute myeloid leukemia and high-risk myelodysplastic syndrome in patients not considered fit for intensive treatment. Cancer. 2007;109(6):1114-24.

[16] Amadori S, Suciu S, Selleslag D, Aversa F, Gaidano G, Musso M, et al.

Gemtuzumab Ozogamicin Versus Best Supportive Care in Older Patients With Newly Diagnosed Acute Myeloid Leukemia Unsuitable for Intensive Chemotherapy: Results of the Randomized Phase III EORTC-GIMEMA AML-19 Trial. J Clin Oncol. 2016;34(9):972-9.

[17] Dombret H, Seymour JF, Butrym A, Wierzbowska A, Selleslag D, Jang JH, et al. International phase 3 study of azacitidine vs conventional care regimens in older patients with newly diagnosed AML with >30% blasts. Blood. 2015;126(3):291-9.

[18] Kantarjian HM, Thomas XG, Dmoszynska A, Wierzbowska A, Mazur G, Mayer J, et al. Multicenter, randomized, open-label, phase III trial of decitabine versus patient choice, with physician advice, of either supportive care or low-dose cytarabine for the treatment of older patients with newly diagnosed acute myeloid leukemia. J Clin Oncol. 2012;30(21):2670-7.

[19] DiNardo CD, Jonas BA, Pullarkat V, Thirman MJ, Garcia JS, Wei AH, et al. Azacitidine and Venetoclax in Previously Untreated Acute Myeloid Leukemia. N Engl J Med. 2020;383(7):617-29.

[20] Giles FJ, Borthakur G, Ravandi F, Faderl S, Verstovsek S, Thomas D, et al. The haematopoietic cell transplantation comorbidity index score is predictive of early death and survival in patients over 60 years of age receiving induction therapy for acute myeloid leukaemia. Br J Haematol. 2007;136(4):624-7.

[21] Deschler B, Ihorst G, Platzbecker U, Germing U, Marz E, de Figuerido M, et al. Parameters detected by geriatric and quality of life assessment in 195 older patients with myelodysplastic syndromes and acute myeloid leukemia are highly predictive for outcome. Haematologica. 2013;98(2):208-16.

[22] Savic A, Kvrgic V, Rajic N, Urosevic I, Kovacevic D, Percic I, et al. The hematopoietic cell transplantation comorbidity index is a predictor of early death and survival in adult acute myeloid leukemia patients. Leuk Res. 2012;36(4):479-82.

[23] Kantarjian H, O'Brien S, Cortes J, Giles F, Faderl S, Jabbour E, et al. Results of intensive chemotherapy in 998 patients age 65 years or older with acute myeloid leukemia or high-risk myelodysplastic syndrome: predictive prognostic models for outcome. Cancer. 2006;106(5):1090-8.

[24] Wheatley K, Brookes CL, Howman AJ, Goldstone AH, Milligan DW, Prentice AG, et al. Prognostic factor analysis of the survival of elderly patients with AML in the MRC AML11 and LRF AML14 trials. Br J Haematol. 2009;145(5):598-605.

[25] Klepin HD, Geiger AM, Tooze JA, Kritchevsky SB, Williamson JD, Pardee TS, et al. Geriatric assessment predicts survival for older adults receiving induction chemotherapy for acute myelogenous leukemia. Blood. 2013;121(21):4287-94.

[26] Rollig C, Thiede C, Gramatzki M, Aulitzky W, Bodenstein H, Bornhauser M, et al. A novel prognostic model in elderly patients with acute myeloid leukemia: results of 909 patients entered into the prospective AML96 trial. Blood. 2010;116(6):971-8.

[27] Krug U, Rollig C, Koschmieder A, Heinecke A, Sauerland MC, Schaich M, et al. Complete remission and early death after intensive chemotherapy in patients aged 60 years or older with acute myeloid leukaemia: a web-based application for prediction of outcomes. Lancet. 2010;376(9757):2000-8.

[28] Yates J, Glidewell O, Wiernik P, Cooper MR, Steinberg D, Dosik H, et al.

Cytosine arabinoside with daunorubicin or adriamycin for therapy of acute myelocytic leukemia: a CALGB study. Blood. 1982;60(2):454-62.

[29] Krug U, Gale RP, Berdel WE, Muller-Tidow C, Stelljes M, Metzeler K, et al. Therapy of older persons with acute myeloid leukaemia. Leuk Res. 2017;60:1-10.

[30] Burnett AK, Milligan D, Goldstone A, Prentice A, McMullin MF, Dennis M, et al. The impact of dose escalation and resistance modulation in older patients with acute myeloid leukaemia and high risk myelodysplastic syndrome: the results of the LRF AML14 trial. Br J Haematol. 2009;145(3):318-32.

[31] Burnett AK, Russell NH, Hills RK, Kell J, Freeman S, Kjeldsen L, et al. Addition of gemtuzumab ozogamicin to induction chemotherapy improves survival in older patients with acute myeloid leukemia. J Clin Oncol. 2012;30(32):3924-31.

[32] Amadori S, Suciu S, Stasi R, Salih HR, Selleslag D, Muus P, et al. Sequential combination of gemtuzumab ozogamicin and standard chemotherapy in older patients with newly diagnosed acute myeloid leukemia: results of a randomized phase III trial by the EORTC and GIMEMA consortium (AML-17). J Clin Oncol. 2013;31(35):4424-30.

[33] Schlenk RF, Weber D, Fiedler W, Salih HR, Wulf G, Salwender H, et al. Midostaurin added to chemotherapy and continued single-agent maintenance therapy in acute myeloid leukemia with FLT3-ITD. Blood. 2019;133(8):840-51.

[34] Ossenkoppele GJ, Breems DA, Stuessi G, van Norden Y, Bargetzi M, Biemond BJ, et al. Lenalidomide added to standard intensive treatment for older patients with AML and high-risk MDS. Leukemia. 2020;34(7):1751-9.

[35] Castaigne S, Pautas C, Terre C, Raffoux E, Bordessoule D, Bastie JN, et al. Effect of gemtuzumab ozogamicin on survival of adult patients with de-novo acute myeloid leukaemia (ALFA-0701): a randomised, open-label, phase 3 study. Lancet. 2012;379(9825):1508-16.

[36] Hills RK, Castaigne S, Appelbaum FR, Delaunay J, Petersdorf S, Othus M, et al. Addition of gemtuzumab ozogamicin to induction chemotherapy in adult patients with acute myeloid leukaemia: a meta-analysis of individual patient data from randomised controlled trials. Lancet Oncol. 2014;15(9):986-96.

[37] Kantarjian H, Ravandi F, O'Brien S, Cortes J, Faderl S, Garcia-Manero G, et al. Intensive chemotherapy does not benefit most older patients (age 70 years or older) with acute myeloid leukemia. Blood. 2010;116(22):4422-9.

[38] Fenaux P, Mufti GJ, Hellstrom-Lindberg E, Santini V, Finelli C, Giagounidis A, et al. Efficacy of azacitidine compared with that of conventional care regimens in the treatment of higher-risk myelodysplastic syndromes: a randomised, open-label, phase III study. Lancet Oncol. 2009;10(3):223-32.

[39] Vardiman JW, Thiele J, Arber DA, Brunning RD, Borowitz MJ, Porwit A, et al. The 2008 revision of the World Health Organization (WHO) classification of myeloid neoplasms and acute leukemia: rationale and important changes. Blood. 2009;114(5):937-51.

[40] Fenaux P, Mufti GJ, Hellstrom-Lindberg E, Santini V, Gattermann N, Germing U, et al. Azacitidine prolongs overall survival compared with conventional care regimens in elderly patients with low bone marrow blast count acute myeloid leukemia. J Clin Oncol. 2010;28(4):562-9.

[41] Blum W, Garzon R, Klisovic RB, Schwind S, Walker A, Geyer S, et al. Clinical response and miR-29b predictive significance in older AML patients treated with a 10-day schedule of decitabine. Proc Natl Acad Sci U S A. 2010;107(16):7473-8.

[42] Ritchie EK, Feldman EJ, Christos PJ, Rohan SD, Lagassa CB, Ippoliti C, et al. Decitabine in patients with newly diagnosed and relapsed acute myeloid leukemia. Leuk Lymphoma. 2013;54(9):2003-7.

[43] Hilberink J, Hazenberg C, van den Berg E, Mulder A, Schuringa JJ, van der Helm L, et al. Not type of induction therapy but consolidation with allogeneic hematopoietic cell transplantation determines outcome in older AML patients: A single center experience of 355 consecutive patients. Leuk Res. 2019;80:33-9.

[44] Short NJ, Kantarjian HM, Loghavi S, Huang X, Qiao W, Borthakur G, et al. Treatment with a 5-day versus a 10-day schedule of decitabine in older patients with newly diagnosed acute myeloid leukaemia: a randomised phase 2 trial. Lancet Haematol. 2019;6(1):e29-e37.

[45] Fenaux P, Gobbi M, Kropf PL, Mayer J, Roboz GJ, Dohner H, et al. Results of ASTRAL-1 study, a phase 3 randomized trial of Guadecitabine (G) vs Treatment choice (TC) in treatment naïve acute myeloid leukemia (TN-AML) not eligible for intensive chemotherapy (IC). HemaSphere. 2019;*Abstract*.

[46] Garcia-Manero G, Griffiths EA, Steensma DP, Roboz GJ, Wells R, McCloskey J, et al. Oral cedazuridine/decitabine for MDS and CMML: a phase 2 pharmacokinetic/pharmacodynamic randomized crossover study. Blood. 2020;136(6):674-83.

[47] Quintas-Cardama A, Ravandi F, Liu-Dumlao T, Brandt M, Faderl S, Pierce S, et al. Epigenetic therapy is associated with similar survival compared with intensive chemotherapy in older patients with newly diagnosed acute myeloid leukemia. Blood. 2012;120(24):4840-5.

[48] Burnett AK, Russell NH, Culligan D, Cavanagh J, Kell J, Wheatley K, et al. The addition of the farnesyl transferase inhibitor, tipifarnib, to low dose cytarabine does not improve outcome for older patients with AML. Br J Haematol. 2012;158(4):519-22.

[49] Burnett AK, Hills RK, Hunter AE, Milligan D, Kell WJ, Wheatley K, et al. The addition of gemtuzumab ozogamicin to low-dose Ara-C improves remission rate but does not significantly prolong survival in older patients with acute myeloid leukaemia: results from the LRF AML14 and NCRI AML16 pick-a-winner comparison. Leukemia. 2013;27(1):75-81.

[50] Burnett AK, Russell NH, Hunter AE, Milligan D, Knapper S, Wheatley K, et al. Clofarabine doubles the response rate in older patients with acute myeloid leukemia but does not improve survival. Blood. 2013;122(8):1384-94.

[51] Dohner H, Lubbert M, Fiedler W, Fouillard L, Haaland A, Brandwein JM, et al. Randomized, phase 2 trial of low-dose cytarabine with or without volasertib in AML patients not suitable for induction therapy. Blood. 2014;124(9):1426-33.

[52] Sekeres MA, Lancet JE, Wood BL, Grove LE, Sandalic L, Sievers EL, et al. Randomized phase IIb study of low-dose cytarabine and lintuzumab versus low-dose cytarabine and placebo in older adults with untreated acute myeloid leukemia. Haematologica. 2013;98(1):119-28.

[53] Heidel F, Cortes J, Rucker FG, Aulitzky W, Letvak L, Kindler T, et al.

Results of a multicenter phase II trial for older patients with c-Kit-positive acute myeloid leukemia (AML) and high-risk myelodysplastic syndrome (HR-MDS) using low-dose Ara-C and Imatinib. Cancer. 2007;109(5):907-14.

[54] Fiorentini A, Capelli D, Saraceni F, Menotti D, Poloni A, Olivieri A. The Time Has Come for Targeted Therapies for AML: Lights and Shadows. Oncol Ther. 2020;8(1):13-32.

[55] Roberts AW, Davids MS, Pagel JM, Kahl BS, Puvvada SD, Gerecitano JF, et al. Targeting BCL2 with Venetoclax in Relapsed Chronic Lymphocytic Leukemia. N Engl J Med. 2016;374(4):311-22.

[56] Stilgenbauer S, Eichhorst B, Schetelig J, Hillmen P, Seymour JF, Coutre S, et al. Venetoclax for Patients With Chronic Lymphocytic Leukemia With 17p Deletion: Results From the Full Population of a Phase II Pivotal Trial. J Clin Oncol. 2018;36(19):1973-80.

[57] Seymour JF, Kipps TJ, Eichhorst B, Hillmen P, D'Rozario J, Assouline S, et al. Venetoclax-Rituximab in Relapsed or Refractory Chronic Lymphocytic Leukemia. N Engl J Med. 2018;378(12):1107-20.

[58] Pan R, Hogdal LJ, Benito JM, Bucci D, Han L, Borthakur G, et al. Selective BCL-2 inhibition by ABT-199 causes on-target cell death in acute myeloid leukemia. Cancer Discov. 2014;4(3):362-75.

[59] Konopleva M, Pollyea DA, Potluri J, Chyla B, Hogdal L, Busman T, et al. Efficacy and Biological Correlates of Response in a Phase II Study of Venetoclax Monotherapy in Patients with Acute Myelogenous Leukemia. Cancer Discov. 2016;6(10):1106-17.

[60] Wei AH, Montesinos P, Ivanov V, DiNardo CD, Novak J, Laribi K, et al. Venetoclax plus LDAC for newly diagnosed AML ineligible for intensive chemotherapy: a phase 3 randomized placebo-controlled trial. Blood. 2020;135(24):2137-45.

[61] Roboz GJ, DiNardo CD, Stein EM, de Botton S, Mims AS, Prince GT, et al. Ivosidenib induces deep durable remissions in patients with newly diagnosed IDH1-mutant acute myeloid leukemia. Blood. 2020;135(7):463-71.

[62] Pollyea DA, Tallman MS, de Botton S, Kantarjian HM, Collins R, Stein AS, et al. Enasidenib, an inhibitor of mutant IDH2 proteins, induces durable remissions in older patients with newly diagnosed acute myeloid leukemia. Leukemia. 2019;33(11):2575-84.

[63] Stone RM, Mandrekar SJ, Sanford BL, Laumann K, Geyer S, Bloomfield CD, et al. Midostaurin plus Chemotherapy for Acute Myeloid Leukemia with a FLT3 Mutation. N Engl J Med. 2017;377(5):454-64.

[64] Irvine DA, Copland M. Targeting hedgehog in hematologic malignancy. Blood. 2012;119(10):2196-204.

[65] Cortes JE, Douglas Smith B, Wang ES, Merchant A, Oehler VG, Arellano M, et al. Glasdegib in combination with cytarabine and daunorubicin in patients with AML or high-risk MDS: Phase 2 study results. Am J Hematol. 2018;93(11):1301-10.

[66] Cortes JE, Heidel FH, Hellmann A, Fiedler W, Smith BD, Robak T, et al. Randomized comparison of low dose cytarabine with or without glasdegib in patients with newly diagnosed acute myeloid leukemia or high-risk myelodysplastic syndrome. Leukemia. 2019;33(2):379-89.

[67] Lancet JE, Cortes JE, Hogge DE, Tallman MS, Kovacsovics TJ, Damon LE, et al. Phase 2 trial of CPX-351, a fixed 5:1 molar ratio of

cytarabine/daunorubicin, vs cytarabine/daunorubicin in older adults with untreated AML. Blood. 2014;123(21):3239-46.

[68] Ritchie EK, Miah SK, Lee S, Curcio T, Desai P, Ball J, et al. CPX-351 as first intensive therapy for elderly patients with AML. Blood. 2019;134.

[69] Lancet JE, Uy GL, Cortes JE, Newell LF, Lin TL, Ritchie EK, et al. CPX-351 (cytarabine and daunorubicin) Liposome for Injection Versus Conventional Cytarabine Plus Daunorubicin in Older Patients With Newly Diagnosed Secondary Acute Myeloid Leukemia. J Clin Oncol. 2018;36(26):2684-92.

[70] Ostronoff F, Othus M, Lazenby M, Estey E, Appelbaum FR, Evans A, et al. Prognostic significance of NPM1 mutations in the absence of FLT3-internal tandem duplication in older patients with acute myeloid leukemia: a SWOG and UK National Cancer Research Institute/Medical Research Council report. J Clin Oncol. 2015;33(10):1157-64.

[71] Buchner T, Berdel WE, Haferlach C, Haferlach T, Schnittger S, Muller-Tidow C, et al. Age-related risk profile and chemotherapy dose response in acute myeloid leukemia: a study by the German Acute Myeloid Leukemia Cooperative Group. J Clin Oncol. 2009;27(1):61-9.

[72] Juliusson G, Karlsson K, Lazarevic V, Wahlin A, Brune M, Antunovic P, et al. Hematopoietic stem cell transplantation rates and long-term survival in acute myeloid and lymphoblastic leukemia: real-world population-based data from the Swedish Acute Leukemia Registry 1997-2006. Cancer. 2011;117(18):4238-46.

[73] Sorror ML, Sandmaier BM, Storer BE, Franke GN, Laport GG, Chauncey TR, et al. Long-term outcomes among older patients following nonmyeloablative conditioning and allogeneic hematopoietic cell transplantation for advanced hematologic malignancies. JAMA. 2011;306(17):1874-83.

[74] Sorror ML, Maris MB, Storb R, Baron F, Sandmaier BM, Maloney DG, et al. Hematopoietic cell transplantation (HCT)-specific comorbidity index: a new tool for risk assessment before allogeneic HCT. Blood. 2005;106(8):2912-9.

[75] Devine SM, Owzar K, Blum W, Mulkey F, Stone RM, Hsu JW, et al. Phase II Study of Allogeneic Transplantation for Older Patients With Acute Myeloid Leukemia in First Complete Remission Using a Reduced-Intensity Conditioning Regimen: Results From Cancer and Leukemia Group B 100103 (Alliance for Clinical Trials in Oncology)/Blood and Marrow Transplant Clinical Trial Network 0502. J Clin Oncol. 2015;33(35):4167-75.

[76] McClune BL, Weisdorf DJ, Pedersen TL, Tunes da Silva G, Tallman MS, Sierra J, et al. Effect of age on outcome of reduced-intensity hematopoietic cell transplantation for older patients with acute myeloid leukemia in first complete remission or with myelodysplastic syndrome. J Clin Oncol. 2010;28(11):1878-87.

[77] Versluis J, Hazenberg CL, Passweg JR, van Putten WL, Maertens J, Biemond BJ, et al. Post-remission treatment with allogeneic stem cell transplantation in patients aged 60 years and older with acute myeloid leukaemia: a time-dependent analysis. Lancet Haematol. 2015;2(10):e427-36.

[78] Farag SS, Maharry K, Zhang MJ, Perez WS, George SL, Mrozek K, et al. Comparison of reduced-intensity hematopoietic cell transplantation with chemotherapy in patients age 60-70 years with acute myelogenous leukemia in first remission. Biol Blood Marrow Transplant. 2011;17(12):1796-803.

Section 4

Stem Cell Transplantation

Chapter 11

Stem Cell Transplantation in Acute Myeloid Laeukemia

Salvatore Leotta, Annalisa Condorelli, Giovanni Schininà, Roberta Sciortino, Alessandra Cupri and Giuseppe Milone

Abstract

Allogeneic hematopoietic stem cell transplantation represents the only potentially curative therapeutic approach for Acute Myeloid Leukemia. The choice to perform an allogeneic hematopoietic transplant is the result of a decision-making process that considers disease-related factors (AML-risk category and the state of disease at the time of transplant), the type of donor available and his characteristics (HLA compatibility, gender, CMV serostatus) and the individual risk associated with the procedure itself. The choice of the appropriate conditioning regimen depends on the patient's age and comorbidities. While the introduction of reduced intensity regimen and the availability of alternative donors allows more patients to be eligible for transplantation, myeloablative conditioning remains the standard of care for fit patients. Disease relapse is the leading cause of treatment failure and new strategies attempting at reducing the relapse incidence post transplantation are currently being investigated.

Keywords: acute myeloid leukemia, allogeneic stem cell transplantation, treatment-related mortality, donor selection, conditioning regimen

1. Introduction

Allogeneic hematopoietic stem cell transplantation (HSCT) represents the only potentially curative therapeutic approach for Acute-Myeloid Leukemias (AML) [1]. This approach is often limited by the patient's transplant-eligibility, which depends on age and comorbidities. Moreover, in patients considered at low risk of relapse, allogeneic transplantation can be offered in case of disease relapse rather than in first complete remission. The high percentage of relapse of leukemia is the leading cause for failure of transplant [2]. The outcome of patients who relapse after transplantation is poor, especially for those who relapse within six months after transplantation for which overall survival at two years is often inferior to 20% [3].

Allogeneic HSCT for AML in first CR is indicated, according to The European Leukemia Network (ELN), when the risk of relapse exceeds 30–40% and the advantage in disease-free survival (DFS) that can derive from it is greater than 10% [4].

The choice to perform an allogeneic hematopoietic transplant is the result of a decision-making process that considers the AML-risk category together with the transplant risk calculated by evaluating both age and comorbidities. In adjunct, the decision-making process comprises the assessment of the disease-status at the moment in which the patient comes to the observation of the transplant-physician.

For patients in complete remission of the disease, also, the status of minimal residual disease must be considered [5] so that the most appropriate conditioning regimen and modulation of immunosuppressive therapy post-transplant can be chosen.

2. Indications to allogeneic transplantation for acute myeloid leukemia

2.1 AML-risk categories

2.1.1 Low risk, intermediate risk AML and the role of minimal residual disease (MRD)

The European Leukemia Network (ELN) has recently redefined the risk categories for AML into three risk-groups: favourable, intermediate and adverse according to karyotype and somatic mutations harboring prognostic significance (**Table 1**) [6]. The EBMT has provided guidance on indications for transplantation based on clinical evidence and current practice which was updated in 2019 [7]. According to EBMT indications for transplant-eligible patients with favorable risk in first complete remission, the autologous stem cell transplantation may be an option instead of repeated consolidation cycles if MRD is negative. Allogeneic HSCT (from HLA-identical sibling or unrelated donor) remains an option in case of MRD positivity. A growing body of evidence indicates that the pre-transplant evaluation of minimal residual disease (MRD) has a prognostic significance [8–10] and it hasto be considered for the transplant choice. Pre-transplantation positivity of MRD is associated with worse overall survival, disease free-survival and relapse incidence [10]. For Intermediate-risk patients in 1st CR allogeneic transplant from an HLA identical sibling is considered as "standard" while autologous transplantation and HSCT from unrelated-donor and alternative donor are considered clinical options [7]. Mannis et al. retrospectively analyzed data from 334 consecutive adult AML patients who underwent to autologous transplantation between 1988 and 2013. Among these patients, 133 were classified as intermediate-risk according to karyotype. Median relapse-free survival (RFS) was three years and 45% of patients maintain a complete remission at five years. Fifty-four patients relapsed after auto-SCT and of whom 26 underwent to allo-HSCT. Among allografted patients 35% (9/26) died of NRM, 35% (9/26) died of progressive disease, 12% (3/26) lived relapse-free at a

Risk category	Genetic abnormalities
Favourable	t(8;21)(q22;q22.1); RUNX1-RUNX1T1 inv.(16)(p13.1q22) or t(16;16)(p13.1;q22); CBFB-MYH11; Mutated NPM1 without FLT3-ITD or with FLT3-ITDlow; Biallelic mutated CEBPA.
Intermediate	Mutated NPM1 and FLT3-ITDhigh; Wild-type NPM1 without FLT3-ITD or with FLT3-ITDlow (without adverse-risk genetic lesions); t(9;11)(p21.3;q23.3); MLLT3-KMT2A; Cytogenetic abnormalities not classified as favorable or adverse.
Adverse	t(6;9)(p23;q34.1); DEK-NUP214 t(v;11q23.3); KMT2A rearranged t(9;22)(q34.1;q11.2); BCR-ABL1 inv.(3)(q21.3q26.2) or t(3;3)(q21.3;q26.2); GATA2,MECOM(EVI1) 25 or del (5q); 27; 217/abn(17p) Complex karyotype, monosomal karyotype; Wild-type NPM1 and FLT3-ITD high; Mutated RUNX1; Mutated ASXL1; Mutated TP53.

Ref. [6].

Table 1.
ELN Risk stratification by genetics.

follow-up of 3.8 years while the remaining five patients lost at follow-up. The authors conclude that ASCT in 1st CR may cure about 40% of patients affected by intermediate-risk AML. However, the study of Mannis et al. is limited by the absence of mutational testing for FLT3-ITD and NPM1 end CEBPA for the vast majority of patients and the risk stratification is based on cytogenetics only [11]. National Comprehensive Cancer Network (NCCN) guidelines do not recommend ASCT as a treatment option for intermediate-risk AML in 1st CR outside of a clinical trial [12]. The recent GIMEMA AML 1310 study evaluated a risk-oriented treatment in intermediate-risk (IR) patients in 1st CR: the patients underwent to autologous or to allogeneic transplantation according to post-consolidation negative or positive MRD respectively [13]. Overall survival (OS) and disease-free survival (DFS) in intermediate-risk MRD-positive patients who underwent to allo-HSCT were comparable to OS and DFS of favourable-risk (FR) patients that underwent to autologous transplantation (IR-MRD+: OS and DFS 70% and 67% respectively – FR: OS and DFS 74% and 61% respectively). In IR-MRD negative patients who underwent to autologous stem cells transplantation (ASCT) OS and DFS were 79% and 61% respectively [13]. MRD was evaluated by detecting Leukemia-associated phenotype (LAIP) by 8-colour multiparametric flow cytometry and the threshold was 3.5 x 10e-4 leukemic cells.

Based on the GIMEMA AML 1310 trial, the transplant choice in transplant-eligible intermediate-risk AML patients in 1st CR should be taken according to post-consolidation MRD. Some difficulties limit the application of MRD in clinical practice: the cut-off levels, the absence of LAIP or genetic mutations evaluable as MRD-markers in a portion of AML-patients, experience of the laboratory, the method used for molecular MRD assessment. As regard to cut off levels, a consensus from the ELN recommends 0,1% as the threshold level for MRD-positivity [14]. Some studies indicate that also MRD levels inferior to 0.1% are consistent with MRD [15, 16], although residual leukemic cells between 0.01% and 0.1% may define a good-prognosis sub-group of patients. Further studies are needed to address the prognostic significance of very low levels of MRD. As regards to the method used for molecular MRD assessment, the ELN consensus recommends real-time quantitative PCR (RQ-PCR) as the standard. RQ-PCR can detect up to 0.1% residual leukemic cells, although further improvements will come from more advanced approaches based on techniques not yet validated such as next-generation sequencing (NGS) and digital-PCR. Validated markers for MRD are *RUNX1-RUNX1T1*, *CBF-B/MYH11*, *PML-RARα*, *NPM1*-mutation. About 60% of AML-patients lacks a somatic mutation suitable for MRD monitoring and *WT1*is not recommended as a marker for MRD [14]. Mutations interesting *DNMT3A*, *TET2* and *ASXL1* loci may persist in CR without having a defined prognostic significance in terms of increased risk of relapse [17].

2.1.2 High-risk AML

The categories comprising high-risk acute myeloid leukaemias (i.e. AML harboring *FLT3-ITD*, monosomic karyotype or complex karyotype, abn(17p), 5q- or del(5), 7q- or del(7), inv.(3) or t(3;3), t(8;9), t(8;22), AML harboring mutated *RUNX1*, *ASXL1*, *TP53*, secondary and therapy-related AML) have a poor prognosis in the absence of allogeneic hematopoietic transplantation.

As regard to *FLT3*-mutated-AML, the mitigating effect of *NPM-1* mutation on outcome has been established [18, 19]. ELN has distinguished between two categories: AML harboring *NPM1*-mutated and *FLT3-ITD* at high allelic ratio or *FLT3-ITD* at low allelic ratio and wild-type *NPM1* are classified into intermediate-risk AML while AML harboring *FLT3-ITD* at high allelic ratio and wild-type *NPM1* are classified as high-risk AML [6]. Given the high risk of relapse, a recent position-statement by the EBMT recommends allo-HSCT for *FLT3*-mutated AML (also with *NPM*1-mutation) in 1st CR from related or alternative donors. The expert panel also recommends a maintenance treatment with *FLT3*-inhibitor: Sorafenib is the suggested option if the patient is treated outside of a clinical trial [19, 20].

As regards the high-risk categories harboring a particular adverse prognosis AML expressing del(5)/5q-, del(7)/7q-, abn(17p), monosomic karyotype, the EBMT have conducted a retrospective analysis on transplant outcome reporting two-year overall survival and leukaemia-free survival between 27% and 34% and between 20% and 24% respectively [21–23]. The worse outcome was observed in patients expressing both 5q- and abn(17p) [23].

2.1.3 Secondary- and therapy-related AML

Secondary AML (sAML) and therapy-related AML comprise a group of heterogeneous disease that, respect to de novo AML, occur more frequently in elderly patients, most often are chemo-resistant to cytotoxic chemotherapy and have a worse prognosis [24]. Sengsayadeth et al. have conducted a retrospective analysis on 3960 patients affected by sAML undergoing to allo-HSCT between 2000 and 2016. The two years overall survival and disease-free survival were respectively 45% and 39%. The subgroup of patients receiving HSCT not in complete remission experienced the worse outcome (2 years OS and DFS, respectively 35 and 29%) [25]. Recently the Acute Leukemia Working Party of the EBMT published a retrospective registry-based study comparing the outcome of allo-HSCT for sAML and de novo AML patients transplanted in the time interval 2000–2016. The three years overall survival, disease-free survival and cumulative incidence of relapse (CIR) were respectively 60%, 55%, 28% and 46%, 41% and 35% respectively for de novo AML and sAML. In multivariate analysis, sAML was associated with worse OS, DFS and CIR than de novo AML [26]. In patients fit for transplant affected by sAMLallo-HSCT must be offered upfront, preferably in 1st CR. Novel agent CPX351 (liposomal formulation of Cytarabine and Daunorubicine in a 5:1 ratio) has been recently approved as induction treatment for these patients and has demonstrated superiority compared to the conventional "7 + 3" schedule [27].

2.1.4 Chemotherapy-refractory AML

The prognosis of patients who fail to reach complete remission after induction chemotherapy is poor. In these patients, five years survival is <10%. Allogeneic transplantation may improve survival to 25–30% [28].

Jabbour et al. compared outcomes of 28 AML primary-induction failure (PIF) patients who underwent to allo-HSCT to that of 149 PIF patients who were treated with salvage chemotherapy alone: results were dramatically in favour of allo-HSCT with a three years OS rate of 39% for allo-grafted patients versus 2% for chemotherapy-only patients [29].

Ferguson et al. in a retrospective analysis on 8907 patients have found that patients who fail to achieve a reduction of myeloid blasts <50% with >15% residual blasts after one course of induction chemotherapy as well as patients who fail to achieve complete remission after two courses of induction chemotherapy have a very dismal prognosis if treated with further chemotherapy. Allogeneic stem cell transplantation may improve survival of these patients [28].

The FLAMSA regimen has been designed for patients with active disease who undergo allo-HSCT. It comprises an initial debulk with Aracytin, Fludarabine and Amsacrine followed by a reduced-intensity conditioning and HSCT [30, 31].

In summary, allogeneic HSCT may rescue about 30% of patients with primary induction or re-induction failure and the improvements in recent years in HLA-typing, donor availability (i.e. haploidentical donors), conditioning regimen and supportive care expand the possibility to give allogeneic transplantation to this category of patients [32]. In primary refractory disease performing more than two induction courses before allogeneic transplantation has no benefit [28, 30]. Duval et al. developed a prognostic score for the outcome of allo-HSCT performed for AML refractory to chemotherapy (named Duval Score). They analyzed data from 1673 patients from CIBMTR registry and developed a score based on five variables: phase of disease at HSCT (PIF or refractory relapse after CR > 6 months versus refractory relapse after CR < 6 months), cytogenetic class of risk (good/intermediate vs. high), circulating blasts (absent vs. present), HLA match (HLA matched related vs. matched unrelated vs. mismatched unrelated vs. haploidentical) and Karnofsky Score (KS: > 90 vs. < 90). Four class of risk correlated with different survival were identified. Three-years OS varied from 40% for score 0 versus 6% for score ≥ 3 [33].

2.1.5 Transplantation in 2nd CR

The current indications for allo-HSCT in 2nd CR include transplantation-eligible patients affected by low-risk AML relapsed after previous chemotherapy or autologous transplantation [7]. Allo-HSCT in 2nd CR may also be offered to patients for whom this procedure was previously considered not indicated or too risky (for example intermediate-risk AML for whom MRD was absent after consolidation chemotherapy, or patients lacking HLA-identical sibling donors and considered unfit for an alternative donor at the time of 1st CR).

Some retrospective analysis by ALWP of EBMT has addressed the role of allogeneic transplantation in 2nd CR of AML. Christopeit and coll. have analyzed 537 patients who have undergone allograft in 2nd CR or first relapse after ASCT: 3-years overall survival (OS), leukaemia-free survival (LFS) and non-relapse mortality (NRM) were respectively 39.5%, 31.5% and 33%. Cumulative incidence of relapse (CIR) was 34.6%. A longer survival correlated with allo-HSCT performed in complete remission than in chemo-refractory relapse, with favorable-risk cytogenetics and with a longer duration of 1st CR (more than ten months in median).NRM was higher in patients undergoing to allo—HSCT from alternative donors than HLA-identical sibling and in those who received Total-body Irradiation (TBI) as part of the conditioning pre-ASCT [34].

Gilleece and coll. published a registry report by the EBMT on allo-HSCT in 2nd CR of AML including 1879 patients transplanted between 2007 and 2016. The global outcome at 2 years were: LFS: 52%, OS: 58%, Relapse Incidence: 30%. NRM was 20%. The results were split by age < 50 or ≥ 50 years old and by the intensity of conditioning. OS and LFS for <50 yrs. old were 61% and 54% respectively (without differences due to conditioning regimen). For ≥50 years old OS was respectively 58% and 54% for myeloablative (MAC) and reduced-intensity conditioning (RIC) and LFS was 50% for both conditioning regimens. In multivariate analysis, the intensity of the conditioning regimen did have an impact on NRM that was lower for RIC in patients aged ≥50 years (HR 0.54, $p < 0.001$). Overall Survival, LFS, CIR and Graft-relapse free survival (GRFS) were better in patients with longer intervals from diagnosis to allo-HSCT. Performance status (PS) and the cytogenetic class of risk at diagnosis (good, intermediate and adverse) also correlated with outcome [35].

Halaburda K et al. retrospectively analyzed 631 patients affected by Core-binding factor (CBF) AML who were allo-grafted in 2nd CR and reported to the EBMT registry between 2000 and 2014. Five-years OS and LFS were respectively 58% and 54% while relapse and NRM at were 22.5% and 23%. The composite end-point of Graft-relapse free survival (GRFS) at 2 and 5 years was 40 and 34% respectively. In multivariate analysis, GRFS was associated with three or more additional cytogenetic abnormalities and in vivo T-cell depletion (HR 1.6, P = 0.03). A trend for a better GRFS was associated with a transplant from a CMV-seronegative donor and for MRD –negative status at allo-HSCT [36].

Passweg and coll. conducted a retrospective study to compare the impact of a previous ASCT versus chemotherapy consolidation without ASCT on the outcome of allo-HSCT performed in 2nd CR. The study included 2619 allo-grafted patients in 2nd CR between 2000 and 2017. Of these, 417 were previously treated in 1st CR with ASCT and 2202 with chemotherapy consolidation respectively. The patients were not evenly distributed among the two cohorts because patients treated with ASCT respect to those treated with chemotherapy consolidation were younger, had undergone transplantation earlier, had more often an unfavorable karyotype, more often received allo-HSCT from alternative donors than from HLA matched siblings and more often received a RIC than a MAC regimen. Two-years OS, LFS, GRFS and NRM were respectively 58, 50, and 21% for chemotherapy consolidations and 55, 46, 35 and 25% for ASCT-patients. In multivariate analysis risk of NRM, LFS and GRFS were higher for previous ASCT-patients than for previous chemotherapy consolidation patients. As well as in the study of Christopeit NRM of the allogeneic transplant was higher for patients in whom TBI was included in the pre-ASCT conditioning [37]. However, after first relapse, the attempt of a second complete remission is not always successful and if outcome is measured from the time-point of relapse, the overall results are very poor. Infact, only 10% of all AML patients that relapse and are treated with re-induction chemotherapy and subsequently with allogeneic hematopoietic transplantation are survivors at 5 years [38].

In summary, about 50% of patients in 2nd CR of AML, if eligible to transplantation, may be rescued by allo-graft, particularly when 1st CR has been longer than six months [33]. The chance to achieve a second remission after a first relapse is, however, limited. Furthermore, prior autologous transplantation is associated with an increased risk of NRM post allogeneic transplantation and this must be considered when choosing auto-transplantation in 1st CR, in particular for low and intermediate-risk AML.

3. Risk assessment

Allogeneic Hematopoietic Stem Cell Transplantation remains a procedure associated with significant mortality and morbidity.

Once the bone marrow transplant has been established as a therapeutic indication, the candidate has to be evaluated in order to define eligibility for treatment and to choose the most appropriate conditioning regimen.

The study of the factors related to the disease, to the donor characteristics and to the patient's general health allows us to evaluate the probability of post-HSCT non-relapse mortality (NRM).

Here we describe the predictive models used in the clinical practice that quantify the post-HSCT risk profile by integrating all these different factors and therefore predict tolerability to allogeneic BM transplant.

3.1 Disease risk index (DRI)

The score arises from the evidence that the outcome of HCT depends on the state of the disease at the time of transplantation. Armand et al. led to the development of the Disease Risk Index, conducting a retrospective study involving 1539 patients analyzing information about the disease and its status [39].

It does not take into account factors like age and comorbidities. It categorizes patients into four risk groups with different OS and PFS based on differences in the relapse risk as described in **Tables 2** and **3**.

3.2 HSCT-Comorbidity Index (HCT-CI)

Sorror et al., through a retrospective analysis study, developed the Hematopoietic cell transplantation-specific comorbidity index (HCT-CI) (**Table 4**) [40]. Initially developed in 2005, as an adaptation of the Charlson Comorbidity Index to HSCT, it was revised in 2014 to include the age variable [41]. Compared to the previous scores, the HCT-CI places much emphasis on the patient's general health and organ dysfunctions, analyzing 17 comorbidities as described in **Table 2**. It defines 3 risk groups: score 0 (low risk), score 1–2 (intermediate risk), >= 3 (high risk).HSCT-CI was subsequently validated in an independent cohort of patients by Raimondi et al. in 2012 [42]. It is an independent predictor of both NRM and OS. 2 years NRM is 14.7%, 21.3%, and 27.3% in patients having ad HSCT score of 0, 1–2 and > 3 respectively and OS was 56.4%, 21.3% and 41.3% respectively. Patients with low scores should be enrolled in randomized clinical trials or undergoing high intensity conditioning regimens (total busulfan dose>8 mg / kg, or cyclophosphamide dose>120 mg / kg or > 60 mg/kg in combination with other drugs, or melphalan dose>140 mg/mq or total body irradiation dose>6 Gy), while patients with a high score should be candidates for the reduced intensity/non myeloablative conditioning regimens.

3.3 EBMT score

Another score widely used in transplantation practice is the EBMT risk score [43]. It was introduced more than ten years ago initially for patients with chronic myeloid leukaemia (CML), the most frequent indication for allogeneic stem cell transplantation in those years, and subsequently extended to other haematological diseases. Each of the five factors taken into consideration has the same "weight" and importance on the global risk: age, stage of the disease, time from diagnosis, donor type and donor-recipient gender. The score allows us to predict approximately the 5-year probability of OS and TRM for any disease. The novelty, compared to the HSCT-CI, is the introduction of the concept of the disease stage to improve the score predictivity.

1. By age, 3 categories are identified: <20 years (0 score points), 20–40 years (1 score point) and > 40 years (2 score points). The introduction of low-intensity conditioning regimes has opened access to allogeneic transplantation also to elderly patients, but this does not take away the fact that mortality is higher in this category of patients.

2. For disease stage, three categories are defined: early disease stage (0 score point) represented by acute leukaemia in first CR, intermediate disease stage (1 score point) in which acute leukaemia in second CR and late-stage disease (2 score points) are included with advanced leukaemia.

3. The time interval from diagnosis to transplant provides a cut-off of 12 months. If the elapsed time is <12 months 0 score points if>12 months one score point. For acute leukaemias in the first CR we arbitrarily set as 0.

Disease		Disease risk
AML favorable cytogenetics		Low
CLL		
CML		
Indolent B-cell NHL		
ALL		Intermediate
AML intermediate cytogenetics		
MDS intermediate cytogenetics		
Myeloproliferative neoplasms		
Multiple Myeloma		
Hodgkin lymphoma		
DLBCL/Transformed indolent B-NHL		
Mantle cell lymphoma		
T-cell lymphoma, nodal		
AML adverse cytogenetics		High
MDS adverse cytogenetics		
T-cell lymphoma, extranodal		
Stage		**Stage risk**
1st Complete Remission		Low
2nd or subsequent CR		
1st PR		
Untreated		
Chronic Phase CML		
2nd or subsequent PR **(if RIC)**		
2nd or subsequent PR **(if MAC)**		High
Induction Failure		
Active Relapse		
Accelerated or Blast Phase CML		
Overall assignment		
Disease risk	**Stage risk**	**DRI assignment**
Low	Low	Low
Low	High	Intermediate
Intermediate	Low	
Intermediate	High	High
High	Low	
High	High	Very high

DLBCL, diffuse large B cell lymphoma; RIC, reduced intensity conditioning; MAC, myeloablative conditioning; other abbreviations are as in ***Table 1.***
Ref. [39].

Table 2.
Summary of disease and stage risk groups from original DRI.

Disease	Stage	No. of patients	HR*	Original DRI	Percentage of patients	New DRI Group	2-y OS (%)	95% CI
Hodgkin lymphoma CR		126	0.36	Int	14	Low	66	63–68
CLL CR		81	0.47	Low		Low		
Mantle cell lymphoma CR		160	0.51	Int		Low		
Indolent NHL CR		183	0.53	Low		Low		
AML favorable cytogenetics CR		190	0.64	Low		Low		
Indolent NHL PR		276	0.71	Low		Low		
CLL PR		400	0.78	Low		Low		
CML chronic phase 1/2		390	0.82	Low		Low		
CML advanced phase		69	0.92	Int	63	Int	51	50–52
Mantle cell lymphoma PR		149	0.95	Int		Int		
Myeloproliferative neoplasm	Any	426	0.98	Int		Int		
AML intermediate cytogenetics CR		3611	Ref	Int		Int		
ALL CR1		1023	1.00	Int		Int		
T-cell NHL CR		171	1.00	Int		Int		
Multiple myeloma CR/VGPR/PR		339	1.03	Int		Int		
Aggressive NHL CR		181	1.05	Int		Int		
Low-risk MDS adverse cytogenetics	Early†	103	1.06	High		Int		
T-cell NHL PR		164	1.06	Int		Int		
Low-risk MDS Intermediate cytogenetics	Early†	516	1.09	Int		Int		
HL PR		225	1.09	Int		Int		
Low-risk MDS intermediate cytogenetics	Advanced†	235	1.18	Int		Int		
Indolent NHL	Advanced†	128	1.21	Int		Int		
CLL	Advanced	265	1.22	Int		Int		
High-risk MDS intermediate cytogenetics	Early	364	1.24	Int		Int		
Aggressive NHL PR		205	1.26	Int		Int		
T-cell NHL	Advanced†	93	1.41	High	20	High	33	31–35
AML favorable cytogenetics	Advanced†	34	1.42	Int		High		
HL	Advanced†	85	1.48	High		High		

Disease	Stage	No. of patients	HR*	Original DRI	Percentage of patients	New DRI Group	2-y OS (%)	95% CI
High-risk MDS intermediate cytogenetics	Advanced†	179	1.56	Int		High		
High-risk MDS adverse cytogenetics	Early	80	1.58	High		High		
ALL CR2		407	1.58	Int		High		
AML adverse cytogenetics CR		175	1.59	High		High		
Mantle cell lymphoma	Advanced†	46	1.59	High		High		
High-risk MDS adverse cytogenetics	Advanced†	30	1.59	Very high		High		
BL‡ CR		23	1.65	NA		High		
Multiple myeloma	Advanced†	150	1.65	High		High		
ALL CR3		61	1.70	Int		High		
Low-risk MDS adverse cytogenetics	Advanced†	32	1.86	Very high		High		
AML Intermediate cytogenetics	Advanced	1227	1.89	High		High		
CML blast phase		52	2.02	Int	4	Very high	23	20–27
ALL	Advanced†	235	2.23	High		Very high		
Aggressive NHL	Advanced†	154	2.54	High		Very high		
AML adverse cytogenetics	Advanced†	76	2.83	Very High		Very high		
BL‡ PR	Advanced†	12	5.21	NA		Very high		

Int, intermediate. Ref. [39].
**Hazard ratio for mortality compared with AML intermediate cytogenetics in CR1.*
†Advanced stage refers to induction failure or active relapse, including stable or progressive disease for NHL, HL, and CLL.
‡Those categories were not included in the original DRI.

Table 3.
Refinement of DRI.

4. Concerning the type of donor, the identical sibling donors will have a 0 point score, while the unrelated ones will have one score point. It is interesting to note how the impact of donor typer is different for different pathologies, having a significant impact on aplastic anaemia and the least of all for acute lymphoblastic leukaemia.

5. Last but not least, the gender difference between recipient and donor. Female donor for male recipient (1 score point) as it has been noted that it leads to a higher NRM, due to increased incidence of acute and chronic GVHD.

Also donor or recipient cytomegalovirus (CMV) seropositivity has a prognostic impact: recently a study showed that, compared to CMV-seronegative recipients who

Comorbidity	*HCT-CI score*	N	%
Arrhytmia	1	7	3
Cardiac	1	18	9
Inflammatory bowel disease	1	1	0.5
Diabetes	1	5	2
Cerebrovascular disease	1	1	0.5
Psychiatric disturbance	1	10	5
Hepatic-mild	1	10	5
Obesity	1	14	7
Infection	1	28	14
Rheumatologic	2	2	1
Peptic ulcer	2	2	1
Moderate/severe renal	2	8	4
Moderate pulmonary	2	30	15
Prior solid malignancy	3	12	6
Heart valve disease	3	4	2
Severe pulmonary	3	49	24
Moderate/severe hepatic	3	2	1
No comorbidities	0	65	32

Abbreviation: HCT-CI, hematopoietic cell transplantation comorbidity index; N, *number of patients. Ref. [40].*

Table 4.
Definitions of comorbidities included in the HCT-CI score.

underwent allograft from a CMV-seronegative donor, cases of CMV seropositivity of the donor and/or the recipient showed a significantly decreased 2-year leukemia-free survival (44% vs. 49%, $P < .001$) and overall survival (50% vs. 56%, $P < .001$), and increased nonrelapse mortality (23% vs. 20%, $P < .001$) [44]. In a CIBMTR analysis early CMV-reactivation was associated with lower overall survival (HR: 1.27) and it was confirmed as a poor risk factor for post-transplant outcome [45].

Also cytokine's encoding gene polymorphisms seem to have a prognostic impact. It has been shown that single nucleotide polymorphisms (SNPs) in the IL-6 encoding gene influence outcome after allogeneic stem cell transplantation as described by Tvedt et al. [46].

4. Donor selection

The selection of a donor is a critical element contributing to the success of hematopoietic cell transplantation (HCT).

Among the many factors that influence the outcome of hematopoietic stem cell transplantation, polymorphism of the classical human leukocyte antigen represents the most important barrier [47]. The human Major Histocompatibility Antigens is located on the short arm of chromosome 6. The MHC falls into three main regions, class I, II and III. The most relevant genes for transplantation belong to class I (*HLA-A*, *HLA-B* and *HLA-C*) and class II (*HLA-DR*, *HLA-DQ* and *HLA-DP*). MCH genes are inheritedin a co-dominant manner following Mendelian rules. Therefore, the probability for siblings to be HLA-identicalis 25% [48]. HLA compatibility with the donor is usually defined by high-resolution typing (four digits) for ten alleles, *HLA-A*, *HLA-B*, *HLA-C*, *HLA-DR* and *HLA-DQ*, but there is increasing evidence supporting the relevance of *DPB1* matching [49]. An HLA–identical sibling donor is generally considered the best donor for allo-HSCT; however, less than a third of patients will have one available. For the remaining 70% of patients, alternative sources of stem cells are a matched unrelated adult volunteer donor, a haploidentical donor or a cord blood unit. The probability of identifying a highly matched unrelated donor depends on the frequency of the patient's HLA haplotypes and ethnic origin. 1–5% of patients do not have a single potentially matched donor upon direct interrogation of the BMDW database because the large majority of donors registered in the database are of Western European ancestry. In European countries, 45–65% of patients will eventually have a 10/10 matched donor, and a 9/10 matched donor may be identified for an additional 20–30% of patients [50]. There is a consensus that single *HLA-A*, *B* or *C* allele mismatches and double *HLA-DRB1* mismatches are associated with increased mortality in non-T-cell-depleted bone marrow transplantation [51]. Disparities in *HLA-DQB1*, as well as C-allele disparities in C 03:03 vs. 03:04, have been reported to be permissive with no adverse effects on the outcome [52]. Disparities in *HLA-DPB1* are observed in the majority of *HLA-A*, *HLA-B*, *HLA-C* and *HLA-DQB1* (10/10) MUD transplants [53]. Different studies have demonstrated that biological models can be used to identify selected, permissive *DPB1* mismatches combination, associated with lower clinical risks compared to their high risk, non-permissive, counterparts. There are five different biological models for the assignment of *DPB1* permissiveness that have been identified to date, three of which are based on functional T-cell epitopes (TCE) [54]. A study shows that survival probabilities can be significantly increased by selecting donors with TCE4- permissive *HLA-DPB1* disparities, with a significant association with NRM and OS in 10/10 and 9/10 matched transplantation. Therefore, the UD searches should be directed up-front toward the identification of a 10/10 or 9/10 matched donor presenting TCE4-permissive *HLA-DPB1* disparities [55].

Whenever two or more 10/10 matched donors are available, other factors are studied. We have to evaluate the presence of HLA-antibodies in the recipient and select a donor for whom there are no recipient donor-specific anti HLA antibodies (DSA). An essential element is the donor age with priority for the youngest. Another factor is the matching for patient/recipient CMV serostatus with the best scenario be a seronegative patient receiving from a seronegative donor. Donor gender is also considered with priority for the male donor since female donor can immunize post-pregnancy. Another factor to be considered is AB0-matching, even though the impact of blood group compatibility on outcome has been reported to be modest [56]. Other factors to be considered include NK cell alloreactivity and KIR haplotype matching and non-inherited maternal HLA antigens (NIMA) mismatching [57].

Many advances in MUD HCT have occurred over the past 20 years and several studies suggest that transplantation from fully Matched Unrelated Donor (8/8 or 10/10) and Matched Sibling Donor results in similar survival times for patients with AML [58]. The study of Center for International Blood and Marrow Transplant Research analyzed outcomes of 2223 adult acute myelogenous leukaemia patients who underwent allogeneic HCT between 2002 and 2006 (HLA-Matched related donor MRD, n = 624; 8/8 HLA locus matched MUD, n = 1193; 7/8 MUD, n = 406). The 100-day cumulative incidence of GVHD was significantly lower in MRD HCT recipients than in 8/8 MUD and 7/8 MUD HCT recipients (33%, 51% and 53% respectively; $P < .001$). In multivariate analysis, 8/8 MUD HCT recipients had a similar survival rate compared with MRD HCT recipients. 7/8 MUD HCT recipients had higher early mortality than MRD HCT recipients, but beyond six months after

HCT, their survival rates were similar [58].Another study compared the outcomes of the unrelated donor (URD, n = 385) with human leukocyte antigen (HLA)-matched sibling donor (MSD, n = 226) transplantation in patients with acute myeloid leukaemia in first complete remission (CR1) having unfavourable cytogenetics at diagnosis. Three-year leukaemia-free survival (LFS) for MSD was 42% compared with 34% for HLA-well-matched URD and 29% for partially matched URD. In multivariate analysis, HLA-well-matched URD and MSD yielded similar LFS and OS. LFS and OS were significantly inferior for HLA-partially matched URD recipients, those with prior myelodysplastic syndrome, and those older than 50 years. Patients with chronic GVHD had a significantly lower risk of relapse [59].

If 10/10 matched unrelated donor is not available, an alternative donor has to be considered: HLA 9/10 matched unrelated donor; haploidentical donor; HLA mismatched unrelated donor; cord blood unit.

A haploidentical related donor is defined by the sharing of one haplotype (or a single identical copy of chromosome 6) with the patient containing the HLA region involving class I and class II histocompatibility genes (patient's parents or sons; sometimes brothers or sisters or cousins). A significant advantage of haploidentical transplantation is the rapid access to a donor which is of crucial importance for patients with high-risk AML since a delay in transplantation due to the donor issues can result in a poor outcome. Today primary prevention and treatment of GVHD have been a major challenge in this peculiar HLA-mismatched setting [60]. Two main platforms have been developed: ex vivo T cell depletion, which is used in a few centers because it is expensive and it needs highly specialized laboratories [61, 62], and unmanipulated graft transplantation, which is way more used since the introduction of Post-transplant Cyclophosphamide (PT-CY) (that will be discussed in the chapter on conditioning regimens). Several studies found that the OS secondary outcomes of patients with AML who received haplo-HSCT were not significantly different from MSD-HSCT and MUD-HSCT [63].

Another alternative source of stem cells is the cord blood unit (UCB). It has been established that a single UCB unit contains sufficient numbers of HSCs for durable engraftment in most patients.

Thanks to immunological immaturity, an advantage of UCB is its apparent reduced alloreactive response as compared with bone marrow. The data would suggest that UCB, despite HLA mismatching, is associated with low GVHD risk. Disadvantages of Umbilical Cord Blood Transplantation are slower engraftment, higher risk of non-immunological rejection (graft failure), remote possibility of transmission of a genetic disease, more significant delay in immune reconstitution, no possibility of donor lymphocyte infusion [64, 65].

A retrospective analysis including 106,188 adult patients with haematological malignancies who underwent allogeneic hematopoietic stem cell transplantation studied overall survival at three years. The results showed: 54.6% for a matched sibling, 51.6% for a matched unrelated donor, 41.3% for a mismatched unrelated donor, 44.2% for haploidentical and 43.7% for cord blood [66]. OS following HSCT is improving with substantial progress among recipients of haploidentical and cord blood HSCT, but the traditional donor hierarchy of matched sibling donors followed by matched unrelated donors and then other donors hold [66].

5. Conditioning regimens

Conditioning is the treatment used to prepare patients undergoing hematopoietic bone marrow transplantation. The role of conditioning is to eradicate the residual haematological disease from the bone marrow, to provide room in the host bone marrow for the donor stem cells and to have an immunosuppressive effect in order to ensure engraftment.

Conditioning regimens can include Total Body Irradiation (TBI) or they can be radiation-free and be based only on chemotherapy. They usually consist of a myeloablative compound (such as Busulfan or Melphalan) and an immunosuppressive agent (such as Fludarabine or Cyclophosphamide).

Conditioning regimens have been classified into three categories based on the duration of the induced pancytopenia and the requirement for stem cells support [67]:

Myeloablative conditioning (MAC): *a combination of agents expected to produce irreversible pancytopenia; stem cells support is required to rescue marrow function;*

Non-myeloablative conditioning (NMA): *a regimen that will cause minimal cytopenia and does not require stem cells support;*

Reduced-intensity conditioning (RIC): *a regimen that cannot be classified as NMA or MA; it can cause pancytopenia which may be prolonged and do require stem cells support; cytopenia may not be irreversible; RIC regimens differ from MA conditioning because of the dose that must be reduced by at least 30%.*

Traditionally, the two most important myeloablative regimens were TBI/Cyclophosphamide (Cy) (TBI 12 Gy, Cy 60 mg/kg × 2 days) and BU (Busulfan)/Cy (BU 4 mg/kg × 4 days and CY 60 mg/kg × 2 days). In AML, different studies showed the equivalence between these regimens in terms of Leukemia Free Survival (LFS) and Overall Survival (OS) [68, 69]. Cyclophosphamide is often replaced by Fludarabine, a purine analogue with antineoplastic and immunosuppressive effect and a better toxicity profile. The combination BU-FLU (BU 4 mg/kg × 4 days and FLU 40 mg/m^2/day for four consecutive days) has been demonstrated to be as effective as the regimen BU-CY but with a lower Transplant Related Mortality (TRM) [70, 71]. Thiotepa (TT), an alkylating compound with antineoplastic and myeloablative activity, can be added to these combinations in order to reduce the risk of relapse [72].

In the last two decades, the introduction of RIC regimens has revolutionized the transplant landscape by allowing more patients to be eligible for transplantation. RIC transplantation relies more on the graft versus leukaemia (GvL) effect than a cytotoxic action for efficacy. RIC regimens are a good treatment option in older patients (age > 60 years) or younger patients with comorbidities that are ineligible for a MAC regimen [73]. These regimens usually combine Fludarabine with an alkylating agent (like Busulfan or Thiothepa) or TBI in reduced doses. Many studies in the literature comparing MAC and RIC regimens in AML showed a comparable survival; even though a higher relapse rate was observed in RIC regimen, it was balanced by a lower TRM [74–78]. To address this question, a phase III randomized trial comparing MAC with RIC in patients with acute myeloid leukaemia or myelodysplastic syndromes was performed. In this study, RIC resulted in lower TRM but higher relapse rates compared with MAC, with a statistically significant advantage in LFS with MAC. These data support the use of MAC as the standard of care for fit patients with acute myeloid leukaemia [79].

Intermediate-intensity conditioning has been developed to reduce the relapse incidence (RI) while maintaining a reduced TRM after RIC transplantation. The FLAMSA regimen has been designed for patients with active disease who undergo allo-HSCT. It comprises an initial debulk with Aracytin, Fludarabine and Amsacrine followed by a reduced-intensity conditioning and HSCT [80–81]. Schmid and coll. employed the FLAMSA regimen on 75 consecutive high-risk patients, 27 of whom affected by primary refractory AML and 22 by untreated relapse of AML, and reported a one-year non-relapse mortality of 33% and a 2-years DFS of 40%. This regimen also includes the use of prophylactic donor-leukocyte infusions (pDLI) in the absence of Graft-Versus-Host Disease (GVHD). The authors describe a better survival in patients who experienced a mild chronic GVHD respect to no GVHD or severe GVHD [82].

The Baltimore group has pioneered Post-transplant Cyclophosphamide (PT-CY) on day +3 and +4 after the transplant in the contest of haploidentical donor transplantation and it reduces the incidence of GVHD [83–86]. PT-CY prevents GVHD by killing alloreactive T cells of the donor and host origin with preservation of regulatory T cells; on the other hand, stem cells are protected by the drug because of their high level of aldehyde dehydrogenase which converts Cy to a non-toxic metabolite [87]. Since its advent, the transplant from a haploidentical donor has become one of the most commonly used alternative donor strategies. In the study by Ciurea et al. clinical outcomes of patients diagnosed with AML undergoing SCT from MUD or haploidentical donor with PT-CY were evaluated and overall survival resulted comparable in two groups with a lower incidence of GVHD in the haploidentical donor group [85]. The introduction of this strategy allowed even minor transplant centers to be able to perform haploidentical donor transplantation by omitting the need for ex vivo T cell depletion, which is an expensive procedure that requires dedicated laboratories. Because of the success demonstrated at preventing GVHD in the haploidentical setting, its role is now being also evaluated in the other settings—Matched unrelated donor, HLA identical donor [86, 88]—and it might be the strategy allowing calcineurin inhibitors and mTOR inhibitors-free GvHD prophylaxis [89].

Comparable results at preventing GVHD in the unmanipulated HSCT setting were obtained with another strategy based on the use of BM cells harvested from donors primed with low dose G-CSF (4 μg/kg/day) and on the administration of either MAC or RIC preparative regimen and an intensive GVHD prophylaxis consisting of a combination of five drugs: ATG, CSA, MTX, MMF and Basiliximab [90]. G-CSF stimulation increases the number of BM $CD34^{+}$ cells [91] and has an intense immunoregulatory effect on BM T cells by down-regulating the expression of adhesion and CD28/B7 molecules and by favouring a T-cell shift from Th1- to Th2-type cells and inducing a higher production of IL-4 and IL-10 anti-inflammatory cytokines [92].

T-cell depletion to prevent GVHD remains an option in the haploidentical setting and the lack of extensive prospective studies comparing it with the unmanipulated graft transplantation leave the choice to the experience of the SCT center. This modality has been associated with a higher leukaemia relapse incidence - since T cells are responsible for the graft versus leukaemia effect - and higher TRM due to slower engraftment and a higher incidence of opportunistic infections [93]. New methods of graft manipulation have been developed in order to address these problems. A promising approach is the graft depletion of B cells and T cells carrying the γδ chains of T cell receptor (TCR), being responsible for GVHD, while keeping αβ T cells and Natura Killer (NK) cells that play an essential role in anti-tumour surveillance and the antiviral immunity (TCR γδ/CD19 negative selection) [94]. A different strategy recently presented by the Perugia group is the infusion of donor regulatory T cells at day – 4 followed by the infusion of a megadose of CD34+ and conventional T cells on day 0 and no use of pharmacological post-transplant immunosuppression. This method resulted in a significant reduction in the incidence of leukaemia relapse, suggesting that regulatory T cells limit GVHD with no loss of GvL [95].

Disease recurrence remains the leading cause of treatment failure [96]. In order to reduce the RI post allogeneic stem cell transplantation (allo-SCT), studies including cellular therapies (DLI) [97, 98] and new drugs that seem to enhance the GvL effect like *FLT-3* inhibitors, immune checkpoint inhibitors [99] and epigenetic therapies in the post-transplantation setting are ongoing. In the RICAZA trial azacitidine was administrated for the first year after transplantation in 51 patients affected by AML undergoing allogeneic SCT and it showed a reduced risk of disease relapse [100].

Acknowledgements

We wish to thank all nurses who care for the patients receiving bone marrow transplant in our Unit.

Conflict of interest

"The authors declare no conflict of interest."

Author details

Salvatore Leotta[1], Annalisa Condorelli[1], Giovanni Schininà[1], Roberta Sciortino[1], Alessandra Cupri[1] and Giuseppe Milone[1,2]*

1 Division of Hematology, Bone Marrow Transplantation Unit, University Hospital, Polyclinic of Catania, Italy

2 Istituto Oncologico del Mediterraneo, Bone Marrow Transplantation Unit, Viagrande, Italy

*Address all correspondence to: giuseppe.milone@gmail.com

References

[1] Gupta V, Tallman MS, Weisdorf DJ. Allogeneic hematopoietic cell transplantation for adults with acute myeloid leukaemia: myths, controversies, and unknowns. Blood. 2011

[2] Tsirigotis P, Byrne M, Schmidt C et al. Relapse of AML after hematopoie tic stem cell transplantation: methods of monitoring and preventive strategies. A review from the ALWP of the EBMT. Bone Marrow Transplant. 2016 Nov;.

[3] Thanarajasingham G, Kim HT, Cutler C et al. Outcome and prognostic factors for patients who relapse after allogeneic hematopoietic stem cell transplantation. Biol Blood Marrow Transplant. 2013 Dec;.

[4] Cornelissen JJ, Gratwhol A, Schlenk RF, et al. The European Leukemia Net AML Working Party consensus statement on allogeneic HSCT for patients with AML in remission: an integrated risk-adapted approach. Nature Reviews. Clinical Oncology. 2012a;**9**:579-590

[5] Buccisano F, Hourigan C, Walter R. The prognostic significance of measurable ("Minimal") residual disease in Acute Myeloid Leukemia. CurrOpinMalig Rep. 2017

[6] Dohner H, Estey E, Grimwade D, et al. Diagnosis and management of _ AML in adults: 2017 ELN recommendations from an international expert panel. Blood. 2017

[7] Duarte R, Labopyn M, Bader P, et al. Bone MarrowTransplant. 2019:2019

[8] Buccisano F, Maurillo L. Spagnoli A et al. Blood: Cytogenetic and molecular diagnostic characterization combined to post-consolidation minimal residual disease assessment by flow cytometry improves risk stratification in adult acute myeloid leukaemia; 2010

[9] Zhou Y, Othus M, Araki D et al. Pre- and post-transplant quantification of measurable ("minimal") residual disease via multiparameter flow cytometry in adult acute myeloid leukaemia. Leukemia 2016;.

[10] Buckley SA, Wood BL, Othus M, et al. Minimal Residual Disease prior to allogeneic hematopoietic cell transplantation in acute myeloid leukaemia: a meta-analysis. Haematologica. 2017

[11] Mannis G, Martin TG III. Damon LE et al. Leuk Lymph: Long-term outcomes of patients with intermediate-risk acute myeloid leukaemia treated with autologous hematopoietic cell transplant in first complete remission; 2016

[12] National Comprehensive Cancer Network clinical practice guidelines in oncology – Acute Myeloid Leukemia version 2014.

[13] Venditti A, Piciocchi A, Candoni A, et al. GIMEMA AML1310 trial of risk-adapted. Blood: MRD-directed therapy for young adults with newly diagnosed acute myeloid leukaemia; 2019

[14] Schuuruis GJ, Heuser M, Freeman S, et al. Minimal/measurable residual disease in AML: a consensus document from the European Leukemia Net MRd Working Party. Blood. 2018

[15] Walter R, Buckley S. Pagel JM et al. Blood: Significance of minimal residual disease before myeloablative allogeneic hematopoietic cell transplantation for AML in first and second complete remission; 2013

[16] Quek L, Otto GW, Garnett C, et al. Genetically distinct leukemic stem cells in human CD34+ acute myeloid leukaemia are arrested at a hematopoietic precursor-like stage. The Journal of Experimental Medicine. 2016

[17] Jongen-Lavrencic M, Grob T, Hanekamp D, Kavelaars FG, Al Hinai A, Zeilemaker A, Erpelinck-Verschueren CAJ, Gradowska PL, Meijer R, Cloos J, Biemond BJ, Graux C, van MarwijkKooy M, Manz MG, Pabst T, Passweg JR, Havelange V, Ossenkoppele GJ, Sanders MA, Schuurhuis GJ, Löwenberg B, Valk PJM. Molecular Minimal Residual Disease in Acute Myeloid Leukemia. N Engl J Med. 2018

[18] Pratcorona M, Brunet S, Nomdede' J et al.; GrupoCooperativo Para elEstudio y Tratamiento de lasLeucemiasAgudasMieloblasticas. Favourable outcome of patients with acute myeloid leukaemiaharbouring a low-allele burden FLT3-ITD mutation and concomitant NPM1 mutation: relevance to post-remission therapy. Blood. 2013;

[19] Gale RE, Green C, Allen C, et al. Medical Research Council Adult Leukaemia Working Party The impact of FLT3 internal tandem duplication mutant level, number, size, and interaction with NPM1 mutations in a large cohort of young adult patients with acute myeloid leukaemia. Blood. 2008

[20] Bazarbachi A, Bug G, Baron F, et al. Clinical practice recommendation on hematopoietic stem cell transplantation for acute myeloid leukaemia patients with FLT3-internal tandem duplication: a position statement from the Acute Leukemia Working Party of the European Society for Blood and Marrow Transplantation. Haematologica. 2020

[21] Poiret X, Labopin M, Cornelissen JJ, et al. Outcome of conditioning intensity in acute myeloid leukaemia with monosomal karyotype in patients over 45-year-old: A study from the acute leukaemia working party (ALWP) of the European group of blood and marrow transplantation (EBMT). American Journal of Hematology. 2015

[22] Poiret X, Labopin m, Maertens J et al. Allogeneic stem cell transplantation in adult patients with acute myeloid leukaemia and 17p abnormalities in first complete remission: a study from the Acute Leukemia Working Party (ALWP) of the European Society for Blood and MarrowTransplantation (EBMT). J HematolOncol 2017;

[23] Poiret X, Labopin M, Polge E, et al. Allogeneic stem cell transplantation using HLA-matched donors for acute myeloid leukaemia with deletion 5q or monosomy 5: a study from the Acute Leukemia Working Party of the EBMT. Haematologica. 2020

[24] Oliai C, Schiller G. How to address second and therapy-related acute myelogenous leukaemia. British Journal of Hematology. 2020;**188**:116-128

[25] Sengsayadeth S, Labopin M, Boumendil A et al. Transplant Outcomes for Secondary Acute Myeloid Leukemia: Acute LeukemiaWorking Party of the European Society for Blood and Bone Marrow Transplantation Study. Biol Blood Marrow Transplant 24 2018

[26] Schmaelter A-K, Labopin M, Socié G et al. Inferior outcome of allogeneic stem cell transplantation for secondary acute myeloid leukaemia in first complete remission as compared to de novo acute myeloid leukaemia. Blood Cancer Journal (2020).

[27] Lancet TE, Uy GL, Cortes JE, et al. CPX-351 (Cytarabine and Daunorubicin) liposome for injection versus conventional cytarabine plus daunorubicin in older patients with newly diagnosed secondary acute myeloid leukaemia. Journal of Clinical Oncology. 2018

[28] Ferguson P, Hills RK, Grech A et al. An operational definition of primary refractory acute myeloid leukaemia allowing early identification of patients

who may benefit from allogeneic stem cell transplantation. Haematologica 2016 Nov;

[29] Jabbour E, Daver N, Champlin R et al. Allogeneic stem cell transplantation as initial salvage therapy for patients with acute myeloid leukaemia refractory to high-dose cytarabine-based induction chemotherapy. Am J Hematol 2104;

[30] Schmid C, Schleuning M, Schwerdtfleger R et al. Long-term survival in refractory acute myeloid leukaemia after sequential treatment with chemotherapy and reduced-intensity conditioning for allogeneic stem cell transplantation. Blood 2006;

[31] Schmid C, Scheluning M, Ledderose G, et al. Sequential regimen of chemotherapy, reduced-intensity conditioning for allogeneic stem-cell transplantation, and prophylactic donor lymphocyte transfusion in high-risk acute myeloid leukaemia and myelodysplastic syndrome. Journal of Clinical Oncology. 2005

[32] Gyurkozca B, Lazarus HM, Giralt S. Allogeneic hematopoietic transplantation in patients with AML not achieving remission: potentially curative therapy. Bone Marrow Transplantation. 2017

[33] Duval M, Klein JP, He W, et al. Hematopoietic stem cell transplantation for acute leukemia in relapse or primary induction failure. Journal of Clinical Oncology. 2010

[34] Christopeit M, Labopin M, Gorin N-C et al. Allogeneic stem cell transplantation following relapse post autologous stem cell transplantation in adult patients with acute myeloid leukaemia: a retrospective analysis of 537 patients from the Acute Leukemia Working Party of the EBMT. Am J Hematol 2018;

[35] Gillece MH, Labopin M, Savani BN, et al. Allogeneic haemopoietic transplantation for acute myeloid leukaemia in second complete remission: a registry report by the Acute Leukaemia Working Party of the EBMT. Leukaemia. 2020

[36] Halaburda K, Labopin M, Mailhol A, et al. Allogeneic stem cell transplantation in second complete remission for core-binding factor acute myeloid leukaemia: a study from the Acute Leukemia Working Party of the European Society for Blood and Marrow Transplantation. Haematologica. 2020

[37] Passweg JR, Labopin M, Christopeit M et al. Postremission Consolidation by Autologous Hematopoietic Cell Transplantation (HCT) for Acute Myeloid Leukemia in First Complete Remission (CR) and Negative Implications for Subsequent Allogeneic HCT in Second CR: A Study by the Acute Leukemia Working Party of the European Society for Blood and Marrow Transplantation (EBMT). Biol Blood and Marrow Transplant 26 2020

[38] Forman SJ. Rowe JM. Blood: The myth of the second remission of acute leukemia in the adult; 2013 Feb 14

[39] Armand P, Kim HT, Logan BR, et al. Validation and refinement of the Disease Risk Index for allogeneic stem cell transplantation. *Blood*. 2014;

[40] Sorror ML, Maris MB, Storb R, et al. Hematopoietic cell transplantation (HCT)-specific comorbidity index: a new tool for risk assessment before allogeneic HCT. Blood. 2005

[41] Sorror ML, Storb RF, Sandmaier BM, et al. Comorbidity-age index: a clinical measure of biologic age before allogeneic hematopoietic cell transplantation. J ClinOncol. 2014

[42] Roberto Raimondi, Alberto Tosetto, Rosi Oneto, Riccardo Cavazzina,

Francesco Rodeghiero, Andrea Bacigalupo, Renato Fanin, Alessandro Rambaldi, Alberto Bosi; Validation of the Hematopoietic Cell Transplantation-SpecificComorbidity Index: a prospective, multicenter GITMO study. Blood 2012;

[43] Gratwohl A. The EBMT risk score. Bone Marrow Transplantation. 2012

[44] Martin Schmidt-Hieber, Myriam Labopin, Dietrich Beelen, LiisaVolin, Gerhard Ehninger, Jürgen Finke, Gerard Socié, Rainer Schwerdtfeger, Nicolaus Kröger, Arnold Ganser, DietgerNiederwieser, Emmanuelle Polge, Igor W. Blau, Mohamad Mohty; CMV serostatus still has an important prognostic impact in de novo acute leukemia patients after allogeneic stem cell transplantation: a report from the Acute Leukemia Working Party of EBMT. Blood 2013;

[45] Pierre Teira, MinooBattiwalla, MuthalaguRamanathan, A. John Barrett, KwangWooAhn, Min Chen, Jaime S. Green, Ayman Saad, Joseph H. Antin, Bipin N. Savani, Hillard M. Lazarus, Matthew Seftel, WaelSaber, David Marks, Mahmoud Aljurf, MaximNorkin, John R. Wingard, Caroline A. Lindemans, Michael Boeckh, Marcie L. Riches, Jeffery J. Auletta; Earlycytomegalo virus reactivation remains associated with increased transplant-related mortality in the current era: a CIBMTR analysis. *Blood* 2016;

[46] Tvedt THA, Hovland R, Tsykunova G, Ahmed AB, Gedde-Dahl T, Bruserud Ø. A pilot study of single nucleotide polymorphisms in the interleukin-6 receptor and their effects on pre- and post-transplant serum mediator level and outcome after allogeneic stem cell transplantation. Clinical and Experimental Immunology. 2018

[47] Petersdorf EW. Genetics of graft-versus-host disease: The major histocompatibility complex. *Blood Rev*; 2013

[48] M. Martin, D. Mann, and M. Carrington, "Recombination rates across the HLA complex: Use of microsatellites as a rapid screen for recombinant chromosomes," *Human Molecular Genetics*. 1995.

[49] K. Fleischhauer and B. E. Shaw, "HLA-DP in unrelated hematopoietic cell transplantation revisited: Challenges and opportunities," *Blood*. 2017.

[50] Tiercy J-M. Unrelated Hematopoietic Stem Cell Donor Matching Probability and Search Algorithm. *Bone Marrow Res*; 2012

[51] Morishima Y et al. Biological significance of HLA locus matching in unrelated donor bone marrow transplantation. *Blood*; 2015

[52] Pidala J et al. Nonpermissive HLA-DPB1 mismatch increases mortality after myeloablative unrelated allogeneic hematopoietic cell transplantation. *Blood*; 2014

[53] Lee SJ et al. High-resolution donor-recipient HLA matching contributes to the success of unrelated donor marrow transplantation. *Blood*; 2007

[54] F. Lorentino *et al.*, "Comparative evaluation of biological HLA-DPB1 mismatch models for survival and graft versus host disease prediction after unrelated donor hematopoietic cell transplantation," *Haematologica*. 2020.

[55] Crocchiolo R et al. Nonpermissive HLA-DPB1 disparity is a significant independent risk factor for mortality after unrelated hematopoietic stem cell transplantation. *Blood*; 2009

[56] Kollman C et al. The effect of donor characteristics on survival after unrelated donor transplantation for hematologic malignancy. *Blood*; 2016

[57] Y. J. Chang, L. Luznik, E. J. Fuchs, and X. J. Huang, "How do we choose the best donor for T-cell-replete, HLA-haploidentical transplantation?," *Journal of Hematology and Oncology*. 2016.

[58] Saber W, Opie S, Rizzo JD, Zhang MJ, Horowitz MM, Schriber J. Outcomes after matched unrelated donor versus identical sibling hematopoietic cell transplantation in adults with acute myelogenous leukemia. *Blood*; 2012

[59] Gupta V et al. Comparable survival after HLA-well-matched unrelated or matched sibling donor transplantation for acute myeloid leukemia in first remission with unfavorable cytogenetics at diagnosis. *Blood*; 2010

[60] C. J. Lee *et al.*, "Haploidentical hematopoietic cell transplantation for adult acute myeloid leukemia: A position statement from the acute leukemia working party of the European society for blood and marrow transplantation," *Haematologica*. 2017.

[61] Aversa F et al. Successful engraftment of T-cell-depleted haploidentical 'three-loci' incompatible transplants in leukemia patients by addition of recombinant human granulocyte colony-stimulating factor-mobilized peripheral blood progenitor cells to bone marrow inoculum. *Blood*; 1994

[62] André-Schmutz I et al. Immune reconstitution without graft-versus-host disease after haemopoietic stem-cell transplantation: A phase 1/2 study. *Lancet*; 2002

[63] Kunacheewa C, Ungprasert P, Phikulsod P, Issaragrisil S, Owattanapanich W. Comparative Efficacy and Clinical Outcomes of Haploidentical Stem Cell Transplantation to Other Stem Sources for Treatment in Acute Myeloid Leukemia and Myelodysplastic Syndrome Patients: A Systematic Review and Meta-Analysis. *Cell Transplant*; 2020

[64] Wagner JE et al. Transplantation of unrelated donor umbilical cord blood in 102 patients with malignant and nonmalignant diseases: Influence of CD34 cell dose and HLA disparity on treatment-related mortality and survival. *Blood*; 2002

[65] Brunstein CG et al. Alternative donor transplantation after reduced intensity conditioning: Results of parallel phase 2 trials using partially HLA-mismatched related bone marrow or unrelated double umbilical cord blood grafts. *Blood*; 2011

[66] Shouval R et al. Outcomes of allogeneic haematopoietic stem cell transplantation from HLA-matched and alternative donors: a European Society for Blood and Marrow Transplantation registry retrospective analysis. *Lancet Haematol*; 2019

[67] Bacigalupo A et al. Defining the Intensity of Conditioning Regimens: Working Definitions. Biology of Blood and Marrow Transplantation. 2009; **15**(12):1628-1633

[68] Nagler A et al. Allogeneic hematopoietic stem-cell transplantation for acute myeloid leukaemia in remission: Comparison of intravenous busulfan plus cyclophosphamide (Cy) versus total-body irradiation plus cy as conditioning regimen-A report from the acute leukaemia working. Journal of Clinical Oncology. 2013;**31**(28): 3549-3556

[69] Bredeson C et al. Prospective cohort study comparing intravenous busulfan to total body irradiation in hematopoietic cell transplantation. Blood. 2013;**122**(24):3871-3878

[70] Rambaldi A et al. Busulfan plus cyclophosphamide versus busulfan plus

fludarabine as a preparative regimen for allogeneic haemopoietic stem-cell transplantation in patients with acute myeloid leukaemia: An open-label, multicentre, randomised, phase 3 trial. The Lancet Oncology. 2015;**16**(15): 1525-1536

[71] Ben-Barouch S, Cohen O, Vidal L, Avivi I, Ram R. Busulfan fludarabine vs busulfan cyclophosphamide as a preparative regimen before allogeneic hematopoietic cell transplantation: Systematic review and meta-analysis. Bone Marrow Transplantation. 2016; **51**(2):232-240

[72] Eder S et al. Thiotepa-based versus total body irradiation-based myeloablative conditioning prior to allogeneic stem cell transplantation for acute myeloid leukaemia in first complete remission: A retrospective analysis from the Acute Leukemia Working Party of the Euro. European Journal of Haematology. 2016;**96**(1): 90-97

[73] Devine SM et al. Phase II study of allogeneic transplantation for older patients with acute myeloid leukaemia in first complete remission using a reduced-intensity conditioning regimen: Results from Cancer and Leukemia Group B 100103 (Alliance for Clinical Trials in Oncology). Journal of Clinical Oncology. 2015;**33**(35): 4167-4175

[74] Massenkeil G et al. Survival after reduced-intensity conditioning is not inferior to standard high-dose conditioning before allogeneic haematopoietic cell transplantation in acute leukaemias. Bone Marrow Transplantation. 2005;**36**(8):683-689

[75] Sébert M et al. Equivalent outcomes using reduced intensity or conventional myeloablative conditioning transplantation for patients aged 35 years and over with AML. Bone Marrow Transplantation. 2015;**50**(1):74-81

[76] Flynn CM et al. Reduced-intensity compared with high dose conditioning for allotransplantation in acute myeloid leukaemia and myelodysplastic syndrome: A comparative clinical analysis. American Journal of Hematology. 2007;**82**(10):867-872

[77] A. EP *et al.*, "Impact of Conditioning Regimen Intensity on Outcome of Allogeneic Hematopoietic Cell Transplantation for Advanced Acute Myelogenous Leukemia and Myelodysplastic Syndrome," Biology of Blood and Marrow Transplantation, vol. 12, no. 10, pp. 1047–1055, 2006.

[78] Ringdén O et al. Reduced-intensity conditioning compared with myeloablative conditioning using unrelated donor transplants in patients with acute myeloid leukaemia. Journal of Clinical Oncology. 2009;**27**(27): 4570-4577

[79] Scott BL et al. Myeloablative versus reduced-intensity hematopoietic cell transplantation for acute myeloid leukaemia and myelodysplastic syndromes. Journal of Clinical Oncology. 2017;**35**(11):1154-1161

[80] Malard F et al. Sequential Intensified Conditioning Regimen Allogeneic Hematopoietic Stem Cell Transplantation in Adult Patients with Intermediate- or High-Risk Acute Myeloid Leukemia in Complete Remission: A Study from the Acute Leukemia Working Party of the European Gr. Biology of Blood and Marrow Transplantation. 2017;**23**(2): 278-284

[81] Saure C et al. Upfront Allogeneic Blood Stem Cell Transplantation for Patients with High-Risk Myelodysplastic Syndrome or Secondary Acute Myeloid Leukemia Using FLAMSA-Based High-Dose Sequential Conditioning Regimen. Biology of Blood and Marrow Transplantation. 2012;**18**(3):466-472

[82] Schmid C, Scheluning M, Ledderose G, et al. Sequential regimen of chemotherapy, reduced-intensity conditioning for allogeneic stem-cell transplantation, and prophylactic donor lymphocyte transfusion in high-risk acute myeloid leukaemia and myelodysplastic syndrome. Journal of Clinical Oncology. 2005;**23**:5675-5687

[83] Munchel A et al. Nonmyeloablative, HLA-haploidentical bone marrow transplantation with high dose, post-transplantation cyclophosphamide. Pediatr. Rep. 2011;**3**(2S):43-47

[84] Kasamon YL et al. Nonmyeloablative HLA-Haploidentical Bone Marrow Transplantation with High-Dose Posttransplantation Cyclophosphamide: Effect of HLA Disparity on Outcome. Biology of Blood and Marrow Transplantation. 2010; **16**(4):482-489

[85] Ciurea SO et al. Haploidentical transplant with posttransplant cyclophosphamide vs matched unrelated donor transplant for acute myeloid leukaemia. Blood. 2015;**126**(8): 1033-1040

[86] M. M. *et al.*, "Posttransplantation cyclophosphamide for prevention of graft-versus-host disease after HLA-matched mobilized blood cell transplantation," Blood, vol. 127, no. 11, pp. 1502–1508, 2016.

[87] Moreb JS. Aldehyde dehydrogenase as a marker for stem cells. Current Stem Cell Research & Therapy 2008 Dec;3 (4):237–246. doi: 10.2174/ 157488808786734006. PMID: 19075754.

[88] Moiseev IS et al. Graft-versus-Host Disease Prophylaxis in Unrelated Peripheral Blood Stem Cell Transplantation with Post-Transplantation Cyclophosphamide, Tacrolimus, and Mycophenolate Mofetil. Biology of Blood and Marrow Transplantation. 2016;**22**(6):1037-1042

[89] L. Williams, F. Cirrone, K. Cole, M. Abdul-Hay, L. Luznik, and A. S. Al-Homsi, "Post-transplantation Cyclophosphamide: From HLA-Haploidentical to Matched-Related and Matched-Unrelated Donor Blood and Marrow Transplantation," *Frontiers in Immunology*, vol. 11. 2020.

[90] Di Bartolomeo P et al. Haploidentical, unmanipulated, G-CSF-primed bone marrow transplantation for patients with high-risk hematologic malignancies. Blood. 2013;**121**(5): 849-857

[91] Shier LR, Schultz KR, Imren S, Regan J, Issekutz A, Sadek I, Gilman A, Luo Z, Panzarella T, Eaves CJ, Couban S. Differential effects of granulocyte colony-stimulating factor on marrow- and blood-derived hematopoietic and immune cell populations in healthy human donors. Biology of Blood and Marrow Transplantation 2004 Sep;10(9):624–634. doi: 10.1016/j.bbmt.2004.05.009. PMID: 15319774.

[92] Chang YJ, Zhao XY, Huo MR, Huang XJ. Expression profiles of adhesion molecules on naïve T cells in bone marrow grafts of healthy donors treated with granulocyte colony-stimulating factor. Transplant Immunology. 2009;**21**(4):228-233

[93] Reisner Y, Hagin D, Martelli MF. Haploidentical hematopoietic transplantation: Current status and future perspectives. Blood. 2011; **118**(23):6006-6018

[94] Airoldi I et al. γδ T-cell reconstitution after HLA-haploidentical hematopoietic transplantation depleted of TCR-αβ+/CD19+ lymphocytes. Blood. 2015;**125**(15):2349-2358

[95] Martelli MF et al. HLA-haploidentical transplantation with regulatory and conventional T-cell adoptive immunotherapy prevents

acute leukaemia relapse. Blood. 2014; **124**(4):638-644

[96] Cornelissen JJ *et al*,. "The European LeukemiaNet AML Working Party consensus statement on allogeneic HSCT for patients with AML in remission: an integrated-risk adapted approach", *Clin Oncol*. 2012.

[97] Jaiswal SR, Zaman S, Chakrabarti A, Sen S, Mukherjee S, Bhargava S, Ray K, O'Donnell PV, Chakrabarti S. Improved Outcome of Refractory/Relapsed Acute Myeloid Leukemia after Post-Transplantation Cyclophosphamide-Based Haploidentical Transplantation with Myeloablative Conditioning and Early Prophylactic Granulocyte Colony-Stimulating Factor-Mobilized Donor Lymphocyte Infusions. Biol Blood Marrow Transplant. 2016 Oct

[98] F. J. *et al.*, "Full donor chimerism without graft-versus-host disease: The key factor for the maximum benefit of pre-emptive donor lymphocyte infusions (pDLI)," *Bone Marrow Transplant.*, vol. 50, pp. S125–S126, 2015.

[99] Soiffer RJ, Davids MS, Bin Chen Y. Tyrosine kinase inhibitors and immune checkpoint blockade in allogeneic hematopoietic cell transplantation. Blood. 2018;**131**(10):1073-1080

[100] Craddock C et al. Tolerability and Clinical Activity of Post-Transplantation Azacitidine in Patients Allografted for Acute Myeloid Leukemia Treated on the RICAZA Trial. Biology of Blood and Marrow Transplantation. 2016;**22**(2):385-390

Chapter 12

Consolidation: Autologous Stem Cell Transplantation in Acute Leukemia

Fatma Keklik Karadağ, Fahri Şahin and Güray Saydam

Abstract

The goal of complete remission (CR) in acute leukemias could be achieved with intensive induction chemotherapy however patients need post remission consolidation strategies such as high-dose chemotherapy, or autologous (ASCT) or allogeneic (allo-SCT) hematopoetic stem cell transplantation for durable response. However, Allo-SCT is getting more attention in last decades because of improvements of conditioning regimens and graft versus host disease (GVHD) prohylaxis strategies and alternatively available donor sources, it is not suitable for all leukemia patients. The patients who would benefit from Allo-SCT or ASCT could be defined more easily by using risk stratification systems and minimal residual disease (MRD) monitoring. ASCT is considered a treatment option even if its use is declining in the world. Herein, we tried to summarize the studies that report the outcomes of ASCT in acute myeloid leukemia (AML) and acute, lymphoblastic leukemia and describe the patients who would be good candidate for ASCT.

Keywords: autologous stem cell, transplantation, acute leukemia, adult, lymphoblastic leukemia, myeloid leukemia

1. Introduction

Standard chemotherapy regimens are the first step for the treatment of acute leukemias. However, the complete remission could be achieved with intensive chemotherapy, durable remission is not common and patients will relapse within months unless additional therapy is given. There is an extensive debate about post remission therapy. There is no consensus about intensive chemotherapy as a consolidation and/or stem cell transplantation (SCT) after first remission (CR1). Allogeneic stem cell transplantation (Allo-SCT) for acute leukemias has been increased due to the developments of allo-SCT techniques. Availability of alternative donor sources (including haploidentical, matched unrelated donors and umbilical cord blood), improvements of graft versus host disease (GVHD) prophylaxis strategies and reduced-intensity conditioning (RIC) regimens are developed in last decades and Allo-SCT has been used widely all over the world. However, lower incidence of relapse rates after allo-SCT because of graft versus leukemia effect makes allo-SCT more popular, high morbidity rates due to chronic GVHD, secondary graft failure and high treatment related mortality (TRM) rates in the patients who underwent Allo-SCT should be considered and it is not recommended for the patients with good risk. Allo-SCT is not available for elderly patients and

IntechOpen

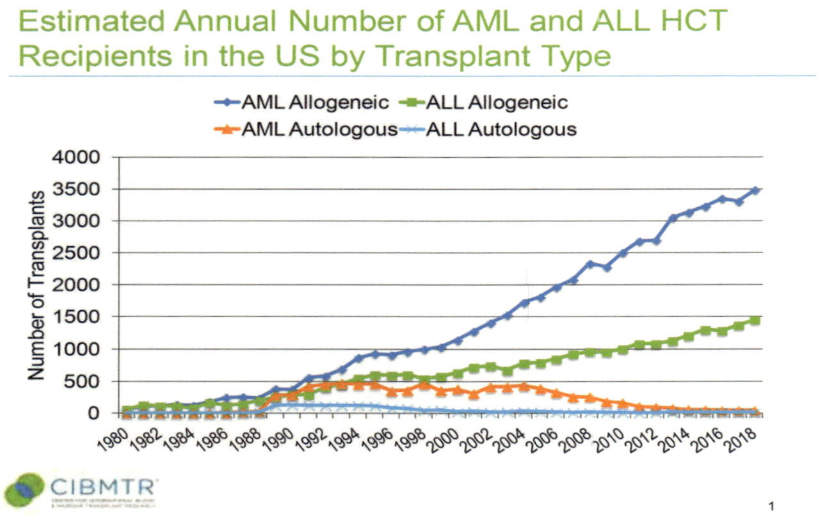

Figure 1.
The rates of autologous stem cell transplantation (ASCT) and allogeneic stem cell transplantation in acute myeloid leukemia (AML) and acute lymphoblastic leukemia (ALL). (*Data presented in table is kindly provided by CIBMTR).*

the patients who do not have HLA-matched related or unrelated donor. Autologous stem cell transplantation (ASCT) is an alternative and valuable treatment option with acceptable long term outcomes and lower TRM rates for the patients with low and intermediate risk after CR1 and the patients who are not eligible for Allo-SCT. Center for International Blood and Marrow Transplantation Research (CIBMTR) showed the rates of ASCT and Allo-SCT in acute myeloid leukemia (AML) and acute lymphoblastic leukemia (ALL) in the USA (**Figure 1**).

2. ASCT for acute myeloid leukemia

More than half of AML patients achieved complete remission after standard induction therapy but 60–70% of patients will relapse without consolidation therapy. ASCT, an effective therapy for AML was started to use in 1980's for consolidation in AML patients [1–5]. Since then, it is a challenge to define the patients who would benefit from ASCT. Bone marrow (BM) initially preferred source of stem cells for ASCT. After hematopoietic growth factors provided the possibility to use peripheral blood stem cells (PBSC) grafts after intensive chemotherapy courses since 1994, the treatment compliance of ASCT has improved and the treatment-related mortality (TRM) has been reduced due to accelerated hematopoietic reconstitution [6]. Mobilized PBCS have replaced bone marrow because of the main advantages of PBSCs as a stem cell source are markedly faster neutrophil and platelet recovery times than bone marrow, with consequently reduced infection, bleeding and hospitalization risks. The PBSC target dose is considered an amount of CD34+ cells $\geq 2 \times 10^6$/kg body weight. There is numerous clinical studies compare ASCT with chemotherapy or Allo-SCT in AML patients according to cytogenetic risk groups and CR1 or second remission (CR2). National Comprehensive Cancer Network (NCCN) and European leukemia network (ELN) divided patients with AML into three risk status groups: good/favorable, intermediate, and poor/adverse risk by genetic abnormality in 2017 (**Table 1**) [7]. The 'favorable' group includes patients with either inv.(16), t(16;16), t(8; 21), mutated NPM1 without FLT3

Risk category	Cytogenetic abnormality
Favorable	t(8;21)(q22;q22): *RUNX1-RUNX1T1*
	inv(16)(p13.1q22) or t(16;16)(p13.1;q22): *CBFB-MYH11*
	Mutated *NPM1* without *FLT3*-ITD or with *FLT3*-ITD^{low}
	Biallelic mutated *CEBPA*
Intermediate	Mutated *NPM1* and *FLT3*-ITD^{high}
	Wild type *NPM1* without *FLT3*-ITD or with *FLT3*-ITD^{low}
	t(9;11)(p21.3;q23.3); *MLLT3-KMT2A*
	Cytogenetic abnormalities not classified as favorable or adverse
Adverse	t(6;9)(p23;q34): *DEK-NUP214*
	t(v;11)(v;q23): *KMT2A* rearranged
	t(9;22)(q34.1;q11.2); *BCR-ABL1*
	−7
	Complex karyotype
	Monosomal karyotype
	Wild type *NPM1* and *FLT3*-ITD^{high}
	Mutated *RUNX1*
	Mutated *ASXL1*

Table 1.
Genetic risk stratification according to the ELN-2017.

ITD (internal tandem duplications) (NPM+/FLT3 ITD−) or mutated CEBPA. An 'adverse' group consists of patients with inv. (3) or t (3;3), t(6;9), t(v;11) either −5 or del (5q), −7, abn (17p) or ⩾3 cytogenetic abnormalities not including translocations (complex karyotype). An intermediate-1 group comprises patients with a normal karyotype (NK) and with the other genotypic combinations of NPM1 and FLT3 ITD (+/+, −/−, −/+) and an intermediate-2 group consists of patients with t (9;11) and cytogenetic abnormalities not noted above. Good-risk AML patients qualify for chemotherapeutic consolidation, but recent reports suggested favorable outcome for good-risk patients with ASCT, which provides a possible option in that category of patients [8, 9]. The survival outcomes of patients with good-risk or intermediate-risk AML who underwent ASCT as postremission therapy were favorable—probably due to the use of PBSC rather than instead of BM, which may decrease the risk of transplant-related complications—but that the survival outcomes of similarly treated poor-risk AML patients were not.

Gruppo Italiano Trapianto di Midollo Osseo (GITMO) analyzed 809 AML patients who were autografted in CR1 retrospectively [10]. Two year leukemia free survival (LFS) and Overall Survival (OS) rates were found 51% and 65%, respectively and it was reported that survival was significantly influenced by cytogenetic risk. Patients with good risk group had remarkable better outcomes in this study. The 2 year cumulative incidence of relapse was higher in poor risk patients (28 ± 7% for good risk group vs. 48 ± 8% for poor risk group, p < 0,0002). Patients with CEBPA double mutated (CEBPAdm) and nucleophosmin-1 (NPM) mutated AML have better outcome with ASCT [9, 11]. It has been already demonstrated that the subset of patients with *NPM1*$^{+}$ mutations without fms-related tyrosine kinase 3 gene *(FLT3)* internal tandem duplications (*FLT3-ITD*) derive no survival benefit from allo-SCT [12].

Several historical randomized trials have reported that ASCT can significantly reduce the relapse rates compare with conventional chemotherapy alone. The study performed by the Dutch–Belgian Hemato-Oncology Cooperative Group/Swiss Group for Clinical Cancer Research (HOVON-SAKK) Cooperative Consortium compared the outcomes of ASCT with chemotherapy including 517 patients who were randomly recorded between 1995 and 2006 [1]. Rates of relapse after chemotherapy vs. after ASCT were 70% vs. 58%, respectively (P = .02), 5 year follow up and no significant difference in LFS of 29% vs. 38% (P = .065). OS did not differ between these two groups and was estimated to be 41% vs. 44%, respectively, at 5 years from randomization. TRM was higher in ASCT group than chemotherapy group (4% vs. 1% respectively).

A meta-analysis which included 11 studies compared survival outcomes of alloSCT from matched sibling donor (MSD) or matched unrelated donor (MUD) versus ASCT in intermediate-risk AML and demonstrated alloSCT from MSDs rather than MUDs was associated with better OS than that with ASCT [13] however recent retrospective trials reported similar survival rates for AML patients who underwent autoSCT and allo-SCT from MSDs and MUDs [3, 14, 15].

The treatment options are not well defined in older patients with leukemia. Higher incidence of AML secondary to previous myelodysplastic syndrome (MDS), adverse mutation pattern and karyotype and poor performance status are the reasons of poor outcomes in older AML patients [16–18]. They usually do not have MSD and available regimens are limited due to many of comorbidities especially cardiovascular disease. ASCT may be used in patients up to age 70 years with an acceptable TRM of approximately 8%, which compares favorably to 17% as was observed after RIC alloHSCT.

Several reports from EBMT and CIBMTR showed long-term leukemia free survival (LFS) rates are 45–55% in patients transplanted in CR 1 and 25–35% for those transplanted in CR2 [19–21]. The patients who are not eligible for Allo-SCT ASCT may be an acceptable post-remission therapy in CR1 [14]. Allo-SCT still remains first line treatment for poor risk patients while ASCT is getting attention for good risk and especially intermediate risk patients who have favorable prognostic factors, including MRD negativity after the imitation of induction chemotherapy, a WBC count of <20,000/μL at time of the diagnosis, an FAB classification of M1–5, and ≥ 50% MPO positivity. Decision-making might benefit from taking minimal residual disease (MRD) into account [22, 23]. Real-time quantitative PCR (qPCR) and multiparameter flow cytometry (MFC) are effective techniques for monitoring MRD before and after ASCT in patients with AML, and MRD status pre-ASCT is an independent prognostic factor for both OS and LFS after ASCT [24, 25]. Whereby MRD-negative patients may be consolidated by ASCT and MRD-positive patients may proceed to allo-SCT. ASCT is generating new interest, especially in intermediate-risk patients who became MRD negative upon induction chemotherapy [26].

The traditional conditioning regimens before ASCT that are mostly myeloablative and based on busulfan; combination of busulfan/ cyclophosphamide (BUCY), busulfan/etoposide, cyclophosphamide/Total body irradiation (TBI), Busulfan/ high dose melphalan. Different regimens such as modifications of the BCNU, etoposide, cytarabine, melphalan (BEAM) regimen, busulfan/etoposide/ cytarabine, TBI/cytarabine/melphalan could be used in different centers. Three large retrospective studies showed that busulfan/high dose melphalan regimen has better outcomes than BUCY [27–29]. Although both oral and intravenous busulfan were used in various regimens, it has become clear that the intravenous administration of busulfan should be preferred because of fewer complications [30]. Favorable long-term LFS after auto-SCT using a high-dose cytarabine-containing regimen has been showed. The most common treatment related complication of ASCT is mucositis and mucositis are usually more frequent in the patients who were treated with oral busulfan than ıv busulfan.

3. ASCT for acute promyelocytic leukemia

Acute promyelocytic leukemia (APL) accounts 10–15% of AML in adults. It is highly curable disease and remission is achieved in 90% of APL patients after anthracycline-based induction therapy plus ATRA and recently arsenic trioxide (ATO). The combination of ATRA and anthracyclines remains the gold standard for high risk patients. There is not a role for stem cell transplantation in APL in CR1, independently from any initial risk category. ELN suggested that patients who relapsed after ATRA plus chemotherapy should be treated with an ATRA plus ATO based approach as salvage therapy until achievement of MRD negativity. Despite of SCT is accepted treatment for the 10–20% patients who relapsed, the choice of ASCT vs. Allo-SCT remains controversial.

EBMT reviewed 625 APL patients transplanted ASCT or Allo-SCT, lower relapse rates and higher 5 year LFS reported in Allo-SCT group. Although TRM was higher in Allo-SCT patients, Allo-SCT was recommended in CR2 when a sibling donor was available in this study [31]. Holter et al. reported OS was better after ASCT than after chemotherapy and ATO. ASCT was the preferred therapy for patients with CR2 status, and survival outcomes were superior in patients who received ASCT compared with those who received ATO-based consolidation therapy [32]. Besides ASCT is superior than allo-SCT in relapsed APL due to low TRM and durable remission, pre-SCT bone marrow cytogenetic and molecularly evaluation is important. It was recommended allogeneic HCT if the pre-HCT marrow was cytogenetically or molecularly positive [33]. ASCT is less toxic than allo-SCT, and appears equally potent particularly when a negative *PML-RARA* status is achieved before transplantation.

4. ASCT for acute lymphocytic leukemia

ALL is divided into tumors of B cell and T cell lineage and it is the most common cause of leukemia in children however up to 20% of the cases of ALL occur in adults. Despite of the developments of induction chemotherapy regimen, relapse rates and mortality still remain high in this century. Most of studies were designed according to risk stratification and categorized patients into standard, intermediate or poor risk. Poor risk criteria are cytogenetic abnormalities t(9;22), t(4;11), or t(1;19); pro–B-cell immunophenotype; high WBC (i.e., > 30×10^9/L in case of B-ALL; > 100×10^9/L in case of T-cell ALL [T-ALL]) at the time of diagnosis. Although the introduction of more aggressive chemotherapy regimens has reduced the need for allo-HSCT in patients younger than 35 years of age, allo-HSCT remains the standard of care for high-risk patients and relapse after CR1. SCT is still a debate in ALL patients without poor-risk features however Allo-SCT is highly recommended in poor risk ALL patients in CR1. Allo-SCT is not certainly suggested in ALL patients without poor risk to avoid the unnecessary risks of transplantation procedure-related mortality and GVHD to patients, who may be cured with chemotherapy alone and to postpone allo-SCT to an eventual relapse. The standard risk patients rather than the high-risk patients, older patients and the patients who are not eligible for Allo-SCT may be the ones who are most likely to benefit from ASCT in first remission. MRD has emerged as a prognostic marker that can define patients to high-risk, making them candidates for Allo-SCT.

Several studies have been published about the experience of ASCT in ALL. The results of some recent trials are summarized in **Table 2**. Data from three prospective trials of the French group have failed to demonstrate any significant superiority of ASCT over chemotherapy, even in a subset of high-risk patients [39–41]. Conversely, it has been reported that ASCT may be an effective treatment for ALL patients who experienced an isolated extramedullary relapse. A recent randomized study of 433 adult standard risk ALL patients showed that LFS at 5 years was significantly better in patients who underwent allo-HSCT compared with ASCT (60% vs. 42%, $P = 0.01$). In a large study which is comparing chemotherapy and autologous transplantation in ALL patients, the LFS and OS were found superior for chemotherapy group [34]. In the LALA-87 trial, results in standard-risk ALL were similar for Allo-SCT [37] and for chemotherapy or ASCT and then the same group reported no benefit of ASCT for ALL in all risk groups [42].

The Philadelphia chromosome (Ph) translocation (9; 22) is the most common chromosomal abnormality seen in adult patients with ALL. The t(9;22) is observed

Reference	Patient number	Period	Age (years)	Study design	Outcomes
Goldstone et al. 2008 [34]	1929	1993–2006	15–59	Ph- ALL patients divided groups; with donor vs. no donor chemotherapy vs. ASCT group	5-year OS is better in donor group, 53% versus 45% (P = .01), and lower the relapse rate in donor group (P < or = .001) OS is better in Chemotherapy group than ASCT group (46% [95% CI = 39–53%] vs. 37% [95% CI = 31–44%]; *P* = .03)
Thomas et al. 2004 (LALA94 study) [35]	922	1994–2002	15–55	ASCT vs. chemotherapy	ASCT did not show superiority over chemotherapy in high-risk ALL patients.
Hunault et al. 2003 (GOELAMS) [36]	198	1994–1998	15–59	Allo-SCT vs. ASCT	OS and LFS is better in Allo-SCT (75% vs. 39% *P* = .0027 and 72% vs. 32% *P* = .0004 respectively) relapse rates higher in ASCT
Fiere et al. 1993 [37]	572	1986–1991	15–60	ASCT vs. consolidative chemotherapy	Not significantly benefit of ASCT over chemotherapy
Powles et al. 2002 [38]	77	1984–1998	16–59	All patients underwent ASCT	10-year LFS and OS rates are 50% (95% CI, 38–62%) and 53% (95% CI, 41–65%), respectively

Table 2.
Summaries of studies on autologous stem cell transplantation in ALL.

in 2 to 5% of children with ALL and 30% percent of adults. Historically, Ph-positive ALL (Ph + ALL) was considered a very high-risk subtype and Allo-SCT was highly recommended for all eligible patients. After the introduction of tyrosine kinase inhibitors (TKIs) (first TKI, imatinib; second-generation TKIs such as dasatinib or nilotinib; the third-generation TKI, ponatinib) which could be successfully used both as salvage therapy and upfront in combination with intensive chemotherapy, complete remission is achieved in 90% of Ph + ALL patients [43]. The critical role of MRD prior to ASCT was already confirmed in Ph-negative ALL and may also be important in the Ph + setting [44]. Results of ASCT for Ph + ALL improved markedly in recent years with more than half of patients being alive and leukemia-free at 2 years [43, 45, 46]. The role of biologic response modifiers such as α-interferon (α-IFN and interleukin-2) in Ph + ALL is analyzed and it was reported that combination of α-IFN with maintenance chemotherapy and ASCT improves the outcomes in Ph + ALL [47, 48].

5. Conclusion

According to NCCN guidelines; Patients with good-risk AML are recommended to undergo high-dose cytarabine-based chemotherapy. Patients with poor-risk AML are recommended to undergo allogeneic stem cell transplantation (alloSCT). However, the best post remission therapy for patients with intermediate-risk AML in first complete remission (AML/CR1) is still uncertain. ASCT would be an option in CR1 and MRD negative. ASCT is a kind of standard treatment of CR2 in APL patients. There is no benefit of ASCT in Ph negative ALL patients however ASCT is a therapeutic option for relapsed Ph + ALL. Although the main disadvantages of ASCT are the possibility of contamination of leukemic cells in the stem cell product and the absence of graft-versus-leukemia effect, which lead to a higher relapse rates than that of Allo-SCT, ASCT should be considered a standard therapy in acute leukemia patients who are not eligible Allo-SCT and MRD negative in CR1 and the patients without poor risk.

Author details

Fatma Keklik Karadağ, Fahri Şahin and Güray Saydam*
Ege University, School of Medicine, Hematology, Izmir, Turkey

*Address all correspondence to: guraysaydam@gmail.com

References

[1] Vellenga E, van Putten W, Ossenkoppele GJ, Verdonck LF, Theobald M, Cornelissen JJ, et al. Autologous peripheral blood stem cell transplantation for acute myeloid leukemia. Blood. 2011;**118**(23):6037-6042

[2] Fernandez HF, Sun Z, Litzow MR, Luger SM, Paietta EM, Racevskis J, et al. Autologous transplantation gives encouraging results for young adults with favorable-risk acute myeloid leukemia, but is not improved with gemtuzumab ozogamicin. Blood. 2011;**117**(20):5306-5313

[3] Mizutani M, Hara M, Fujita H, Aoki J, Kanamori H, Ohashi K, et al. Comparable outcomes between autologous and allogeneic transplant for adult acute myeloid leukemia in first CR. Bone marrow transplantation. 2016;**51**(5):645-653

[4] Czerw T, Labopin M, Gorin NC, Giebel S, Blaise D, Meloni G, et al. Long-term follow-up of patients with acute myeloid leukemia surviving and free of disease recurrence for at least 2 years after autologous stem cell transplantation: A report from the acute leukemia working Party of the European Society for blood and marrow transplantation. Cancer. 2016;**122**(12):1880-1887

[5] Yanada M, Takami A, Mizuno S, Mori J, Chou T, Usuki K, et al. Autologous hematopoietic cell transplantation for acute myeloid leukemia in adults: 25 years of experience in Japan. International journal of hematology 2020;111(1):93-102.

[6] Reiffers J, Labopin M, Sanz M, Korbling M, Blaise D, De La Rubia J, et al. Autologous blood cell vs marrow transplantation for acute myeloid leukemia in complete remission: An EBMT retrospective analysis. Bone marrow transplantation. 2000;**25**(11):1115-1119

[7] Döhner H, Estey E, Grimwade D, Amadori S, Appelbaum FR, Büchner T, et al. Diagnosis and management of AML in adults: 2017 ELN recommendations from an international expert panel. Blood. 2017;**129**(4): 424-447

[8] Usuki K, Kurosawa S, Uchida N, Yakushiji K, Waki F, Matsuishi E, et al. Comparison of autologous hematopoietic cell transplantation and chemotherapy as postremission treatment in non-M3 acute myeloid leukemia in first complete remission. Clinical lymphoma, myeloma & leukemia. 2012;**12**(6):444-451

[9] Schlenk RF, Taskesen E, van Norden Y, Krauter J, Ganser A, Bullinger L, et al. The value of allogeneic and autologous hematopoietic stem cell transplantation in prognostically favorable acute myeloid leukemia with double mutant CEBPA. Blood. 2013;**122**(9):1576-1582

[10] Saraceni F, Bruno B, Lemoli RM, Meloni G, Arcese W, Falda M, et al. Autologous stem cell transplantation is still a valid option in good- and intermediate-risk AML: A GITMO survey on 809 patients autografted in first complete remission. Bone marrow transplantation. 2017;**52**(1):163-166

[11] Gorin NC, Labopin M, Meloni G, Pigneux A, Esteve J, Mohamad M, et al. Impact of FLT3 ITD/NPM1 mutation status in adult patients with acute myelocytic leukemia autografted in first remission. Haematologica. 2013;**98**(2):e12-e14

[12] Falini B, Bolli N, Liso A, Martelli MP, Mannucci R, Pileri S, et al. Altered nucleophosmin transport

in acute myeloid leukaemia with mutated NPM1: Molecular basis and clinical implications. Leukemia. 2009;**23**(10):1731-1743

[13] Li Z, Liu Y, Wang Q, Chen L, Ma L, Hao S. Autologous stem cell transplantation is a viable postremission therapy for intermediate-risk acute myeloid leukemia in first complete remission in the absence of a matched identical sibling: A meta-analysis. Acta haematologica. 2019;**141**(3):164-175

[14] Keating A, DaSilva G, Perez WS, Gupta V, Cutler CS, Ballen KK, et al. Autologous blood cell transplantation versus HLA-identical sibling transplantation for acute myeloid leukemia in first complete remission: A registry study from the Center for International Blood and Marrow Transplantation Research. Haematologica. 2013;**98**(2):185-192

[15] Gorin NC, Labopin M, Pabst T, Remenyi P, Wu D, Huynh A, et al. Unrelated matched versus autologous transplantation in adult patients with good and intermediate risk acute myelogenous leukemia in first molecular remission. American Journal of Hematology. 2017;**92**(12):1318-1323

[16] Ossenkoppele G, Löwenberg B. How I treat the older patient with acute myeloid leukemia. Blood. 2015;**125**(5):767-774

[17] Ferrara F, Barosi G, Venditti A, Angelucci E, Gobbi M, Pane F, et al. Consensus-based definition of unfitness to intensive and non-intensive chemotherapy in acute myeloid leukemia: A project of SIE, SIES and GITMO group on a new tool for therapy decision making. Leukemia. 2013;**27**(5):997-999

[18] Ye X, Chen D, Zheng Y, Wu C, Zhu X, Huang J. The incidence, risk factors, and survival of acute myeloid leukemia secondary to myelodysplastic syndrome: A population-based study. Hematological oncology. 2019;**37**(4):438-446

[19] Gorin NC, Labopin M, Reiffers J, Milpied N, Blaise D, Witz F, et al. Higher incidence of relapse in patients with acute myelocytic leukemia infused with higher doses of CD34+ cells from leukapheresis products autografted during the first remission. Blood. 2010;**116**(17):3157-3162

[20] Wang J, Ouyang J, Zhou R, Chen B, Yang Y. Autologous hematopoietic stem cell transplantation for acute myeloid leukemia in first complete remission: A meta-analysis of randomized trials. Acta haematologica. 2010;**124**(2):61-71

[21] Meloni G, Vignetti M, Avvisati G, Capria S, Micozzi A, Giona F, et al. BAVC regimen and autograft for acute myelogenous leukemia in second complete remission. Bone marrow transplantation. 1996;**18**(4):693-698

[22] Jourdan E, Boissel N, Chevret S, Delabesse E, Renneville A, Cornillet P, et al. Prospective evaluation of gene mutations and minimal residual disease in patients with core binding factor acute myeloid leukemia. Blood. 2013;**121**(12):2213-2223

[23] Walter RB, Gooley TA, Wood BL, Milano F, Fang M, Sorror ML, et al. Impact of pretransplantation minimal residual disease, as detected by multiparametric flow cytometry, on outcome of myeloablative hematopoietic cell transplantation for acute myeloid leukemia. Journal of clinical oncology : official journal of the American Society of Clinical Oncology. 2011;**29**(9):1190-1197

[24] Percival MM, Estey EH. Current treatment strategies for measurable residual disease in patients with acute myeloid leukemia. Cancer. 2019;**125**(18):3121-3130

[25] Jentzsch M, Schwind S, Bach E, Stasik S, Thiede C, Platzbecker U. Clinical Challenges and Consequences of Measurable Residual Disease in Non-APL Acute Myeloid Leukemia. Cancers. 2019;11(11).

[26] Cornelissen JJ, Blaise D. Hematopoietic stem cell transplantation for patients with AML in first complete remission. Blood. 2016;**127**(1):62-70

[27] Gorin NC, Labopin M, Czerw T, Pabst T, Blaise D, Dumas PY, et al. Autologous stem cell transplantation for adult acute myelocytic leukemia in first remission-better outcomes after busulfan and melphalan compared with busulfan and cyclophosphamide: A retrospective study from the acute leukemia working Party of the European Society for blood and marrow transplantation (EBMT). Cancer. 2017;**123**(5):824-831

[28] Gorin NC, Labopin M, Blaise D, Dumas PY, Pabst T, Trisolini SM, et al. Optimizing the pretransplant regimen for autologous stem cell transplantation in acute myelogenous leukemia: Better outcomes with busulfan and melphalan compared with busulfan and cyclophosphamide in high risk patients autografted in first complete remission: A study from the acute leukemia working party of the EBMT. American Journal of Hematology. 2018;**93**(7):859-866

[29] Lemoli RM, D'Addio A, Marotta G, Pezzullo L, Zuffa E, Montanari M, et al. BU/melphalan and auto-SCT in AML patients in first CR: A 'Gruppo Italiano Trapianto di Midollo Osseo (GITMO)' retrospective study. Bone marrow transplantation. 2010;**45**(4):640-646

[30] Ferrara F, Mele G, Palmieri S, Pedata M, Copia C, Riccardi C, et al. Continuous infusion idarubicin and intravenous busulphan as conditioning regimen to autologous stem cell transplantation for patients with acute myeloid leukaemia. Hematological oncology. 2009;**27**(4):198-202

[31] Sanz MA, Labopin M, Gorin NC, de la Rubia J, Arcese W, Meloni G, et al. Hematopoietic stem cell transplantation for adults with acute promyelocytic leukemia in the ATRA era: A survey of the European cooperative Group for Blood and Marrow Transplantation. Bone marrow transplantation. 2007;**39**(8):461-469

[32] Holter Chakrabarty JL, Rubinger M, Le-Rademacher J, Wang HL, Grigg A, Selby GB, et al. Autologous is superior to allogeneic hematopoietic cell transplantation for acute promyelocytic leukemia in second complete remission. Biology of blood and marrow transplantation : journal of the American Society for Blood and Marrow Transplantation. 2014;**20**(7):1021-1025

[33] Meloni G, Diverio D, Vignetti M, Avvisati G, Capria S, Petti MC, et al. Autologous bone marrow transplantation for acute promyelocytic leukemia in second remission: Prognostic relevance of pretransplant minimal residual disease assessment by reverse-transcription polymerase chain reaction of the PML/RAR alpha fusion gene. Blood. 1997;**90**(3):1321-1325

[34] Goldstone AH, Richards SM, Lazarus HM, Tallman MS, Buck G, Fielding AK, et al. In adults with standard-risk acute lymphoblastic leukemia, the greatest benefit is achieved from a matched sibling allogeneic transplantation in first complete remission, and an autologous transplantation is less effective than conventional consolidation/ maintenance chemotherapy in all patients: Final results of the international ALL trial (MRC UKALL XII/ECOG E2993). Blood. 2008;**111**(4):1827-1833

[35] Thomas X, Boiron JM, Huguet F, Dombret H, Bradstock K, Vey N, et al. Outcome of treatment in adults with acute lymphoblastic leukemia: Analysis of the LALA-94 trial. Journal of clinical oncology : official journal of the American Society of Clinical Oncology. 2004;**22**(20):4075-4086

[36] Hunault M, Harousseau JL, Delain M, Truchan-Graczyk M, Cahn JY, Witz F, et al. Better outcome of adult acute lymphoblastic leukemia after early genoidentical allogeneic bone marrow transplantation (BMT) than after late high-dose therapy and autologous BMT: A GOELAMS trial. Blood. 2004;**104**(10):3028-3037

[37] Fière D, Lepage E, Sebban C, Boucheix C, Gisselbrecht C, Vernant JP, et al. Adult acute lymphoblastic leukemia: A multicentric randomized trial testing bone marrow transplantation as postremission therapy. The French group on therapy for adult acute lymphoblastic leukemia. Journal of clinical oncology : official journal of the American Society of Clinical Oncology. 1993;**11**(10):1990-2001

[38] Powles R, Sirohi B, Treleaven J, Kulkarni S, Tait D, Singhal S, et al. The role of posttransplantation maintenance chemotherapy in improving the outcome of autotransplantation in adult acute lymphoblastic leukemia. Blood. 2002;**100**(5):1641-1647

[39] Gorin NC. Autologous stem cell transplantation in acute lymphocytic leukemia. Stem Cells. 2002;**20**(1):3-10

[40] Patel B, Rai L, Buck G, Richards SM, Mortuza Y, Mitchell W, et al. Minimal residual disease is a significant predictor of treatment failure in non T-lineage adult acute lymphoblastic leukaemia: Final results of the international trial UKALL XII/ECOG2993. British journal of haematology. 2010;**148**(1):80-89

[41] Dhedin N, Dombret H, Thomas X, Lheritier V, Boiron JM, Rigal-Huguet F, et al. Autologous stem cell transplantation in adults with acute lymphoblastic leukemia in first complete remission: Analysis of the LALA-85, −87 and −94 trials. Leukemia. 2006;**20**(2):336-344

[42] Dhédin N, Dombret H, Thomas X, Lhéritier V, Boiron JM, Rigal-Huguet F, et al. Autologous stem cell transplantation in adults with acute lymphoblastic leukemia in first complete remission: Analysis of the LALA-85, −87 and −94 trials. Leukemia. 2006;**20**(2):336-344

[43] Giebel S, Labopin M, Gorin NC, Caillot D, Leguay T, Schaap N, et al. Improving results of autologous stem cell transplantation for Philadelphia-positive acute lymphoblastic leukaemia in the era of tyrosine kinase inhibitors: A report from the acute leukaemia working Party of the European Group for blood and marrow transplantation. European journal of cancer. 2014;**50**(2):411-417

[44] Giebel S, Stella-Holowiecka B, Krawczyk-Kulis M, Gökbuget N, Hoelzer D, Doubek M, et al. Status of minimal residual disease determines outcome of autologous hematopoietic SCT in adult ALL. Bone marrow transplantation. 2010;**45**(6):1095-1101

[45] Wetzler M, Watson D, Stock W, Koval G, Mulkey FA, Hoke EE, et al. Autologous transplantation for Philadelphia chromosome-positive acute lymphoblastic leukemia achieves outcomes similar to allogeneic transplantation: Results of CALGB study 10001 (Alliance). Haematologica. 2014;**99**(1):111-115

[46] Giebel S, Labopin M, Potter M, Poire X, Sengeloev H, Socie G, et al. Comparable results of autologous and allogeneic haematopoietic stem

cell transplantation for adults with Philadelphia-positive acute lymphoblastic leukaemia in first complete molecular remission: An analysis by the acute leukemia working party of the EBMT. European journal of cancer. 2018;**96**:73-81

[47] Visani G, Martinelli G, Piccaluga P, Tosi P, Amabile M, Pastano R, et al. Alpha-interferon improves survival and remission duration in P-190BCR-ABL positive adult acute lymphoblastic leukemia. Leukemia. 2000;**14**(1):22-27

[48] Piccaluga PP, Martinelli G, Isidori A, Malagola M, Rondoni M, Paolini S, et al. Long-term molecular complete remission with IFN-alpha in Ph+ adult acute lymphoid leukemia patients. Leukemia. 2008;**22**(8):1617-1618

Chapter 13

Molecular Monitoring in Acute Myeloid Leukemia Patients Undergoing Matched Unrelated Donor: Hematopoietic Stem Cell Transplantation

Irina Panovska-Stavridis

Abstract

Minimal residual disease (MRD) in acute myeloid leukemia (AML) is a complex, multi-modality assessment and much as its clinical implications at different points are extensively studied, it remains even now a challenging area. It is the disease biology that governs the modality of MRD assessment; in patients harboring specific molecular targets, high sensitivity techniques can be applied. In AML patients undergoing allogenic hematopoietic stem cell transplantation (alloHSCT), relapse in considered as leading cause for treatment failure. In post-transplant setting, regular MRD status assessment enables to identify patients at risk of impending relapse when early therapeutic intervention may be beneficent. We analyzed data of AML patients who underwent matched unrelated donor (MUD) HSCT since the introduction of this procedure in the Republic of North Macedonia. Chimeric fusion transcripts were identified in three patients; two of them positive for RUNX-RUNX1T1 transcript and one for CBFB-MYH11. One patient harbored mutation in the transcription factor CCAAT/enhancer binding protein α (*CEBPA*). Post-transplant MRD kinetics was measured by quantitative polymerase chain or multiplex fluorescent-PCR every three months after the transplantation during the first two years after the transplant. MRD negativity was achieved in three patients by the sixth month of HSCT, who were pre-transplant MRD positive. They sustained hematological and molecular remission for 19, 9 and 7 months, respectively. The forth patient died due to transplant-related complication. Our experience suggests, when molecularly-defined AML patients undergo HSCT, regular MRD monitoring helps predict impending relapse and direct future treatment strategies.

Keywords: minimal residual disease (MRD), molecular monitoring, matched unrelated donor (MUD) hematopoietic stem cell transplantation (HSCT), acute myeloid leukemia (AML)

1. Introduction

1.1 Acute myeloid leukemia (AML)

Acute myeloid leukemia (AML) is a heterogeneous malignant disease of the hematopoietic system, marked by mutational arrest of myeloid lineage precursor cells and limited myeloid differentiation capacity [1]. Theoretically, malignant transformation can arise at any level at which cell precursors are capable of self-renewal. However, the hematopoietic precursors are typically arrested in the earliest stages of myeloid maturation pathway - myeloblasts or promyelocytes. The malignant cells suppress the normal hematopoiesis by accumulating in the bone marrow and displacing the normal hematopoietic stem cells, resulting in depletion of normal blood cells. The presence of more than 20% myeloblasts in the bone marrow or peripheral blood, as assessed by morphological evaluation of blood smears and bone marrow aspirate smears is diagnostic for AML. Morphologically, AML cells resemble normal myeloblasts to some extent, although they are distinguished by specific features, such as Auer Bodies – crystalloid azurophylic granules or Auer Rods – needle-shaped conglomerates of granules. Immunophenotyping, cytogenetics and molecular genetics must be employed to confirm the diagnosis of AML and further characterize the AML subtype [1].

AML is one of the most common types of leukemia in adults, as stated by American Society of Cancer, the second most common, following chronic lymphocytic leukemia (CLL), but the leading cause of mortality of leukemic deaths [2]. The median age at diagnosis is approximately 70 years. The estimated annual age-standardized incidence rate is 4.3 per 100.000, more precisely, from 1.3 per 100.000 in patients younger than 65 years and 12.2 per 100.000 in patients older than 65 [2, 3].

The etiology of de novo cases of AML is quite obscure. Only a small portion of all AML cases - around 10%, are secondary AML, due to transformation of prior hematological malignancy, such as myelodisplastic syndrome (MDS) or myeloproliferative neoplasm (MPN). Around another 10% of all cases arise from suggested DNA damage of known previous factor, as prior therapy with alkylating agents or topoisomerases, or prior radiotherapy [4].

1.2 WHO classification of AML

The revised fourth revision to the World Health Organization classification of Tumors of Hematopoietic and Lymphoid Tissues, published in 2017, distinguishes six AML subtypes and it incorporates cytogenetic and molecular abnormalities into diagnostic algorithms, in contrast to previous classifications of AML, based on morphology and immunophenotype [5]. The entity "AML with recurrent genetic abnormalities" comprises 11 subcategories of AML, with acute promyelocitic leukemia (APL with PML-RARA) included. The abnormalities that are not included in this group are considered to be rare among adult population. Six well-defined recurrent balanced translocations and inversions and their variants are covered within this classification. Two entities included are new provisional subcategories: AML with *BCR-ABL1* fusion gene and AML with mutated *RUNX1*. Although a matter of long-time controversy, de novo BCR-ABL+ AML is now classified as distinct AML subtype. However, current data show that BCR-ABL occur primarily in AML with antecedent myeloid disorder, such as myelodysplasia-related changes [6]. The cytogenetic and molecular abnormalities included in this classification are summarized in **Table 1**.

AML with recurrent genetic abnormalities adapted from 4th revised WHO classification 2017		**Risk group, as per 2017 ELN stratification**
Cytogenetic abnormality	**Molecular abnormality**	
t(8;21) (q22;q22.1)	RUNX1-RUNX1T1- AML	Favorable
inv(16)(p13.1q22) or t(16;16)(p13.1;q22)	CBFB-MYH11- AML	Favorable
t(9;11)(p21.3;q23.3)	MLLT3-KMT2A AML	Intermediate
t(6;9)(p23;q34.1)	DEK-NUP214 AML	Adverse
inv(3)(q21.3q26.2) or t(3;3)(q21.3;q26.2)*	GATA2; MECOM	Adverse
t(1;22)(p13.3;q13.3)	RBM15-MKL1	
	AML with mutated NPM1	*Favorable if without FLT-ITD or with FLT-ITD low* *Intermediate if FLT-ITH high*
	AML with biallelic mutations of CEBPA$	*Favorable*

**Inv(3)(q21.3q26.2) results in reposition of a distal GATA2 enhancer to activate MECOM expression, not a fusion gene.*
$Mutated CEBPA is associated with biallelic mutations of the gene, not a single mutation.

Table 1.
Recurrent cytogenetic and molecular abnormalities in AML (4th revision of WHO classification, published in 2017) and ELN risk categories.

1.3 AML risk categories

Current AML risk categorization follows the latest 2017 European LeukemiaNet (ELN) recommendations and is based on pretreatment genetic abnormalities. It is designed for risk-adapted treatment approach of patients with AML, conforming to their molecular profiles [7]. Three risk categories are recognized: favorable risk, intermediate risk and adverse risk group [7]. However, the prognostic significance of genetic abnormalities should be only analyzed in association/codependence with other patient-related or disease-related prognostic factors. Increasing age is correlated with poor prognosis for two reasons; not only the poorer performance status in older age groups and the increased risk of toxicity and treatment-related mortality, but also the increased probability of previous underlying malignancy such as MDS or MPN, associated with adverse cytogenetic and higher risk of treatment resistance. Furthermore, the presence of two genetic abnormalities simultaneously and their interactions can result in different prognostic impact, depending on the presence or the absence of another. The best studied example is the NPM1-FLT3-ITD interaction. As shown in **Table 1**, mutated NPM1 in the absence of a *FLT3*-ITD or presence of *FLT3*-ITD with a low allelic ratio is related to favorable prognosis, while the high allelic ratio of *FLT3*-ITD relocates it in the intermediate risk group. To the contrary, not mutated NPM1, or wild-type NPM1 in the absence of a *FLT3*-ITD or low allelic ratio *FLT3*-ITD is considered as intermediate risk group and finally, wild-type NPM1 plus high allelic ratio of *FLT3*-ITD carries adverse prognosis [8]. ELN risk categories are presented in **Table 1** in association with WHO classification of AML. In addition to those abnormalities, mutations in RUNX1, mutations in ASXL1 and in TP53 convey particularly poor prognosis [9]. In regards to AML-karyotype, complex karyotypes and monosomal karyotypes, specific aneuploidies, such as deletion of chromosome 5 and chromosome 7 or 5q, 7q deletion, predict adverse prognosis in AML patients. These are often associated with TP53 mutations [10].

2. The role of allogeneic hematopoietic stem cell transplantation (alloHSCT) in AML

Allogeneic hematopoietic stem cell transplantation plays a key role in the management of patients with AML, making it one of the commonest indications for alloHSCT. By overcoming the limitations of donor availability and the increasing pool of donors in the recent decades on one hand and improving the transplant procedures and post-transplant strategies on the other, alloHSCT evolved into a definitive curative option for a significant number of AML patients [11]. The major challenge remains the identifying the allo-mandatory patients who are likely to benefit from an allograft.

2.1 Matched related sibling and unrelated donor SCT in AML

The search for a compatible hematopoietic stem cell donor is based on the human leukocyte antigen (HLA) profile of the patient undergoing SCT. The preferred donor type for SCT is a matched sibling donor (MSD), bearing the most favorable outcome; however only about a third of all patients have an available sibling donor. Histocompatibilty antigens are co-dominantly expressed and are inherited following Mendelian rules of inheritance, which means there is only a 25% likelihood of a patient and their sibling inheriting the same parental haplotypes. Assuming an average of 2 to 3 children per family in European countries it has been estimated that a patient seeking a transplant has a 30% likelihood of having a matched sibling donor and therefore a 70% likelihood that the same patient will need a transplant from an unrelated donor. Since the world's first donor registry was founded in 1974, WMDA nowadays comprises of 75 hematopoietic stem cells donor registries from 53 countries, with more than 33.573.307 volunteer donors listed up to date. (https://statistics.wmda.info). The coordination between the transplant centers is facilitated through donor registries. The unrelated donor search procedure commences with a formal search request which is sent to the national registry, which further undertakes the responsibilities in all steps until the graft distribution [12]. The process of an unrelated donor search and activation is completed in 2 months on the average and up to 10 weeks.

2.1.1 The "ideal" unrelated donor profile

The general recommendation is selection of a 10/10 HLA-matched unrelated donor whenever possible (in loci HLA A, HLA B, HLA C, HLA DR and HLA DQ). The second best choice would be 9/10 identical unrelated donor. HLA typing is necessary to be performed at high-resolution level by using next-generation sequencing (NGS) or sequencing-based typing (SBT) as preferable typing method. As published by Lee et al. 2007, HLA mismatch in any of non-permissive or high-risk alleles: HLA A, B, C and DRB1 results in 10% decrease in survival probabilities for each mismatch in transplanted patients at early disease stage, and even worse at advanced disease stage [13]. Donor associated features may narrow down the choice of suitable unrelated donor. At the time of recruitment, donors are assessed in order to exclude medical conditions or habits that can possibly cause harm to transplant recipient, in particular – their history of infectious diseases, inherited, autoimmune and malignant diseases. According to WMDA recommendations a minimum donor blood-borne infectious disease markers testing is suggested, including serology for hepatitis B and C, HIV, syphilis and HTLV1/2. Those recommendations are adapted in line with local polices as additional endemic transmissible diseases may also be covered [14]. The donor's age is considered an important factor, probably the most powerful one; younger donors are associated with better prognosis with a 5.5% increase in the hazard ratio for overall mortality for every 10-year raise in donor age [15]. Donor registries recruit donors between 16 and 55 years and almost half of the registered donors registered are younger than 35. Diverse data on the impact of sex mismatch and blood group incompatibility are been reported, emphasizing the correlation with other factors, such as conditioning regimen or stem cell source. Donor CMV serum-positivity is a negative prognostic factor for transplant outcome. It appears however, that not the CMV serum-negativity, but a matched patient/donor CMV serum status determines the transplant outcome more significantly [16].

2.2 Haploidentical related donors

The recent improvements in transplant technologies have led to the consideration of using a haploidentical related donor when HLA- matched sibling or HLA-matched unrelated donor is not available. It is estimated that around a half of the patients in need of a transplant have rare haplotypes and HLA-matched donor cannot be found in donor registries. In the past, the major inquiry in terms of haploidentical setting has been the expected high rate of GVHD. On the contrary, over the past few years, the use of post-transplant cyclophosphamide on day +3 and day +4 after the transplant, has significantly decreased the rate of acute and chronic GVHD and nowadays haploidentical HSCT is established transplant method for patients lacking HLA-matched donor [17]. Even more, numerous retrospective studies have shown similar outcomes for MUD – SCT and haploidentical HSCT [18].

2.3 Umbilical cord blood transplantation

The first umbilical cord blood transplantation (UCBT) was successfully performed in 1988, in a 5-year-old child, diagnosed with Fanconi Anemia, using HLA-matched sibling, an older brother. Subsequently, in the following years, UCB transplants were encouraged in the pediatric population for the treatment of malignant and non-malignant hematological diseases, using both related and unrelated donors. Therefore, data on UCBT mainly originate from procedures performed in children. The major limitations of this procedure are delayed engraftment and delayed immune reconstitution, leading to severe and often fatal infections [19]. However, during the past few years, as mismatched transplant activity increases, UCBT is progressively superseded by haploidentical HSCT.

3. The role of minimal residual disease (MRD) in AML

In AML patients, a complete hematological remission is defined as total recovery of blood counts, less than 5% blasts in bone marrow and recovery of heamatopoiesis of all cell lineages, as assessed by cytomorphological examination [20]. Morphological assessment of post-therapy disease status is limited to 100–400 nucleated cells and can identify the presence of leukemic cells to levels of 1:20 white blood cells (WBC). Besides the small number of analyzed cells another limitation of cytomorphology is the subjective component and the inaccuracy in distinguishing normal from leukemic myeloblasts [21]. Limitations of cytomorphological assessment were partially overcome by the introduction of highly sensitive methods able to detect the smallest residual leukemic cells populations or minimal (measurable) disease. *Minimal residual disease (MRD)* indicates presence of leukemic cells at levels of $1{:}10^4$ to $1{:}10^6$ WBC. MRD detection in AML is necessary for various reasons. Firstly, it is an objective, well-defined post-treatment method to establish a remission status at deeper level. Secondly, it is a powerful tool for risk stratification of AML and guiding treatment approach. And finally it enables identifying impending relapse in AML patients in complete remission [22–24]. Several studies have so far reported a positive correlation between the MRD positivity and the risk of relapse and shorter survival rate, compared to MRD negative AML patients. This refers to MRD status during and after post-remission chemotherapy, as well as prior and after SCT [24–33]. However, AML is a malignancy with complex molecular landscape and despite the fact that genetic aberrations are shown to be powerful prognostic determinants none of them have been ascertained to accurately predict the outcome [9]. No guidelines or recommendations are available so far on when and how to implement MRD assessments and on how to apply the results to clinical practice. According to ELN recommendations, during the treatment phase MRD should at least be assessed at the following time points: at the time of diagnosis, after 2 cycles of standard induction/consolidation chemotherapy and after the end of the treatment. For patient candidates for allo-HSCT, an MRD assessment should be carried out after the last chemotherapy, not exceeding 4 weeks of the initiation of the conditioning regimen [22].

3.1 MRD in AML patients undergoing allo-SCT

In a post-transplant setting, the primary importance of MRD evaluation is to detect impending relapse and thus to identify patients who may benefit from early clinical intervention [22–24]. The continual death rate due to relapse after allo-SCT is discouraging, even despite the changing landscape of AML and novel treatment paradigms. Data from the Center for International Blood and Marrow Transplant Research (CIBMTR) report 63% mortality rate in patients undergoing unrelated donor HSCTs due to transplant-related events including graft-vs.-host disease, infection and other causes-organ toxicity or second malignancies, compared to 37% of deaths due to relapse [34]. This high relapse ratio suggests that there are residual leukemic cell populations that have survived therapy, capable of causing relapse, referred to as measurable or minimal residual disease. These cell subsets are believed to be present even up to several months before apparent morphological disease, at a time when they can be solely detected by high sensitivity methods.

3.2 Methods for MRD assessment

A number of methods are employed for MRD measurement but is the biology of the disease itself that governs the modality of MRD assessment. The complexity of AML, the myriad of genetic aberrations and the diversity of immunophenotypes restrain the recognition of uniform approach for MRD detection. In addition, as per Butturini A, the of MRD detection in AML is altered by the size of the tested sample, sample source (blood, bone marrow) and the time point of sample obtaining rather than the sensitivity of the employed method for MRD assessment, due to the heterogeneous distribution of residual leukemic cells and the fluctuating expression of the MRD target [24]. In general, two methods are commonly incorporated into clinical routine: multiparameter flow cytometry (MFC) which allows detection of aberrant immunophenotypes and molecular methods by using tumor-specific molecular primers, such as RT-qPCR or multiplex fluorescent- [22, 24]. MFC affords relative sensitivity of $1{:}10^{-3}$. The main constrains of this method are that not all leukemia cells present aberrant immunophenotypes and that the initial phenotypes may change through disease evolution and clone selection [35].

3.2.1 Molecular MRD in AML patients

Two approaches are available for molecular MRD monitoring. The first one is real-time PCR-based and the second is by using sequencing techniques. PCR-based MRD assessment affords sensitivity of $1{:}10^{-5}$ to $1{:}10^{-6}$, which means 100–1000 fold greater than other methods applied. Therefore, it is the ELN-recommended platform for molecular monitoring in AML due to the established high sensitivity [22, 24]. However, considering the molecular heterogeneity of AML, it is restricted to less than half of patients (35% in older patients as their frequency decreases with age); those harboring specific molecular targets that can be tracked for MRD monitoring, including mutations, translocations, inversions, deletions and polymorphisms. More precisely, PCR-based MRD monitoring is proposed for AML with validated molecular markers, such as mutations in the gene encoding nucleophosmin (NPM1) and the chimeric fusion genes RUNX1- RUNX1T1, CBFB-MYH11 and PML-RARA [24, 25]. For these mutations, standardized PCR-assays are employed with well-defined threshold levels [36]. In contrast, the use of the mutations in FLT3-ITD, FLT3-TKD, NRAS, KRAS, DNMT3A, ASXL1, IDH1, IDH2, MLL-PTD, EVI1 and WT1 as single MRD markers is not recommended because of frequent losses or gains of certain mutations at relapse. These markers could be used in combination with a second MRD marker if present [22].

ELN defined the molecular responses for patients in complete hematological remission after completing chemotherapy or after a performed transplant procedure [22]. *Complete molecular remission* is defined by two successive MRD negative samples in an interval of a minimum of 4 weeks. *Molecular persistence at low copy numbers* is defined as presence of 100–200 copies/10^4 ABL copies corresponding to <1–2% of target to reference gene or allele burden; and a copy number or increase of more than 1 log between 2 MRD positive samples. *Molecular progression* is defined as an increase of MRD copy numbers >1 $\log_{10}$ between 2 positive samples. And finally, *molecular relapse* is an increase of MRD copy numbers >1 $\log_{10}$ between 2 positive samples in a patient who previously achieved MRD negativity.

In our practice, MRD assessment, using RT-PCR is routinely performed in AML patients with genetic aberrations. MRD is measured during and after post-remission chemotherapy, and in patients undergoing SCT prior the transplant procedure and at précised time points during the post-transplant period. However, in this paper, we focus on the molecular monitoring in patients undergoing MUD – HSCT, diagnosed with AML with specific genetic aberrations. We present here our findings at four AML patients and our initial experiences. Specific recommendations for molecular follow-up in AML-patients harboring these aberrations and the clinical implication of MRD status in post-transplant period will be discussed in line with our results.

4. Molecular monitoring in patients undergoing allo-SCT: single center experience

4.1 Case definition

Since the introduction of MUD-HSCT in the Republic of North Macedonia in November 2018, 10 AML patients underwent MUD HSCT until June 2020. Of those ten, molecular markers were identified in a total of 4 patients; two patients were positive for RUNX-RUNX1T1 transcript, 1 patient for CBFB-MYH11 transcript and 1 patient had mutation in CEBPA gene. The medical records of these patients were reviewed for initial findings, clinical manifestations, clinical course, treatment regimen and outcome. Patients' individual characteristics are summarized in **Table 2**. Two patients were diagnosed with "de novo" AML and the other two patients had secondary AML evolving from antecedent myelodysplasia and myeloid sarcoma, respectively. All patients were transplanted in first complete hematological remission. Three patients received conditioning regimen considered myeloablative [37] with Bu-Cy + ATG and the one patient received reduced intensity chemotherapy regimen with Bu-Flu + ATG [37]. In all patients, peripheral blood stem cells were used as graft source. The patients underwent HSCT between November 2018 and January 2020. During the post-transplant period, bone marrow samples for MRD monitoring were obtained at scheduled time points - the first one within two months of HSCT and thereafter at +3, +6, +9 and + 12 months of HSCT [38] (**Figure 2**). The cut-off date for follow-up was June 30, 2020. Median follow-up time was 8 months (range: 3–19 months).

4.2 Samples

Samples of 5–10 ml of bone marrow aspirate in EDTA were used for PCR based analyses. PCR analyses were performed at the Center for Biomolecular Pharmaceutical Analyses - UKIM-Faculty of Pharmacy – Skopje.

4.2.1 Molecular PCR based methods (RT-PCR and multiplex fluorescent PCR)

Post-transplant MRD kinetics was evaluated by using quantitative polymerase chain reaction (RT-qPCR) or multiplex fluorescent-PCR every three months after the transplantation. Molecular analyses were performed at the Center for Biomolecular Pharmaceutical Analyses, UKIM-Faculty of Pharmacy, Skopje in bone marrow aspirates. RT- PCR is a high sensitivity method to detect the presence of leukemia cells down to levels of $1{:}10^{-5}$ to $1{:}10^{-6}$ white blood cells (WBC) [22, 36]. Mononuclear cells (MNCs) were isolated by Ficoll density gradient. Detailed procedures for MRD

	Patient 1	Patient 2	Patient 3	Patient 4
Age at diagnosis	22	21	58	37
Sex	male	male	female	Female
Comorbidities	no	no	no	No
2017 ELN risk stratification[16]	favorable	favorable	favorable	favorable
Molecular marker	CBFB-MYH11(inv16)	RUNX-RUNX1T1	5 bp deletion in CEBPA	RUNX-RUNX1T1
Number of induction therapies	2	2	3 (2 + 1)	2
Number of consolidation therapies	2	2	2	2
Time to HSCT	6 months	7 months	15 months	6 months
Disease status prior HSCT	CR1	CR1	CR1	CR1
MRD status prior HSCT	MRD + (0.15%)	MRD + (0.20%)	MRD +	MRD + (0.09%)

Table 2.
Individual and clinical pre-HSCT characteristics of analyzed AML patients.

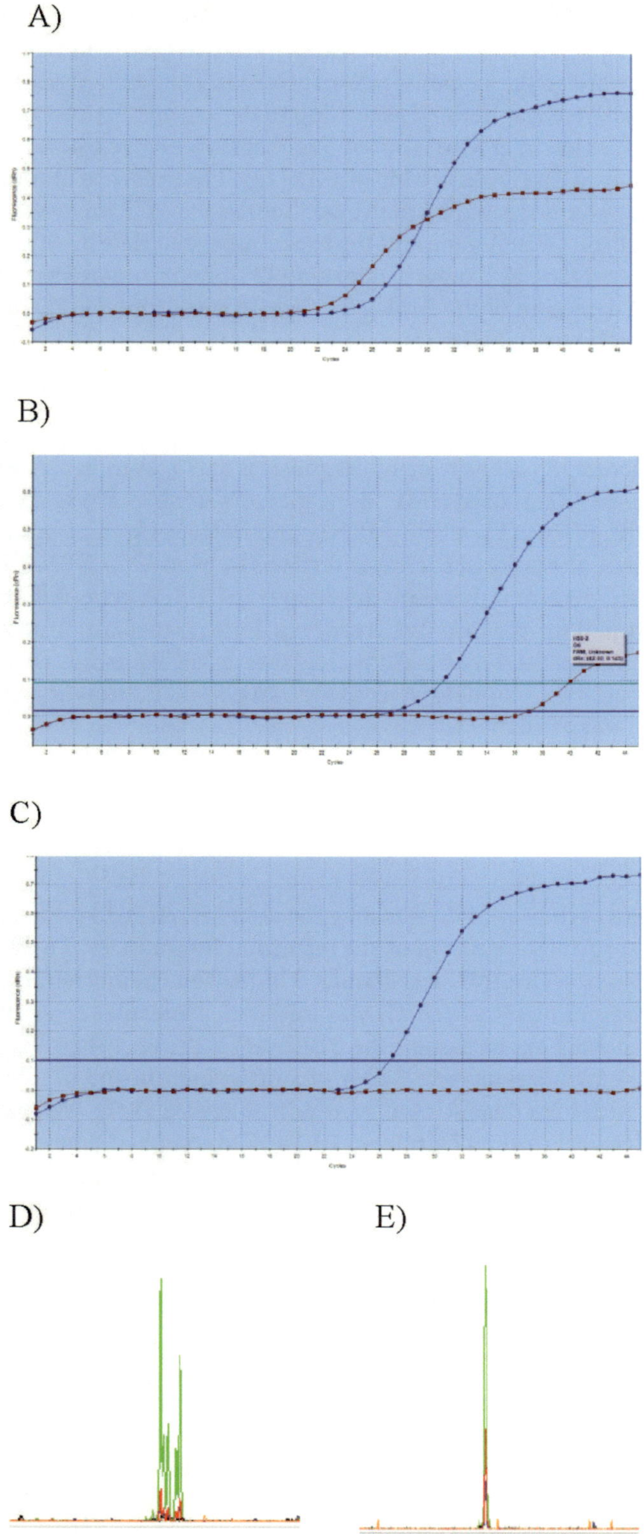

Figure 1.
MRD analyses using the AML-ETO hybrid transcript (A, B, C) or CEBPA mutation (D, E) molecular markers performed at diagnosis (a and D), pre-transplantation (B) and one month after transplantation (C and E). The blue circles and red squares in (A), (B) and (C) indicate the strength of the fluorescent signal generated during the RT/PCR amplification of the internal control ABL and hybrid AML-ETO transcripts, respectively. The arrow in (D) indicates the detection of the 5 bp-del mutant allele in the CEBPA gene.

assays detecting RUNX1-RUNX1T1, CBFB-MYH11 and CEBPA gene mutations have been published by the Europe Against Cancer Initiative [22]. The samples were run in triplicate. The molecular response was expressed as log reduction of transcript levels. MRD positivity was defined according to the Europe Against Cancer Program Criteria (amplification in at least 2 out of 3 replicates with cycle-threshold values of 40 or less, using a threshold setting of 0.1) [22]. The presence of mutations in the CEBPA gene was evaluated by multiplex fluorescent PCR analysis covering the coding region of the CEBPA gene and the exact molecular defects of all additional fragments was analyzed by Sanger sequencing [23]. Representative results of these analyses for the detection of the AML-ETO hybrid transcript and the mutation in the CEBPA gene are shown in **Figure 1**.

4.3 Pre-transplant MRD status

Molecular screening at the time of diagnosis is carried out in almost all our patients with newly diagnosed AML. Bone marrow samples are routinely investigated for RUNX1-RUNX1T1, CBFB-MYH11 and PML-RARα fusion transcripts, as well as single gene alterations, such as insertions in exon 12 in NPM1, FLT3 tandem duplication in exon 12, and deletions/insertions in CEBPA gene. All here presented patients were tested for the initial aberration prior to transplant procedure (median time = 13 days; range: 9–14 days). All patients were MRD positive (0.15%; 0.20% and 0.09% in patient 1, 2 and 4 respectively). In patient 3, presence of 5 bp deletion in CEBPA gene was confirmed.

4.4 Clinical histories

4.4.1 Case I

A young man at the age of 22 was diagnosed in March 2018 with myeloid sarcoma after surgically resection of the intestinal tumor mass. Three months later, the disease progressed in AML and standard induction chemotherapy regimen 3 + 7 DA (anthracycline plus ARA-C) was initiated. Molecular evaluation of the bone marrow showed expression of the CBFB-MYH11 inv.(16) (p13;22) fusion transcript. Remission was achieved after second induction and two consolidation therapies with high dose ARA-C were administered [1, 7]. The patient had a HLA haploidentical sibling. Unrelated 10/10 HLA matched donor, registered to PL-DKMS (Fundacija DKMS) was activated and allo-SCT was performed in November 2018 [14–16]. The patient received myeloablative conditioning regimen with Bu/Cy + ATG and conventional immunosuppressive therapy with cyclosporine and methotrexate was applied [33]. Peripheral blood stem cells (PBSC) were used as graft source at a total dose of $4{,}6 \times 10^6$ CD34+ cells/ kg. In post – transplant period, CBFB-MYH11 inv.(16) (p13;22) was used as a molecular MRD target [22]. On day +45 of HSCT, an increased MRD load, compared to that of pre-transplant MRD was documented. Consequently, the initial dose of 100 mg was reduced to 75 mg per day. On day +90 of HSCT, molecular MRD negativity was confirmed and continuously preserved up to the last evaluation at +15 months after HSCT. Immunosuppression was discontinued in December 2019, after completing one year of HSCT. Molecular MRD kinetics of CBFB-MYH11 inv. (16) (p13;22) in this patient is shown in **Figure 2**. Complete donor chimerism was first documented on day +90 and maintained to follow-up cutoff date. As this patient initially manifested extramyeloid presentation of AML, we did a PET scan assessment, at 12 months after HSCT and no pathological accumulation or activity were observed.

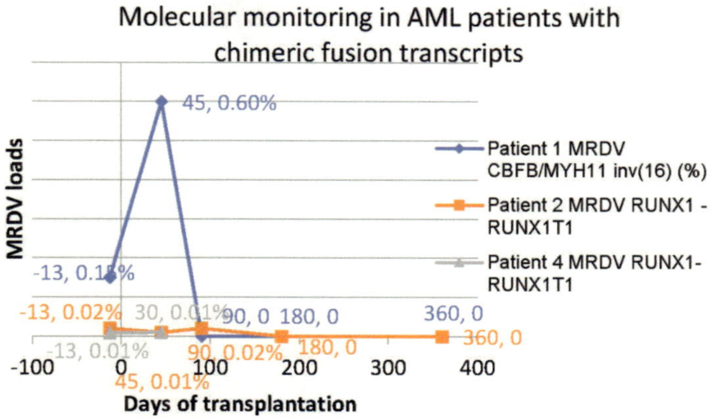

Figure 2.
Molecular MRD monitoring of patients with identified chimeric fusion transcripts. MRD kinetics of patients 1, 2 and 4 is marked with blue, orange and gray curve, respectively.

4.4.2 Case II

A previously healthy young man at the age of 21 was diagnosed with AML in January 2019. Initial findings of bone marrow revealed presence of RUNX1-RUNX1T1 fusion transcript. Remission was achieved after two cycles of standard DA (7 + 3) induction regimen and two consolidation therapies with high dose ARA-C were administered [1, 7]. MUD HSCT was performed in August 2019 after conditioning with Bu/Cy + ATG regimen [37]. Unrelated HLA 10/10 identical donor, signed to the German National Bone Marrow Donor Registry (DE-ZKRD), was activated [14–16]. A total of 5,2 × 10^6 peripheral blood stem cells/ kg were infused. MRD was measured by using RT- PCR, first on day +45 and thereafter at every three months. Up to the sixth month of HSCT, relatively steady kinetics of transcript levels was noted as shown at **Figure 2**. By gradual reduction of immunosupression dose, molecular remission was documented at +6 month of HSCT and at +9 months consecutively. Complete donor chimerism was first documented on day +90 and maintained to the final evaluation at +9 months.

4.4.3 Case III

A 58-year-old woman was diagnosed with refractory anemia-myelodysplastic syndrome (MDS) in July 2018 and rapid progression into overt acute leukemia was demonstrated 4 months later. Initial molecular analysis detected 5 bp deletion in CEBPA gene. Induction chemotherapy (DA 7 + 3) was initiated and bone marrow evaluation showed no signs of remission after two cycles induction chemotherapies [1, 7]. Remission was achieved after one cycle salvage chemotherapy with FLAG-Ida regimen [7, 11]. Two consolidation therapies with high dose ARA-C were administered. MUD HSCT was performed in November 2019. Due to the patient age, reduced intensity chemotherapy (RIC) regimen was preferred, consisting of Busulfan and Fludarabin + ATG (fludarabine 30 mg/m^2 i.v for 5 days – from −8 to −4 and Busulfan 3.5 mg/kg/day for 2 days: day −5 and day −4) [37]. Unrelated HLA 10/10 identical donor from The Italian Bone Marrow Donor Registry (IBMDR) was activated [14–16]. Peripheral blood stem cells were used at a dose of 6,9 × 10^6 CD34+ cells/kg. MRD was first assessed on day +60 and the next one on day +120 with the last one assessed on day +150. Absence of previously detected deletion was confirmed on the first assessment, coupled with complete donor chimerism.

4.4.4 Case IV

A 37-year-old woman was diagnosed with RUNX1-RUNX1T1- mutated AML in July 2019. Treatment was initiated with DA (7 + 3) induction regimen and complete remission was established after two induction cycles [1, 7]. Two consolidation therapies with high dose ARA-C were applied afterwards. Unrelated HLA 10/10 identical donor, recruited through the German National Bone Marrow Donor Registry (DE-ZKRD) was activated and MUD HSCT was performed in January 2020 [14–16]. Peripheral blood stem cells were used as a source and a high number of HSC were harvested - 9×10^5 CD34+ cells/kg. Myeloablative regimen with Bu/Cy + ATG was used [37]. Conventional immunosuppressive therapy with cyclosporine and metothrexate was used. No significant complications were observed in the early post-transplant period [38]. Bone marrow evaluation was performed at +1 month of HSCT when complete donor chimerism was documented. She was MRD positive with MRD loads, nearly equal to those measured in pre-transplant evaluation (MRDv = 0.1% and MRDV = 0.09% respectively). On day +38 of HSCT, she appeared with symptoms of lower gastrtointestinal acute GvHD grade III, subsequently confirmed histologically. Immunosuppressive therapy with high dose methylprednisolone was immediately started. Three days later, she manifested acute severe respiratory symptomatology, leading to respiratory insufficiency and fatal outcome on day +45 of HSCT.

4.5 Post-transplant molecular monitoring

During the post-transplant period, in line with EBMT recommendations [38, 39], chimerism and molecular MRD status were assessed every three months and up to one year of HSCT, starting within two months of HSCT (45 days median time) [7, 24, 25]. In patient 1, a significantly increased MRD load was observed on day +45 of HSCT, compared to pre-transplant MRD load (0,6% and 0,15% respectively) and we reduced the immunosuppression dose. Immunosuppressive therapy is designed to prevent GvHD, but it also inhibits graft-versus leukemia effects (GvL). This patient had no previous signs of GvHD, thus he was carefully monitored for possible occurrence of new ones. Our objective was to enhance GvL effects, without causing serious GVHD, which resulted in achieving MRD negativity at +90 days of HSCT and maintaining it for a year so far in absence of GvHD manifestations. In patient 2, molecular loads kinetics showed a relatively steady curve, almost identical MRD values were measured until the sixth month of HSCT, when molecular negativity was documented. Patients 1, 2 and 3 had been followed up for 19 months of HSCT, 9 and 8 months respectively. They are in complete hematological and molecular remission for 13, 3 and 6 months, as defined by International Working Group for Diagnosis, Standardization of Response Criteria, Treatment Outcomes, and Reporting Standards for Therapeutic Trials in Acute Myeloid Leukemia: completely recovery of peripheral blood cells, <5% blasts in bone marrow, disappearance of the cells with previously documented leukemic immunophenotype and disappearance of previously detected molecular mutation [39]. Patient 4 died on day +45 of HSCT due to transplant-related complication. MRD status was assessed on day +30 of HSCT, when she was MRD positive with low MRD loads, equal to those prior to HSCT. Chimerism analyses in all patients, including patient 4 on day +30 of HSCT, documented early complete donor chimerism, which remained sustained during the follow-up evaluations in the first 3 patients.

5. Discussion

5.1 RUNX1-RUNX1T1- mutated AML

Chimeric fusion genes CBFB-MYH11, RUNX1-RUNX1T1, including PML-RARα, represent about 25% of AML cases, so called core-binding AML. As stated before, *RUNX1-RUNX1T1-mutated AML* is stratified into favorable risk group and therefore, patients harboring this mutation often do not undergo HSCT in first CR. Results from AML Study group show that half of these patients relapse very soon, almost all during the first year of completion of therapy [31]. In comparison, according to a single center study, among transplanted patients with RUNX1-RUNX1T1- AML, only 10–20% are expected to experience relapse [29]. RUNX1-RUNX1T1 transcript is well established powerful marker to predict risk of post-transplant relapse and direct future clinical interventions. In line with the same study [29, 33], RUNX1-RUNX1T1 levels kinetics can accurately predict forthcoming relapse, but not late relapse, due to the narrow time lag from molecular to morphological relapse. For this reason, time intervals between MRD assessments in these patients should not exceed 3 months.

5.2 CBFB-MYH11 - mutated AML

Acute myeloid leukemia (AML) with inv.(16)/ *t*(16,16), leading to specific *CBFB-MYH11* fusion transcript formation is also considered as favorable subtype [32, 33]. Therefore, in terms of transplantation, the same views are held as for RUNX1-RUNX1T1- AML [29–31]. Due to the general low incidence of this subtype, as well asa lower transplant rate in this group, all data originate from small sample-studies. Such limited data suggest that post-transplant MRD is predictive of relapse in contrast to pre-transplant MRD. The strongest predictive value is seen at +3 months of HSCT and it is thought that this period of time reflects the sensitivity of leukemia cells toward the transplant [32]. In regards to the optimal time intervals between MRD assessments in these patients, according to some published data [33], CBFB-MYH11 AML relapses appear to be generally indolent, with the longest delay of 8 months from molecular relapse to hematological evident relapse. However, these findings cannot be taken for granted, as the study involved non-transplanted patients.

5.3 AML with CEBPA aberrations

CEBPA aberrations can be found in up to 10% of patients with AML. Apart from AML, these mutations and deletions can also occur in MDS, multiple myeloma and non-Hodgkin's lymphoma (NHL) patients. CEBPA mutations result in functional block in myeloid differentiation and turning toward the erythroid lineage, with consequent erythroid hyperplasia or dysplasia, as was the case with our patient at the time of initial hematological assessment [40]. The most cases of *CEBPA*-mutant AML are double-mutated and exhibit two mutations and less than one third are single mutants. As per previously published data, double mutants have favorable prognosis, while the prognostic significance of single mutations is still unclear and it is codependent of the presence of additional gene mutations, such as FLT3-ITD and NPM1 and it is influenced by the karyotype [23, 40].

5.4 MRD and chimerism

In addition, in malignant diseases, chimerism kinetics seems to be remarkably correlated to MRD kinetics. Though, chimerism itself cannot be considered as an indirect marker for post-transplant MRD monitoring, it serves more likely as prognostic factor for impending relapse. Therefore, chimerism analyses in bone marrow samples should be combined with MRD assessment in order to optimize the predictive value. As per EBMT recommendations, chimerism status should be evaluated at the same time points as MRD status during the post-transplant follow-up, or more precisely, within the first month of HSCT and at every three months during the first and the second year of HSCT [38, 39].

MRD status can be used to guide future clinical interventions in the post-transplant period. The presence of post-transplant MRD can identify those patients who are unlikely to benefit from re-application of similar therapies, because of selection and expansion of therapy-resistant clones. Different therapy strategies may be adopted in an attempt to eliminate MRD, varying from watchful waiting, through withdrawal of immunosuppression to more aggressive clinical interventions, distinguishing two general approaches - *immunomodulation* and *chemotherapeuteic agents* [41]. Immunomodulation includes donor lymphocyte infusion (DLI), natural killer (NK) cell infusion, both focused on enhancing GvL effects and chimeric antigen receptors (CAR) T-cells. In addition, emerging new chemotherapeutic agents such as DNA hypomethylating agents and targeted therapies could potentially eradicate MRD positivity [42].

6. Conclusion

Since major advancement had been achieved in the field of molecular monitoring, molecular MRD analyses became widely incorporated into the clinical routine and the decision making-process. PCR is currently used in our clinical practice in patients expressing specific molecular targets undergoing both autologous and allogeneic HSCT. Post-transplant molecular monitoring is of twofold significance: predicting impending relapse and guiding future MRD-based decisions and treatment strategies. In patients undergoing allogeneic HSCT, MRD should be evaluated within a month prior to the start of the conditioning regimen. During the follow-up period, MRD should be monitored every three months in a BM sample for at least two years and according to individual risk thereafter. MRD status itself is not a conclusive or a sufficient criterion to decide to intervene therapeutically. The main inquiry remains whether, when and at what thresholds a clinical intervention is required. Well-designed prospective clinical trials are needed to provide answers to these questions and establish MRD- guided clinical protocols.

Author details

Irina Panovska-Stavridis
University Clinic of Hematology, Skopje, Republic of North Macedonia

*Address all correspondence to: dr_irina@yahoo.com

References

[1] Döhner H, Weisdorf DJ, Bloomfield CD. Acute Myeloid Leukemia. N Engl J Med. 2015 Sep 17;373(12):1136-52. doi: 10.1056/NEJMra1406184.

[2] Siegel RL, Miller KD, Jemal A. Cancer statistics, 2019. CA Cancer J Clin. 2019;69(1):7-34. doi:10.3322/caac.21551

[3] De Kouchkovsky I, Abdul-Hay M. 'Acute myeloid leukemia: a comprehensive review and 2016 update'. Blood Cancer J. 2016 Jul 1;6(7):e441. doi: 10.1038/bcj.2016.50.

[4] Shallis RM, Wang R, Davidoff A, Ma X, Zeidan AM. Epidemiology of acute myeloid leukemia: Recent progress and enduring challenges. Blood Rev. 2019;36:70-87. doi:10.1016/j.blre.2019.04.005

[5] Swerdlow SH, Campo E, Harris NL, Jaffe ES, Pileri SA, Stein H, Thiele J, editors. WHO Classification of Tumours of Haematopoietic and Lymphoid Tissues. Revised 4th Edition, Volume 2

[6] Neuendorff NR, Burmeister T, Dörken B, Westermann J. BCR-ABL-positive acute myeloid leukemia: a new entity? Analysis of clinical and molecular features. Ann Hematol. 2016;95(8):1211-1221. doi:10.1007/s00277-016-2721-z

[7] Döhner H, Estey E, Grimwade D, et al. Diagnosis and management of AML in adults: 2017 ELN recommendations from an international expert panel. Blood. 2017;129(4):424-447. doi:10.1182/blood-2016-08-733196

[8] Gale RE, Green C, Allen C, et al; Medical Research Council Adult Leukaemia Working Party. The impact of FLT3 internal tandem duplication mutant level, number, size, and interaction with NPM1 mutations in a large cohort of young adult patients with acute myeloid leukemia. Blood. 2008; 111(5):2776-2784. doi: 10.1182/blood-2007-08-109090

[9] Papaemmanuil E, Gerstung M, Bullinger L, et al. Genomic classification and prognosis in acute myeloid leukemia. N Engl J Med. 2016;374(23):2209-2221. doi: 10.1056/NEJMoa1516192

[10] Bowen D, Groves MJ, Burnett AK, et al. TP53 gene mutation is frequent in patients with acute myeloid leukemia and complex karyotype, and is associated with very poor prognosis. Leukemia. 2009;23(1):203-206. doi: 10.1038/leu.2008.173.

[11] Loke J, Malladi R, Moss P, Craddock C. The role of allogeneic stem cell transplantation in the management of acute myeloid leukaemia: a triumph of hope and experience. Br J Haematol. 2020;188(1):129-146. doi:10.1111/bjh.16355

[12] Evseeva I, Foeken L, Madrigal A. The Role of Unrelated Donor Registries in HSCT. In: Carreras E, Dufour C, Mohty M, et al., editors. The EBMT Handbook: Hematopoietic Stem Cell Transplantation and Cellular Therapies [Internet]. 7th edition. Cham (CH): Springer; 2019. Chapter 3. doi: 10.1007/978-3-030-02278-5_3

[13] Lee SJ, Klein J, Haagenson M, et al. High-resolution donor-recipient HLA matching contributes to the success of unrelated donor marrow transplantation. Blood. 2007;110(13):4576-4583. doi:10.1182/blood-2007-06-097386

[14] Lown RN, Philippe J, Navarro W, et al. Unrelated adult stem cell donor medical suitability: recommendations from the World Marrow Donor Association Clinical Working Group

Committee. Bone Marrow Transplant. 2014;49(7):880-886. doi:10.1038/ bmt.2014.67

[15] Kollman C, Spellman SR, Zhang MJ, et al. The effect of donor characteristics on survival after unrelated donor transplantation for hematologic malignancy. Blood. 2016;127(2):260-267. doi:10.1182/blood-2015-08-663823

[16] Shaw BE, Mayor NP, Szydlo RM, et al. Recipient/donor HLA and CMV matching in recipients of T-cell-depleted unrelated donor haematopoietic cell transplants. Bone Marrow Transplant. 2017;52(5):717-725. doi:10.1038/ bmt.2016.352

[17] Champlin R. Is unrelated donor or haploidentical hematopoietic transplantation preferred for patients with acute myeloid leukemia in remission?. *Haematologica*. 2020;105(2):252-254. doi:10.3324/ haematol.2019.239624

[18] Fuchs EJ. Related haploidentical donors are a better choice than matched unrelated donors: Point. *Blood Adv*. 2017;1(6):397-400. doi:10.1182/ bloodadvances.2016002196

[19] Ballen KK, Gluckman E, Broxmeyer HE. Umbilical cord blood transplantation: the first 25 years and beyond. *Blood*. 2013;122(4):491-498. doi:10.1182/blood-2013-02-453175

[20] Bisel HF. Letter to the editor: criteria for the evaluation of response to treatment in acute leukemia. Blood 1956; 11(7): 676-677.

[21] Hourigan, C., Gale, R., Gormley, N. et al. Measurable residual disease testing in acute myeloid leukaemia. Leukemia 31, 1482-1490 (2017). doi: 10.1038/ leu.2017.113

[22] Schuurhuis GJ, Heuser M, Freeman S, at el. Minimal/measurable residual disease in AML: consensus document from ELN MRD Working Party. Blood. 2018; 131(12):1275-91. doi: 10.1182/blood-2017-09-801498

[23] Claire L. Green, Kenneth K. Koo, Robert K. Hills, Alan K. Burnett, David C. Linch, and Rosemary E. Gale Prognostic Significance of CEBPA Mutations in a Large Cohort of Younger Adult Patients With Acute Myeloid Leukemia: Impact of Double CEBPA Mutations and the Interaction With FLT3 and NPM1 Mutations J Clin Oncol.2010; 28:2739-2747. doi: 10.1200/ JCO.2009.26.2501

[24] Butturini A, Klein J, Gale RP. Modeling minimal residual disease (MRD)-testing. Leuk Res 2003; 27(4): 293-300. doi: 10.1016/ s0145-2126(02)00166-2.

[25] Dillon R, Hills R, Freeman S, et al. Molecular MRD status and outcome after transplantation in NPM1-mutated AML. Blood. 2020;135(9):680-688. doi:10.1182/blood.2019002959

[26] Jentzsch M, Schwind S, Bach E, Stasik S, Thiede C, Platzbecker U. Clinical Challenges and Consequences of Measurable Residual Disease in Non-APL Acute Myeloid Leukemia. Cancers (Basel). 2019;11(11):1625. doi:10.3390/ cancers11111625

[27] Balsat M, Renneville A, Thomas X, et al. Post Induction Minimal Residual Disease Predicts Outcome and Benefit From Allogeneic Stem Cell Transplantation in Acute Myeloid Leukemia With NPM1 Mutation: A Study by the Acute Leukemia French Association Group. J Clin Oncol. 2017;35(2):185-193. doi:10.1200/ JCO.2016.67.1875

[28] Kayser S, Benner A, Thiede C, et al. Pretransplant NPM1 MRD levels predict outcome after allogeneic hematopoietic stem cell transplantation in patients with acute myeloid leukemia. Blood

Cancer J. 2016;6(7):e449. doi:10.1038/bcj.2016.46

[29] Qin YZ, Wang Y, Xu LP, et al. The dynamics of RUNX1-RUNX1T1 transcript levels after allogeneic hematopoietic stem cell transplantation predict relapse in patients with t(8;21) acute myeloid leukemia. J Hematol Oncol. 2017;10(1):44. doi:10.1186/s13045-017-0414-2

[30] Zhu HH, Zhang XH, Qin YZ, et al. MRD-directed risk stratification treatment may improve outcomes of t(8;21) AML in the first complete remission: results from the AML05 multicenter trial. Blood. 2013;121(20):4056-4062. doi:10.1182/blood-2012-11-468348

[31] Rücker FG, Agrawal M, Corbacioglu A, et al. Measurable residual disease monitoring in acute myeloid leukemia with t(8;21)(q22;q22.1): results from the AML Study Group. Blood. 2019;134(19):1608-1618. doi:10.1182/blood.2019001425

[32] Tang FF, Xu LP, Zhang XH, et al. Monitoring of post-transplant CBFB-MYH11 as minimal residual disease, rather than KIT mutations, can predict relapse after allogeneic haematopoietic cell transplantation in adults with inv(16) acute myeloid leukaemia. Br J Haematol. 2018;180(3):448-451. doi:10.1111/bjh.14340

[33] Ommen HB, Schnittger S, Jovanovic JV, et al. Strikingly different molecular relapse kinetics in NPM1c, PML-RARA, RUNX1-RUNX1T1, and CBFB-MYH11 acute myeloid leukemias. Blood. 2010;115(2):198-205. doi:10.1182/blood-2009-04-212530

[34] Horowitz, M., Schreiber, H., Elder, A. et al. Epidemiology and biology of relapse after stem cell transplantation. Bone Marrow Transplant 53, 1379-1389 (2018). doi: 10.1038/s41409-018-0171-z

[35] Bahia DM, Yamamoto M, Chauffaille Mde L, Kimura EY, Bordin JO, Filgueiras MA, et al. Aberrant phenotypes in acute myeloid leukemia: a high frequency and its clinical significance. Haematologica 2001; 86(8): 801-806.

[36] Gabert J, Beillard E, van der Velden VHJ, Bi W, Grimwade D, Pallisgaard N, et al. Standardization and quality control studies of 'real-time' quantitative reverse transcriptase polymerase chain reaction of fusion gene transcripts for residual disease detection in leukemia - a Europe Against Cancer program. Leukemia 2003; 17(12): 2318-2357.

[37] Bacigalupo A, Ballen K, Rizzo D, et al. Defining the intensity of conditioning regimens: working definitions. Biol Blood Marrow Transplant. 2009;15(12):1628-1633. doi:10.1016/j.bbmt.2009.07.004

[38] Rovira M, Suárez-Lledó M. Short- and Long-Term Controls After HSCT. In: Carreras E, Dufour C, Mohty M, Kröger N, eds. The EBMT Handbook: Hematopoietic Stem Cell Transplantation and Cellular Therapies. 7th ed. Cham (CH): Springer; 2019:149-153. doi: 10.1007/978-3-030-02278-5_3

[39] Cheson BD, Bennett JM, Kopecky KJ, et al. Revised recommendations of the International Working Group for Diagnosis, Standardization of Response Criteria, Treatment Outcomes, and Reporting Standards for Therapeutic Trials in Acute Myeloid Leukemia., J Clin Oncol, 2003, vol. 21(pg. 4642-4649). doi: 10.1200/JCO.2003.04.036.

[40] Mannelli F, Ponziani V, Bencini S, et al. CEBPA-double-mutated acute myeloid leukemia displays a unique phenotypic profile: a reliable screening method and insight into biological features. Haematologica.

2017;102(3):529-540. doi:10.3324/haematol.2016.151910

[41] Rein LA, Sung AD, Rizzieri DA. New approaches to manipulate minimal residual disease after allogeneic stem cell transplantation. Int J Hematol Oncol. 2013;2(1):10.2217/ijh.13.4. doi:10.2217/ijh.13.4

[42] Khanal, Nabin & Banskota, Shristi & Bhatt, Vijaya. (2020). Novel treatment paradigms in acute myeloid leukemia. Clinical Pharmacology & Therapeutics. 10.1002/cpt.1962. doi: 10.1002/cpt.1962

Section 5

Targeted Therapies

Chapter 14

Target Therapy in Acute Myeloid Leukemia

Vasko Graklanov

Abstract

Acute myeloid leukemia (AML) is the most common form of acute leukemia in elderly patients. Over the past four decades the basic therapeutic armamentarium was the standard cytotoxic treatment. The new insights in understanding the pathogenesis of AML was the momentum that revolutionized the treatment landscape in AML. The last five years unprecedented growth has been seen in the number of target therapy drugs for the treatment of AML. These new drugs did not just have a clinical benefit as single agents but also have improved AML patient outcomes if combined with conventional cytotoxic therapy. Here, we review recent advances in target-based therapy for patients with AML focusing on their mechanism of action and the results from already published clinical trials.

Keywords: acute myeloid leukemia, target therapy, FLT3 inhibitors, IDH inhibitors, pro-apoptotic agents, smoothened inhibitors, checkpoint inhibitors, CD33-targeted therapy, E-selectin inhibitors, Polo-like kinase inhibitors

1. Introduction

Acute myeloid leukemia (AML) is a heterogeneous malignant disease, characterized by uncontrolled proliferation with impaired differentiation of myeloid progenitor cells and aggressive clinical course. In the past two decades the treatment landscape of AML underwent significant changes due to explosive growth in knowledge of the molecular pathways involved in the AML origin and course evolution. This increased new data and understanding of the pathogenesis of AML, facilitated the development of new drugs in the treatment of AML, particularly the creation of drugs that target the disease on a molecular level. Encouraging efficacy of targeted therapy when combined with the traditional chemotherapy have resulted in big improvement to AML treatment and survival. In this chapter, we will discuss the drugs used in treatment of AML, including targeted treatment strategies that have recently entered the clinical practice.

1.1 Signaling and kinase pathway mutations inhibitors

1.1.1 FLT3 tyrosine kinase inhibitors

Full-length human FLT3 was cloned from a pre-B cell library in 1993 [1], from a CD34+ hematopoietic stem cell-enriched library [2], and is located on chromosome 13q12 [3]. FLT3 is a member of class III receptor tyrosine kinases (RTK) [4] and its activation leads to promotion of cell survival, proliferation, and differentiation

IntechOpen

through various signaling pathways, including PI3K, RAS, and STAT5 [5]. It is present in approximately 20–30% of adult AML patients and 5–15% of pediatric AML patients [6, 7]. FLT3-ITD mutations are associated with higher relapse rate and poorer overall survival, particularly with a high ratio of mutant allelic burden [8, 9]. Several first- and next generation FLT3 inhibitors have been investigated in patients with FLT3-ITD-mutated AML.

1.1.1.1 First-generation FLT3 inhibitors

1.1.1.1.1 Midostaurin

Midostaurin (Rydapt®, Novartis Pharmaceuticals, Inc. (PKC412)) is a multikinase inhibitor, targets wild type FLT3 and mutated FLT3 (ITD and tyrosine kinase domain (TKD)) [10]. Midostaurin also inhibits c-kit, platelet-derived growth factor receptor (PDGFR), vascular endothelial growth factor receptor (VEGFR), and protein kinase C [11]. A phase III international prospective, multinational, randomized, placebo-controlled, double-blind RATIFY study confirmed that, addition of midostaurin to standard induction chemotherapy could significantly increase OS vs. placebo among AML adults with FLT3 mutation (median OS of 74.7 m vs. 25.6 m, HR = 0.78, n = 717). RATIFY enrolled adults aged 18–59 years with newly diagnosed FLT3-mutated (ITD or TKD) AML. Patients were stratified according to FLT3 mutation type (TKD, ITD with a high AR [>0.7], and ITD with a low AR [0.05–0.7]) The addition of midostaurin demonstrated a significant survival benefit in patients with FLT3-mutated AML compared with placebo, with a 22% reduction in the rate of death compared with placebo (hazard ratio [HR], 0.78 [95% CI, 0.63–0.96]; P = 0.009). Although not specifically mandated, allogeneic stem cell transplantation (allo-SCT) was performed in 25% of patients in first complete remission (CR) and 57% of patients overall. Furthermore, patients receiving an allo-SCT in first CR had better outcome if they were treated with midostaurin during induction therapy (P = 0.08), suggesting that the optimal treatment strategy in FLT3-mutated AML would be to move on to allo-SCT early in first CR [12]. Adverse events (AEs) occurring during treatment with midostaurin were common in patients receiving intensive chemotherapy for AML. The most common nonhematologic grade ≥ 3 AEs were febrile neutropenia, infection, lymphopenia, diarrhea, and rash/desquamation. The rates of grade ≥ 3 AEs were largely similar between the midostaurin and placebo groups, with the exceptions of rash/desquamation and anemia (higher in the midostaurin group) and nausea (nearly twice as common in the placebo group) [12, 13]. Other, less common AEs reported with midostaurin included pulmonary AEs (i.e., pneumonitis or pulmonary infiltrate), cardiac AEs (e.g., prolonged corrected QT interval) and hepatic or renal dysfunction [12–14].

1.1.1.1.2 Sorafenib

Sorafenib is a potent first-generation multikinase inhibitor with activity against FLT3/ITD receptor but resistance emerges as FLT3-TKD point mutations [15]. It has been evaluated as either single agent or in combination with chemotherapies in numerous phase I and phase II clinical trials [16–20]. In an early phase clinical trial, sorafenib combined with idarubicin and high dose cytarabine in younger de novo AML patients provided a CR rate of 93% and a 1-year survival rate of 74% in FLT3-ITD positive AML patients [18]. In SORAML study, a placebo-controlled randomized study from Germany in 267 newly diagnosed patients aged 18–60 years. Sorafenib was added to daunorubicin and cytarabine (7 + 3) which resulted in a significantly prolonged 3-year EFS (40 vs. 22%, P = 0.013) and RFS

(56 vs. 38%, P = 0.017) without improvement in OS and CR [21]. Another randomized placebo-controlled trial in 201 older patients aged 61–80 years did not demonstrated improvement in EFS, CR, and OS. The results showed higher early mortality (17 versus 7%, P = 0.052) compared with placebo [22]. In multivariate analysis of retrospective study analysing the effect of sorafenib as post-transplant maintenance in adult patients with FLT3-internal tandem duplication (ITD) acute myeloid leukaemia (AML) in 26 sorafenib patients and 55 controls, sorafenib significantly improved OS [Hazard ratio (HR) 0·26, P = 0·021] and PFS (HR 0·25, P = 0·016). Also there was no difference in 2-year non-relapse mortality (9·8% vs. 9·3%, P = 0·82) or 1-year chronic graft-versus-host disease (55·5% vs. 37·2%, P = 0·28) [23]. The most common adverse events occurring during treatment with sorafenib in SORAML study were fever, infections, pneumonia and pain. Grade 3 or worse adverse events that were significantly more common in the sorafenib group than the placebo group were fever, diarrhea, bleeding, cardiac events, hand-foot-skin reaction and rash [21].

1.1.1.1.3 Sunitinib

Sunitinib is an oral multitargeted kinase inhibitor with selectivity for FLT3, PDGFa/b, VEGF receptor, and Kit receptor tyrosine kinases [24]. Sunitinib induces G1 phase arrest, increases pro-apoptotic molecule expression, and decreases anti-apoptotic molecule expression in AML cells [25]. In a study by O'Farrell and colleagues in 29 AML patients each received a single dose of sunitinib, inhibition of FLT3 phosphorylation was observed in 50% of FLT3 wild-type patients and 100% of FLT3 mutated patients [26]. In another phase I study of sunitinib in 15 patients with refractory AML partial responses were achieved in all 4 patients with FLT3 mutations compared with 2 of 10 in patients with wild-type FLT3. All responses were of short duration and the most frequent grade 2 toxicities were edema, fatigue, and oral ulcerations occurring with a regimen of 50 mg/week [27]. In another phase I/II clinical trial, sunitinib combined with intensive chemotherapy included 22 patients older than 60 years with FLT3/ITD-mutated. Thirteen patients, including 8 patients with FLT3/ITD mutation, achieved CR/CRi. The median overall, relapse-free, and event-free survival of the 17 patients were 1.6, 1.0, and 0.4 years, respectively [28].

1.1.1.1.4 Lestaurtinib

Lestaurtinib (CEP-701) is an orally bioavailable first generation FLT3 inhibitor. It is derived from the bacterial fermentation product K-252a as indolocarbazole alkaloid compound. Except inhibition of FLT3 Lestaurtinib also inhibits JAK2, tropomyosin receptor kinases and neurotrophin receptors [29–33]. In a phase 2 trial lestaurtinib was administered as monotherapy in untreated older patients with AML not considered fit for intensive chemotherapy, irrespective of FLT3 mutation status. This study involved 29 patients with median age of 73 years. Lestaurtinib was administered orally at doses of 60 mg and 80 mg twice daily for 8 weeks. Clinical activity was evident in 8 (30%) patients, including 3 (60%) of 5 FLT3 mutant patients and 5 (23%) of 22 evaluable FLT3 WT patients, the difference in response rates between mutation groups not reaching statistical significance. Lestaurtinib was generally well tolerated. Commonly observed toxicities included mild nausea (8 patients), emesis (5 patients), constipation (5 patients), diarrhea (6 patients), and elevations in alkaline phosphatase concentration (13 patients) [34]. Another phase 1/2 trial in 14 heavily pretreated AML patients treated with CEP-701 at an initial dose of 60 mg orally twice daily, showed clinical evidence of biologic activity and measurable clinical response in 5 patients with significant reductions in bone marrow and peripheral blood blasts and minimal drug related toxicities [35]. A randomized assessment from UK AML 15 and AML 17 trials confirmed no statistically significant benefit observed in the combination of lestaurtinib with standard chemotherapy for newly diagnosed AML patients mostly younger than 60 years.

1.1.1.1.5 Tandutinib

Tandutinib (MLN518) is FLT3, KIT, PDGFR and type III receptor tyrosine kinases inhibitor. Tandutinib induces apoptosis and inhibits FLT3/ITD phosphorylation, cellular proliferation, and signaling of the MAPK and PI3K pathways [36]. In a phase 1 trial tandutinib was given orally (from 50–700 mg twice daily) in 40 patients with either AML or high-risk myelodysplastic syndrome (MDS) with only 8 patients with FLT3-ITD mutations. Even among the patients with FLT3-ITD mutations who were treated at potentially effective doses, response evaluation was often not possible because of rapid disease progression, sudden disease-related clinical deterioration, or tandutinib-related toxicity. Tandutinib treatment was associated muscular weakness, nausea, vomiting and less often diarrhea [37].

1.1.1.2 Second and next generation FLT3 inhibitors

1.1.1.2.1 Quizartinib

Quizartinib (AC220) is a selective and highly potent second-generation class III receptor TKI that selectively inhibits FLT3/STK1, CSF1R/FMS, SCFR/KIT, and PDGFRs in a dose dependent manner [38]. Quizartinib was first tested in phase I dose-escalation trial in patients with relapsed and refractory AML patients irrespective of FLT3 mutation status. Quizartinib was administered orally at escalating doses of 12 to 450 mg/day to 76 patients, with a median of three prior therapies and responses occurred in 23 (30%) of 76 patients, including 10 (13%) complete remissions (CR). The median duration of response was 13.3 weeks and the median survival was 14 weeks. The most common treatment-related adverse events were nausea, vomiting, and prolonged QT interval. The maximum tolerated dose (MTD) was 200 mg/day, and the dose-limiting toxicity was grade 3 QT prolongation [39]. In another 2-part, phase 1, multicenter, open-label, sequential group dose-escalation trial of quizartinib in combination with induction and consolidation chemotherapy in patients with newly diagnosed acute myeloid leukemia a total of 19 patients were enrolled. Sixteen patients (84%) achieved a response; 14 (74%) composite complete response; 2 (11%) morphologic leukemia-free state. Most common grade 3/4 adverse events were febrile neutropenia (47%), neutropenia (42%), thrombocytopenia (32%), and anemia (26%). There were no apparent additional toxicities with addition of quizartinib to chemotherapy although grade ≤ 1 QT prolongation was observed at MTD [40]. In a large phase 2 trial assigning 333 (157 in cohort 1 and 176 in cohort 2) r/r AML patients were enrolled. In cohort 1 56% of FLT3-ITD-positive patients and 36% of FLT3-ITD-negative patients achieved composite complete remission and in cohort 2 46% FLT3-ITD-positive patients achieved composite complete remission whereas 30% of FLT3-ITD-negative patients achieved composite complete remission. Across both cohorts the most common grade 3 or worse treatment-related adverse events were febrile neutropenia, anaemia, thrombocytopenia, QTcF prolongation, neutropenia, leucopenia thrombocytopenia and pneumonia [41]. Preliminary results of a randomized phase 3 study (QuANTUM-R) in patients with FLT3-ITD mutated r/r AML enrolled 367 patients, randomized 2:1 to receive quizartinib or 1 of 3 preselected investigator's choice therapy.(low-dose cytarabine, mitoxantrone, etoposide, and intermediate-dose cytarabine or fludarabine, cytarabine, and granulocyte-colony stimulating factor with idarubicin). The results showed a significantly improved median OS for quizartinib (6.2 vs. 4.7 months; p = 0.017) and an improved cCR rate (48% vs. 27%, p = 0.0001). Rates of treatment-emergent adverse events were comparable between the 2 arms [42].

1.1.1.2.2 Crenolanib

Crenolanib (CP868596) is a benzamidine quinolone derivative, a second generation RTK inhibiting FLT3-ITD and -TKD mutations. It is potent, selective, and invulnerable to resistance-conferring kinase domain mutation. As a type I pan-FLT3 inhibitor crenolanib inhibits FLT3/WT, FLT3/ITD, FLT3-TKD, PDGFRα/β, KIT, and FLT3/D835 [43]. In nearly one third of AML patients treated with FLT3 inhibitors in different clinical trials a resistance point mutations like D835 and F691 are occurring during disease progression [44, 45]. As a more potent RTK inhibitor crenolanib could inhibit both FLT3/ITD and resistant FLT3/D835 mutants and less disruptive of erythroid colony growth, which may result in relatively lessmyelosuppression [46]. In a phase 1 trial of FLT3-ITD positive AML crenolanib was given to 69 patients divided in three cohorts, cohort A patients with R/R FLT3 AML who had not received prior FLT3 inhibitors, cohort B patients progressing on prior TKIs and cohort C patients who developed FLT3 + AML after prior MDS. Crenolanib therapy resulted in a 39% CRi and 11% PR (6 D835, 9 ITD, 3 ITD + D835) amongst the patients in cohort A with an ORR of 50% [47]. In a phase II trial, the tolerability and efficacy of crenolanib combined with standard 7 + 3 induction chemotherapy was examined in 29 patients with newly diagnosed FLT3 mutant AML. 21 of 29 (72%) patients achieved a CR after one cycle of induction with cytarabine/anthracycline/crenolanib. An additional 3 patients achieved a CR either after re-induction (1 patient) or after treatment with HiDAC or HSCT (1 patient each) [48]. In another study with the same inclusion criteria in which 26 patients were enrolled the most common advere events which led to crenolanib dose reductions were periorbital edema, delayed count recovery, LFT elevation, nausea and rash [49]. Also crenolanib was investigated in a patients with a first relapsed/primary refractory AML. The study enrolled 8 patients, received HAM followed by crenolanib. 6 patients were evaluable for responses with a complete remission rate of 67% (2 CR, 2 CRi), including 2 pts who were refractory to front line chemotherapy. 2 of 3 patients with FLT3 activating mutations (1 with ITD and 1 with D835) achieved complete remission with complete count recovery; the third pt (FLT3-ITD) had 10% residual blasts after 1 cycle of induction [50]. Ohanian et al. studied the effect of crenolanib combined with idarubicin and high-dose Ara-C in 13 pts (median age of 51 years) with multiply relapsed/refractory FLT3+ AML. The ORR in 11 pts evaluable for response was 36% (1 CR, 3 CRi; 2 not evaluable because of early discontinuation of therapy). The median OS for all patients was 259 days; median OS by prior therapies was 259 days for patients with ≤2 prior therapies, and 53 days for patients with ≥3 prior therapies. No dose-limiting toxicities were observed at any of the dose levels explored and there were no dose reductions required. Non-hematologic adverse events assessed as possibly or probably related to crenolanib were all grade 1 in severity, including: nausea, vomiting, diarrhea, and abdominal pain [51].

1.1.1.2.3 Gilteritinib

Gilteritinib (ASP2215) is a selective next-generation novel dual FLT3 (to a lesser extent to FLT3-TKD than -ITD)/AXL inhibitor. Gilteritinib was investigated in 252 patients with relapsed or refractory acute myeloid leukaemia in one of seven dose-escalation (n = 23) or dose-expansion (n = 229) cohorts. At least 90% of FLT3 phosphorylation inhibition was seen by day 8 in most patients receiving a daily dose of 80 mg or higher. In the full analysis 249 patients were included, 8% achieved complete remission, 4% complete remission with incomplete platelet recovery, 18% complete remission with incomplete haematological recovery, and 10% partial remission. The most common grade 3–4 adverse events irrespective of relation to treatment were febrile neutropenia (39%), anaemia (24%), thrombocytopenia (13%), sepsis (11%), and pneumonia (11%) [52]. In another open-label phase 1 study in 24 Japanese patients with relapsed/refractory acute myeloid leukemia the ORR among patients with mutated FLT3 was 80% and among FLT wild-type was 36.4%. The MTD was 200 mg/d, dose-limiting toxicities were grade 3 tumor lysis syndrome and grade 3 elevated blood lactate dehydrogenase, amylase, blood creatine phosphokinase levels, and syncope [53]. The phase 3 ADMIRAL trial assessing oral gilteritinib 120 mg per day versus salvage chemotherapy in adult r/r FLT3 mutated AML patients led to an FDA approval for gilteritinib. 369 adults with FLT3 mutated AML in first relapse or refractory to front-line therapy were enrolled. The 21% of patients who achieved had a median time to response of 3.6 months [54].

1.1.1.2.4 Cabozantinib

Cabozantinib is an oral tyrosine kinase inhibitor of multiple receptor tyrosine kinases and exhibits anti-tumor activity in several cancers [55, 56]. It inhibits FLT3, MET, AXL, vascular endothelial growth factor receptor, and KIT. In a study among 18 patients with relapsed/refractory AML, 5 harboring FLT3/ITD mutations no patients had a marrow response according to formal criteria. 4 patients had peripheral blast reductions, 2 of these 4 patients transiently cleared circulating blasts, 1 patient experienced a reduction in marrow blasts, and 1 had stable disease [57] (**Table 1**).

1.2 Mutations in epigenetic modifiers: regulators of DNA methylation and chromatin modification drugs

1.2.1 IDH inhibitors

For the first time IDH1 mutations in AML were identified in 2009 by sequencing an acute myeloid leukemia genome. IDH is an enzyme that catalyzes the oxidative decarboxylation of isocitrate to alpha-ketoglutarate (α-KG). 5-methylcytosine (5mC) coverts to 5-hydroxymethylcytosine (5hmc) as a result of interaction between α-KG and TET2 which promotes DNA and histone demethylation [58]. Approximately 8–19% of AML cases carry IDH2 mutations, with another 7–14% carrying IDH1 mutations [59]. IDH1/2 are found with higher frequency in older patients and patients with a normal karyotype [60, 61]. IDH1 mutations almost exclusively occur at R132 while IDH2 involve substitutions at R140 or R172 [62]. While IDH2-R172 may represent a distinct genomic subgroup, which mutual exclusivity with NPM1 and with a distinct DNA methylation profile [63]. Some studies showed that IDH1 and IDH2-R172 mutation may predict a worse clinical outcome especially in CN-AML, while the IDH2-R140 concomitant NPM1 mutation may be associated with better prognosis in AML [63–65]. More further studies are needed due to the conflicting data about the prognostic impact of IDH1/2 mutations in AML.

Drug Class	Mechanism of action	Agent
Signaling and kinase pathway mutations inhibitors (FLT3 tyrosine kinase inhibitors)		
First-generation FLT3 inhibitors	Inhibition of FLT3	
		Midostaurin (PKC412)
		Sorafenib
		Sunitinib
		Lestaurtinib
		Tandutinib
Second and next generation FLT3 inhibitors		
		Quizartinib
		Crenolanib
		Gilteritinib
		Cabozantinib
Mutations in epigenetic modifiers: Regulators of DNA methylation and chromatin modification drugs (IDH inhibitors)	Inhibition of IDH2	Enasidenib
	Inhibition of IDH1	Ivosidenib
Pro-apoptotic agents (Bcl-2 inhibitors)	Inhibition of BCL2	Venetoclax
Hedgehog Inhibition (Smoothened inhibitors)	inhibition of of HH/GLI signalling	Glasdegib
		Sonidegib
		Vismodegib
Polo-like kinase inhibitors	Inhibition of Plk1	Volasertib
E-selectin inhibitors	Inhibition of E-selectin	Uproleselan
Checkpoint inhibitors	Inhibition of PD-1	Nivolumab Pembrolizumab
	Inhibition of CTLA-4	Ipilimumab
CD33-targeted therapy	Inhibition of CD33	Gemtuzumab Ozogamicin
		Vadastuximab talirine

Table 1.
Selected AML targeted agents.

1.2.1.1 Enasidenib

Enasidenib (AG-221) is the first oral IDH mutation–specific inhibitor. It is a bivalent inhibitor of R140Q and R172K mutated IDH2 and induces terminal differentiation of leukemic blasts into neutrophils in vivo [66]. IDH2 inhibitor enasidenib (AG-221/CC-90007) showed promising activity as a single agent in patients with mutated IDH2 in first-in-human phase 1/2 study with 345 patients enrolled. Median age was 68 years. 214 of 345 patients (62%) with relapsed or refractory (R/R) AML received enasidenib, 100 mg/d. 19.6% attained complete remission, 10.3% proceeded to an allogeneic bone marrow transplant, and the overall response rate was 38.8%. 43.1% red blood cell transfusion–dependent and 40.2% platelet transfusion–dependent patients achieved transfusion independence. Response and survival were comparable among patients with IDH2-R140 or IDH2-R172 mutations. Among all 345 patients, the most common grade 3 or 4 treatment-related adverse events were hyperbilirubinemia (10%), thrombocytopenia (7%), and IDH differentiation syndrome (6%) [67]. These results led to the FDA approval of enasidenib in r/r IDH2 mutated AML patients on 1 August 2017. With regard to predictors of response, the IDH2 mutation allele burden at study entry had no effect on response rate [66]. In a open-label, multicenter, phase 1 study patients 134 newlydiagnosed mIDH1 or mIDH2 AML were treated with induction therapy in combination with either ivosidenib 500 mg once daily (for mIDH1) or enasidenib (mIDH2) 100 mg daily. Among the 77 enasidenib-treated patients evaluable for efficacy, a response of CR, CRi, or CRp was achieved in 73% patients with de novo AML and in 63% patients with sAML. The most frequent co-occurring baseline mutations for patients with IDH2 mutations were DNMT3A, SRSF2 and ASXL1 [68].

1.2.1.2 Ivosidenib

Ivosidenib (AG-120) is a potent and selective IDH1 mutation small-molecule inhibitor. In phase 1, multicenter, open-label, dose-escalation and dose-expansion study 258 patients received ivosidenib orally, daily, in 28-day cycles. In the primary efficacy population (125 patients), the rate of complete remission or complete remission with partial hematologic recovery was 30.4%, the rate of complete remission was 21.6% and the overall response rate was 41.6%. The median durations of these responses were 8.2 months, 9.3 months, and 6.5 months, respectively. No residual detectable IDH1 mutations on digital polymerase-chain-reaction assay were detected in 21% patients who had a complete remission or complete remission with partial hematologic recovery. The most common adverse events (in ≥20% of the patients), irrespective of a relationship to ivosidenib, were diarrhea, leukocytosis, febrile neutropenia, nausea, fatigue, dyspnea, prolongation of the QT interval. Peripheral edema, anemia, pyrexia, cough and and differentiation syndrome [69]. The results of this study led to the FDA approval of ivosidenib in r/r IDH1 mutated AML patients on 2 may 2019. Prescribing information contains a boxed warning about the risk of differentiation syndrome which may be life-threatening or fatal. In a open-label, multicenter, phase 1 study patients 134 newlydiagnosed mIDH1 or mIDH2 AML were treated with induction therapy in combination with either ivosidenib 500 mg once daily (for mIDH1) or enasidenib (mIDH2) 100 mg daily. Among the 41 ivosidenib-treated patients evaluable for efficacy, a response of CR, CRi or CRp was achieved in 93% patients with de novo AML and 46% patients with sAML. Twenty-one patients received ≥1 cycle of consolidation therapy and 11 patients received maintenance after consolidation. Seventeen patients proceeded to HSCT. For patients with IDH1 mutations the most frequent co-occurring baseline mutations were DNMT3A, NPM1 and NRAS. MRD-negative CRs using flow cytometry were observed in 89% of patients with IDH1 positive mutational status [68].

1.3 Pro-apoptotic agents

1.3.1 Bcl-2 inhibitors

Bcl-2 gene is located on chromosome 18q21.33 and it was discovered in 1985 through cloning the breakpoint of a translocation of t(14;18) found in follicular B lymphomas [70]. Bcl-2 is an integral protein of the mitochondrial membrane but has also been identified on endoplasmic reticulum and the nuclear envelope [71]. BCL2 family members are classified into pro and anti-apoptotic proteins. The anti-apoptotic BCL2 family contains 4 proteins: BCL2, BCLXL, BCL-w, and MCL-1. Through direct activation of the effector proteins or antagonizing the effect of antiapoptotic proteins the pro-apoptotic proteins lead to an activation of caspase proteases [72]. Bcl 2 has proven to be major negative regulator in apoptosis, playing key roles in neoplastic transformation and leukemogenesis [73]. Overexpression of anti-apoptotic BCL2 proteins such as BCL2, BCL2L1 and MCL1 is widely associated with tumour initiation, progression and chemo resistance in AML [74].

1.3.1.1 Venetoclax

Venetoclax (ABT-199/GDC- 0199) is a highly selective oral BCL2 inhibitor and does not show significant BCL-XL antagonism [75]. Venetoclax induces apoptosis in AML cell lines, in-vitro patient samples and in mouse xenograft models [75, 76]. In a phase II, single-arm study in 32 patients with high-risk relapsed/refractory AML or unfit for intensive chemotherapy venetoclax was given at a dose of 800 mg daily. The overall response rate was 19%, an additional 19% of patients demonstrated antileukemic activity not meeting IWG criteria (partial bone marrow response and incomplete hematologic recovery). Twelve (38%) patients had IDH 1/2 mutations, of whom 4 (33%) achieved complete response or complete response with incomplete blood count recovery. The responses median progression free interval was 2.5 months. Common adverse events included nausea, diarrhea, febrile neutropenia and hypokalemia. Due to potential tumour lysis syndrome as seen in chronic lymphocytic leukemia, a daily dosing ramp up of venetoclax was executed until 800 mg per day [77]. More effective results were achieved in studies where venetoclax was combined with either low-dose cytarabine (LDAC) or hypomethylating agents (HMAs). In a phase Ib/II study in previously untreated patients with AML venetoclax was combined with low-dose cytarabine in 82 adults 60 years or older. The median age was 74 years, 49% had secondary AML, 29% had prior HMA treatment, and 32% had poor-risk cytogenetic features. 54% achieved complete remission (CR)/CR with incomplete blood count recovery. The median OS was 10.1 months (95% CI, 5.7 to 14.2), and median duration of response (DOR) was 8.1 months (95% CI, 5.3 to 14.9 months). Early (30-day) mortality was 6% [78]. In another phase 1b study of venetoclax plus decitabine or azacitidine in untreated AML patients ≥65 years ineligible for standard induction therapy 145 patients were enrolled. Median age was 74 years, with poor-risk cytogenetics in 49% of patients. With a median time on study of 8.9 months, 67% of patients (all doses) achieved complete remission (CR) + CR with incomplete count recovery (CRi), with a CR + CRi rate of 73% in the venetoclax 400 mg + HMA cohort. No tumor lysis syndrome was observed. Common adverse events (>30%) included nausea, diarrhea, constipation, febrile neutropenia, fatigue, hypokalemia, decreased appetite, and decreased white blood cell count [79]. Due to these marked results venetoclax received FDA approval for combination with low dose cytarabine and HMAs. DiNardo et al. assessed the safety and efficacy of venetoclax in combination with FLAG-IDA in a heavily pre-treated r/r AML patients. Study included 12 patients, of 11 patients, 8 patients (73%) achieved a best response of CR/CRi (7 CR, 1 CRi) with a 6-month survival rate of 67%. Of the 8 responding patients, three patients proceeded to allogeneic SCT [80].

1.4 Hedgehog inhibition

1.4.1 Smoothened inhibitors

The Hedgehog (Hh) family of proteins control cell growth and survival. The Hedgehog signalling pathway (HhP) is essential for embryonic development and usually silenced in adult tissues. Germline mutations that subtly affect Hh pathway activity are associated with developmental disorders, whereas somatic mutations activating the pathway have been linked to multiple forms of human cancer [81–83]. Aberrant activation of the HhP has been implicated in the maintenance of leukaemia stem cells in several model systems. Overexpression of various HH/GLI components have been found in chemotherapy resistant myeloid blasts and subsequent inhibition of the HH/GLI pathway revised the sensitivity to chemotherapy [84, 85].

1.4.1.1 Glasdegib

Glasdegib (PF-913) is an oral, potent, selective, small molecule inhibitor of HH/GLI signalling, which binds to the smoothened (SMO) receptor [86]. In vitro treatment with Glasdegib induced a decrease in the quiescent cell population and in vivo treatment attenuated the leukemia-initiation potential of AML cells in a serial transplantation mouse model [87]. An open-label, dose-finding, phase 1 study of glasdegib in 47 adult patients with myeloid malignancies (AML, n = 28) found 400 mg once daily as the MTD and a minor response was achieved (over 25% decrease from baseline in BM blasts) or better in more than 30% of AML patients. The most common treatment-related adverse events included dysgeusia, decreased appetite, and alopecia [88]. Based on this study a phase II, randomized, open-label, multicenter study evaluated the efficacy of glasdegib plus low-dose cytarabine (LDAC) in patients with AML or high-risk myelodysplastic syndrome unsuitable for intensive chemotherapy. Glasdegib 100 mg was administered orally in 28-day cycles. Eighty-eight and 44 patients were randomized to glasdegib/LDAC and LDAC, respectively. Median overall survival was 8.8 (6.9–9.9) months with glasdegib/LDAC and 4.9 (3.5–6.0) months with LDAC. Fifteen (17.0%) and 1 (2.3%) patients in the glasdegib/LDAC and LDAC arms, respectively, achieved complete remission ($P < 0.05$) [89]. Based on this study the FDA approved glasdegib in combination with low dose cytarabine for AML patients unfit for IC. Another phase-II study to evaluate glasdegib from day 3 plus standard-induction chemotherapy for untreated and fit AML or high-risk MDS patients revealed that 46.4% of patients achieved CR. Among all 69 patients, median OS was 14.9 (80% CI 13.4–19.3) months, with 12-month survival probability 66.6%. The most common treatment-related adverse events (≥50% patients) were diarrhea and nausea [90].

1.4.1.2 Sonidegib

Sonidegib (LDE225) is a specific SMO inhibitor and in refractory AML cells increased cell apoptosis and the efficacy of Adriamycin against tumor cells and lowered the expression of the targeted protein [91]. In a phase I/Ib study of azacitidine and sonidegib in myeloid malignancies the best response outcome for untreated AML/MDS patients was 23.1% and for rel/ref 7.1%. However, the rate of SD was remarkably high particularly in the rel/ref AML population at 76%. The most common Gr 3/4 AEs were: thrombocytopenia, neutropenia, anemia and leukopenia [92].

1.4.1.3 Vismodegib

Vismodegib (GDC-0449) safety and efficacy were evaluated in a phase Ib trial in patients with relapsed/refractory acute myeloid leukaemia. All enrolled patients had received prior cancer therapy; most had received more than one therapy, including hypomethylating agents, immunomodulators and targeted signalling pathway inhibitors. 38 received at least one dose of vismodegib but the study was terminated by the sponsor because of lack of efficacy [93].

1.5 Polo-like kinase inhibitors

Polo-like kinases (Plks) are a family of 5 highly conserved serine/threonine protein kinases. They play a key role in mitotic checkpoint regulation and cell division. Plk1 has been shown to be overexpressed in a range of human cancers, including non-small cell lung cancer, prostate, ovarian, breast, and colorectal cancer as well as AML [94–96].

1.5.1 Volasertib

Volasertib (BI 6727) is a low-molecular-weight, adenosine triphosphate–competitive kinase inhibitor that potently inhibits Plk1 [97]. In a randomized, phase 1/2, open-label, multicenter trial of low-dose cytarabine with or without volasertib in patients with AML ineligible for intensive induction therapy eighty-seven patients (median age 75 years) received LDAC or LDAC + volasertib. The result confirmed greater clinical efficacy in the combination arm, statistically significant in CR (30 vs. 13.3%, P = 0.052). Median overall survival was 8.0 vs. 5.2 months, respectively. LDAC + volasertib led to an increased frequency of adverse events that was most pronounced for neutropenic fever/infections and gastrointestinal events [98].

1.6 E-selectin inhibitors

The endothelial cell adhesion molecule E-selectin is a key component of the bone marrow hematopoietic stem cell (HSC) vascular niche regulating balance between HSC self-renewal and commitment. E-selectin is expressed transiently in the normal vasculature during an inflammatory response and constitutively in the bone marrow. E-selectin directly triggers signaling pathways that promote malignant cell survival and regeneration. In vivo AML blasts with highest E-selectin binding potential are 12-fold more likely to survive chemotherapy and main contributors to disease relapse [99, 100].

1.6.1 Uproleselan

Uproleselan (GMI-1271) is a novel antagonist of E-selectin that down-regulates cell survival pathways and enhances chemotherapy response. In a single arm phase I/II trial of 47 adults with relapsed/refractory AML were treated with GMI-1271 in combination with MEC chemotherapy. GMI-1271 was given 24 hrs prior, then every 12 hrs during and for 48 hrs post induction/consolidation. With a median follow-up of 11 months, the ph 1 median leukemia free survival was not reached and overall survival was 7.6 months. ORR (CR/CRi/MLFS/PR) was evaluable in 21 patients was 50%. Remission rate (CR/CRi) was 45%.Common Gr 3/4 AEs were febrile neutropenia, sepsis, bacteremia, hypoxia. 30 and 60 day mortality were 0 and 7%, respectively [101]. A pivotal phase 2/3 study (NCT03616470) is underway to assess the efficacy and safety of uproleselan with standard salvage chemotherapy in R/R AML. The study is a global, randomized, double-blind, phase 3 trial in adults aged 18–75 years with R/R AML and fit for chemotherapy [102].

1.7 Checkpoint inhibitors

The development of immune checkpoint inhibitors (ICIs) is a revolutionary milestone in the field of immuno-oncology. Immune checkpoint blockade removes inhibitory signals of T-cell activation, which enables tumor-reactive T cells to overcome regulatory mechanisms and mount an effective antitumor response [103–105].

Recent studies suggest a novel mechanism that tumor cells might evade host immune attack through increased expression of PD-L1 [106]. Immune checkpoint inhibitor treatment involves programmed cell death protein 1 (PD1) and cytotoxic Tlymphocyte- associated antigen 4 (CTLA4), both of which have been used in preclinical AML models [107].

1.7.1 Nivolumab

Nivolumab (BMS-936558, ONO-4538, or MDX1106) is the first-in-human immunoglobulin G4 (IgG4) PD-1 immune checkpoint inhibitor antibody that disrupts the interaction of the PD-1 receptor with its ligands PD-L1 and PD-L2, thereby inhibiting the cellular immune response [108, 109]. In a phase IB/II study of nivolumab in combination with azacytidine in patients (pts) with relapsed AML 51 patients with a median age of 69 years (range 45–90) were included. From 35 patients evaluable for response, 6 (18%) achieved complete remission (CR)/(CRi) (3 CR, 3 CRi), 5 (15%) had hematologic improvement (HI), 9 (26%) had 50% BM blast reduction,3 pts. (9%) had stable disease >6 months, and 12 (34%) had progression. In the subgroup of patients who did not receive HMA prior treatment, the superiority of new regimen was even more evident with ORR at 52–22%. The median overall survival for the 35 evaluable pts was 9.3 months (range, 1.8–14.3). Grade 3/4 and Grade 2 immune mediated toxicities were observed in 7 (14%) and 6 (12%) patients, which included pneumonitis, nephritis, transaminitis, and skin rash. Steroids took effect on 88% of the patients who suffered from drug-related toxicities [110]. A single-arm, phase 2 part of the phase 1–2 study of nivolumab in combination with idarubicin and cytarabine was conducted in 44 patients with newly diagnosed acute myeloid leukaemia or high-risk myelodysplastic syndrome. The median overall survival was 18.54 months and median event-free survival was not reached. Among the 44 evaluable patients, the ORR was 77% including 63% CR and 14% CRi. Concerning drug toxicities, the grade 3–4 adverse events were observed in six patients, including rash, colitis, pancreatitis and transaminitis [111]. Using nivolumab in post-transplantation setting showed limited efficacy. Among three relapsed AML patients after allo-HSCT treated with nivolumab, one achieved CR, one experienced stabilization, and the third failed to respond [112].

1.7.2 Pembrolizumab

Pembrolizumab (MK-3475) is another drug that blocks PD-1. In a multicenter phase II study pembrolizumab was administered after high-dose cytarabine salvage chemotherapy in 26 R/R AML patients with median age of 54. The overall response rate was 42% with 9 CR/CRi, one PR, and one patient with morphologic leukemia free state. The median OS was 10.5 months. Most frequently observed grade 3 AEs included hepatitis, rash, and epigastric pain [113]. In another single center, single arm trial of pembrolizumab followed by decitabine in 10 patients R/R AML patients with median age of 62, the ORR was 20% with one patient achieving MRD-negative CR. With a median follow-up of 13 months, the mOS was 7 months [114].

1.7.3 Ipilimumab

Ipilimumab is a human IgG1 monoclonal antibody, CTLA-4 antagonist. In a phase I/Ib, open label, multicenter study of treating patients with relapsed hematological malignancies after allo-SCT with ipilimumab 12 AML patients were enrolled. Complete response was observed in five patients (23%) and the 1-year survival rate was 49%. Immune-related adverse events occurred in three patients. Response was associated with in situ infiltration of CD8+ T cells as well as enrichment of effector T cell subsets [115].

1.8 CD33-targeted therapy

The CD33 antigen is expressed on the blast cells (85–90%) of most cases of acute myeloid leukemia [116–118]. CD33 seems to be much less expressed on normal hematopoietic stem cells and has decreased expression during the differentiation of the myeloid lineage. Mature granulocytes do not express a significant amount of CD33. That makes CD33 an promising target for AML targeted therapy [119, 120]. The only non-haematopoietic cells expressing CD33 are hepatocytes, which explains to some extent hepatic toxicity induced by anti CD33 antibodies [121, 122].

2. Gemtuzumab ozogamicin (GO)

Gemtuzumab ozogamicin (Mylotarg) is a humanized anti-CD33 IgG4 monoclonal antibody conjugated to a cytotoxic agent N-acetyl gamma calicheamicin via an acid-labile hydrazone linker. After GO binds to CD33, calicheamicin is being released and generates single and double strand breaks with subsequent cellular death [123]. In a phase I dose escalation study of an anti-CD33 calicheamicin immunoconjugate 40 patients with relapsed or refractory CD33(+) AML were treated. Leukemia was eliminated from the blood and marrow of 8 (20%) of the 40 patients and the MTD was determined to be 9 mg/m^2 [124]. After the encouraging results from three open label phase II studies, the FDA approved GO for the treatment of patients with CD33-positive AML in first relapse who were ≥ 60 years and not suitable for intensive chemotherapy. 142 patients with AML in first relapse were enrolled in the studies with median age of 61 years. All patients received Mylotarg as a 2-hour intravenous infusion, at a dose of 9 mg/m^2, at 2-week intervals for two doses. 30% of patients obtained complete morphological remission. High incidences of myelosuppression, grade 3 or 4 hyperbilirubinemia, and elevated hepatic transaminase levels were registered [125]. In a post-approval phase III trial gemtuzumab ozogamicin was administred during induction and postconsolidation therapy in younger patients with acute myeloid leukemia. 637 patients were randomly assigned to receive daunorubicin, cytarabine, and GO vs. standard induction therapy with daunorubicin and cytarabine alone. The CR rate was 69% for DA + GO and 70% for DA (P = 0.59). In this study, the addition of GO to induction or post-consolidation therapy failed to show improvement in CR rate, disease-free survival, or overall survival. Also addition of GO was associated with a higher early mortality during induction (5.5% vs. 1.4%). Major causes of death were fatal hemorrhage and infection. Based on these negative results GO was withdrawn from the market in 2010 [126]. In a subsequent trials different schedules of GO were investigated. Phase 3, open-label study enrolled 280 patients aged 50–70 years with previously untreated de novo AML. Patients were randomly assigned in a 1:1 ratio to standard treatment (control group) with or without five doses of intravenous gemtuzumab during induction and day 1 of each of the two consolidation chemotherapy courses. Although the CR rates were similar between the two arms, IC plus GO provided a significantly improved median event free survival (EFS) (19.6 vs. 11.9 months, p = 0.00018) and median OS (34 vs. 19.2 months, p = 0.046). Haematological toxicity, particularly persistent thrombocytopenia, was more common in the GO group than in the control group, without an increase in the risk of death from toxicity [127]. A meta-analysis of five open label, phase 3 trials comprising 3325 AML patients found that the addition of gemtuzumab ozogamicin significantly reduced the risk of relapse and improved overall survival at 5 years without increased toxicity for GO treatment [128]. Based on these results FDA approved GO for the treatment of adults with newly diagnosed CD33-positive AML on 1 September 2017, and also approved Mylotarg for the treatment of patients aged 2 years and older with relapsed or refractory CD33-positive AML.

3. Vadastuximab talirine

Vadastuximab talirine (SGN-CD33A) is a novel anti-CD33 mAb conjugated to 2 molecules of pyrrolobenzodiazepine (PBD). After internalization vadastuximab where transported to the lysosomes where the PBD dimer is released via proteolytic cleavage of the linker, crosslinking DNAand leading to apoptosis. Vadastuximab is highly stable in circulation with relatively less off-target toxicity compared to GO [129]. In a dose-escalation phase 1 study 27 treatment naive patients with CD33 positive AML and median age of 74 years were treated with vadastuximab talirine. Of the 26 efficacy evaluable treatment naive patients, 6 patients achieved CR, 8 patients CRi, and 5 patients achieved a morphologic leukemia-free state [130]. In another phase 1 trial of vadastuximab talirine as monotherapy in patients with CD33-positive AML a total of 131 patients, median age, 73 years were enrolled. The CR + CRi rate was 28%, 50% of patients who responded achieved minimal residual disease negativity. Most AEs were consistent with myelosuppression, nonhematological included fatigue, nausea, and diarrhea [131]. Also vadastuximab talirine was added to a 7 + 3 induction therapy in a phase 1b study in 42 patients with a median age of 45.5 years. The CR/CRi rate was 78%. Twenty-three of 31 (74%) patients attaining CR or CRi achieved MRD negative status. No 30-day mortality or significant hepatotoxicity was observed [132]. Fathi et al. combined vadastuximab talirine with hypomethylating agents in patients with CD33-positive AML. Among 53 patients treated, the median age was 75 years. The CR + CRi rate was 70% and 51% of remissions with minimal residual disease-negative status by flow cytometry. The majority of adverse events were a result of myelosuppression, with some causing therapy delays [133]. A phase III trial (CASCADE, NCT02785900) comparing HMA with or without SGN-CD33A in elderly patients with newly diagnosed AML was terminated because of due to safety reasons, specifically a higher rate of deaths, including fatal infections, in the SGN33A arm versus the control arm.

4. Future perspectives

The great advances in understanding molecular mechanisms of AML as well as their prognostic significance have changed the therapeutic armamentarium against AML. The drugs discussed in this chapter and many novel molecules being evaluated in clinical trials are on their way to change the current standard of treatment in AML. Ongoing efforts to understand the heterogeneity of AML, the constantly changing genomic landscape, the mechanisms of resistance/refractoriness will be very important in the development of new drugs. The rational use of these drugs, their potency that might be improved by combining them with other modes of therapy will hopefully increase long-term benefits for patients with AML. Furthermore, the development of novel ultrasensitive methods for minimal residual disease detection will also refine the treatment decision making process and probably improve the survival rates. However, new issues such as extrapolation of the results from the clinical trials enrolling carefully selected patients to general practice, the access and cost of these new drugs must be considered in the treatment decision process. It is a question of time whether personally tailored therapeutic era is going to be the new standard in the treatment of AML. Till then an increased enrolment of patients with AML into clinical trials evaluating the safety and efficacy of these new drugs and combinations is strongly encouraged and recommended.

Declaration of conflicting interest

The authors declare that there is no conflict of interest.

Author details

Vasko Graklanov
First Department of Internal Diseases, Clinic of Clinical Hematology, Medical University-Plovdiv, UMHAT "St. George", Plovdiv, Bulgaria

*Address all correspondence to: dr.grklanov@yahoo.com

References

[1] Rosnet O, Schiff C, Pébusque MJ, Marchetto S, Tonnelle C, Toiron Y, et al. Human FLT3/FLK2 gene: cDNA cloning and expression in hematopoietic cells. Blood. 1993;**82**:1110-1119

[2] Small D, Levenstein M, Kim E, Carow C, Amin S, Rockwell P, et al. STK-1, the human homolog of Flk-2/Flt-3, is selectively expressed in CD34+ human bone marrow cells and is involved in the proliferation of early progenitor/stem cells. Proc Natl Acad Sci USA. 1994;**91**:459-463

[3] Rosnet O, Matteï MG, Marchetto S, Birnbaum D. Isolation and chromosomal localization of a novel FMS-like tyrosine kinase gene. Genomics. 1991;**9**:380-385. DOI: 10.1016/0888-7543(91)90270-O

[4] Kelly LM, Gilliland DG. Genetics of myeloid leukemias. Annual Review of Genomics and Human Genetics. 2002;**3**:179-198

[5] Grafone T, Palmisano M, Nicci C, Storti S. An overview on the role of FLT3-tyrosine kinase receptor in acute myeloid leukemia: biology and treatment. Oncology Reviews. 2012;**6**:e8

[6] Levis M. FLT3 mutations in acute myeloid leukemia: what is the best approach in 2013? Hematol Am Soc Hematol Educ Program. 2013;**2013**:220-226

[7] Pui CH, Carroll WL, Meshinchi S, et al. Biology, risk stratification, and therapy of pediatric acute leukemias: an update. Journal of Clinical Oncology. 2011;**29**:551-565

[8] Schlenk RF, Kayser S, Bullinger L, Kobbe G, Casper J, Ringhoffer M, et al. Differential impact of allelic ratio and insertion site in FLT3-ITD-positive AML with respect to allogeneic transplantation. Blood. 2014;**124**:3441-3449

[9] Wang Y, Xu Y, Li S, Liu J, Xing Y, Xing H, et al. Targeting FLT3 in acute myeloid leukemia using ligand-based chimeric antigen receptor-engineered T cells. Journal of Hematology & Oncology. 2018;**11**:60

[10] Wang Y, Yin OQ, Graf P, Kisicki JC, Schran H. Dose- and time-dependent pharmacokinetics of midostaurin in patients with diabetes mellitus. Journal of Clinical Pharmacology. 2008;**48**:763-775

[11] Stein EM, Tallman MS. Emerging therapeutic drugs for AML. Blood. 2016;**127**:71-78

[12] Stone RM, Mandrekar SJ, Sanford BL, Laumann K, Geyer S, Bloomfield CD, et al. Midostaurin plus chemotherapy for acute myeloid leukemia with a FLT3 mutation. The New England Journal of Medicine. 2017;**377**:454-464

[13] Rydapt (midostaurin) [package insert]. (2017)

[14] Strati H, Kantarjian F, Ravandi A, Nazha G, Borthakur N, Daver, et al. Phase I/II trial of the combination of midostaurin (PKC412) and 5-azacytidine for patients with acute myeloid leukemia and myelodysplastic syndrome. American Journal of Hematology. 2015;**90**:276-281

[15] Pratz KW et al. A pharmacodynamic study of sorafenib in patients with relapsed and refractory acute leukemias. Leukemia. 2010;**24**:1437-1444

[16] Borthakur G et al. Phase I study of sorafenib in patients with refractory or relapsed acute leukemias. Haematologica. 2011;**96**:62-68

[17] Ravandi F et al. Final report of phase II study of sorafenib, cytarabine and idarubicin for initial therapy in

younger patients with acute myeloid leukemia. Leukemia. 2014;**28**:1543-1545

[18] Ravandi F et al. Phase I/II study of combination therapy with sorafenib, idarubicin, and cytarabine in younger patients with acute myeloid leukemia. Journal of Clinical Oncology. 2010;**28**:1856-1862

[19] Widemann BC et al. A phase I trial and pharmacokinetic study of sorafenib in children with refractory solid tumors or leukemias: a Children's Oncology Group Phase I Consortium report. Clinical Cancer Research. 2012;**18**:6011-6022

[20] Man CH et al. Sorafenib treatment of FLT3-ITD(+) acute myeloid leukemia: favorable initial outcome and mechanisms of subsequent nonresponsiveness associated with the emergence of a D835 mutation. Blood. 2012;**119**:5133-5143

[21] Röllig C, Serve H, Hüttmann A, Noppeney R, Müller-Tidow C, Krug U, et al. Addition of sorafenib versus placebo to standard therapy in patients aged 60 years or younger with newly diagnosed acute myeloid leukaemia (SORAML): a multicentre, phase 2, randomised controlled trial. The Lancet Oncology. 2015;**16**:1691-1699

[22] Serve H, Krug U, Wagner R, Sauerland MC, Heinecke A, Brunnberg U, et al. Sorafenib in combination with intensive chemotherapy in elderly patients with acute myeloid leukemia: results from a randomized, placebo-controlled trial. Journal of Clinical Oncology. 2013;**31**:3110-3118

[23] Brunner AM, Li S, Fathi AT, Wadleigh M, Ho VT, Collier K, et al. Haematopoietic cell transplantation with and without sorafenib maintenance for patients with FLT3-ITD acute myeloid leukaemia in first complete remission. British Journal of Haematology. 2016;**175**:496-504

[24] Yee K, Schittenhelm M, O'Farrell A-M, Town A, McGreevey L, Bainbridge T, et al. Synergistic effect of SU11248 with cytarabine or daunorubicin on FLT3 ITD-positive leukemic cells. Blood. 2005;**104**:4202-4209. DOI: 10.1182/blood-2003-10-3381

[25] Teng CLYC, Hwang WL, Tsai JR, Liu HC, Hwang GY, Hsu SL. Effector mechanisms of sunitinib-induced G1 cell cycle arrest, differentiation, and apoptosis in human acute myeloid leukaemia HL60 and KG-1 cells. Annals of Hematology. 2013;**92**(3):301-313

[26] O'Farrell AM, Foran JM, Fiedler W, et al. An innovative phase I clinical study demonstrates inhibition of FLT3 phosphorylation by SU11248 in acute myeloid leukemia patients. Clinical Cancer Research. 2003;**9**:5465-5476

[27] FIedler W, Serve H, Döhner H, et al. A phase 1 study of SU11248 in the treatment of patients with refractory or resistant acute myeloid leukemia (AML) or not amenable to conventional therapy for the disease. Blood. 2005;**105**:986-993

[28] Fiedler WKS, Kebenko M, Janning M, Krauter J, Schittenhelm M, Gotze K, et al. A phase I/II study of sunitinib and intensive chemotherapy in patients over 60 years of age with acute myeloid leukaemia and activating FLT3 mutations. British Journal of Haematology. 2015;**169**(5):694-700

[29] Marshall JLKH, Deeken J, Bhargava P, Vogelzang NJ, Rizvi N, Luhtala T, et al. Phase I trial of orally administered CEP-701, a novel neurotrophin receptor-linked tyrosine kinase inhibitor. Investigational New Drugs. 2005;**23**(1):31-37

[30] Levis MAJ, Tse KF, Zheng R, Baldwin BR, Smith BD, Jones-Bolin S, et al. A FLT3-targeted tyrosine kinase

inhibitor is cytotoxic to leukemia cells in vitro and in vivo. Blood. 2002;**99**(11):3885-3891

[31] Hexner EOMJ, Prchal J, Roboz GJ, Baer MR, Ritchie EK, Leibowitz D, et al. Phase I dose escalation study of lestaurtinib in patients with myelofibrosis. Leukemia & Lymphoma. 2015;**56**(9):2543-2551

[32] Lee LY, Hernandez D, Rajkhowa T, Smith SC, Raman JR, Nguyen B, et al. Preclinical studies of gilteritinib, a next-generation FLT3 inhibitor. Blood. 2017;**129**:257-260

[33] Hexner EO, Serdikoff C, Jan M, Swider CR, Robinson C, Yang S, et al. Lestaurtinib (CEP701) is a JAK2 inhibitor that suppresses JAK2/STAT5 signaling and the proliferation of primary erythroid cells from patients with myeloproliferative disorders. Blood. 2008;**111**:5663-5671

[34] Knapper SBA, Littlewood T, Kell WJ, Agrawal S, Chopra R, Clark R, et al. A phase 2 trial of the FLT3 inhibitor lestaurtinib (CEP701) as firstline treatment for older patients with acute myeloid leukemia not considered fit for intensive chemotherapy. Blood. 2006;**108**(10):3262-3270

[35] Smith BDLM, Beran M, Giles F, Kantarjian H, Berg K, Murphy KM, et al. Single-agent CEP-701, a novel FLT3 inhibitor, shows biologic and clinical activity in patients with relapsed or refractory acute myeloid leukemia. Blood. 2004;**103**(10):3669-3676

[36] Kelly LMYJ, Boulton CL, Apatira M, Li J, Sullivan CM, Williams I, et al. CT53518, a novel selective FLT3 antagonist for the treatment of acute myelogenous leukemia (AML). Cancer Cell. 2002;**1**(5):421-432

[37] DeAngelo DJSR, Heaney ML, Nimer SD, Paquette RL, Klisovic RB, Caligiuri MA, et al. Phase 1 clinical results with tandutinib (MLN518), a novel FLT3 antagonist, in patients with acute myelogenous leukemia or high-risk myelodysplastic syndrome: safety, pharmacokinetics, and pharmacodynamics. Blood. 2006;**108**(12):3674-3681

[38] Kampa-Schittenhelm KMHM, Akmut F, Dohner H, Dohner K, Schittenhelm MM. Quizartinib (AC220) is a potent second generation class III tyrosine kinase inhibitor that displays a distinct inhibition profile against mutant- FLT3, -PDGFRA and -KIT isoforms. Molecular Cancer. 2013;**12**:19

[39] Cortes JE, Kantarjian H, Foran JM, et al. Phase I study of quizartinib administered daily to patients with relapsed or refractory acute myeloid leukemia irrespective of FMS-like tyrosine kinase 3-internal tandem duplication status. Journal of Clinical Oncology. 2013;**31**(29):3681-3687

[40] Altman JK, Foran JM, Pratz KW, Trone D, Cortes JE, Tallman MS. Phase 1 study of quizartinib in combination with induction and consolidation chemotherapy in patients with newly diagnosed acute myeloid leukemia. American Journal of Hematology. 2018;**93**(2):213-221. DOI: 10.1002/ajh.24974

[41] Cortes J, Perl AE, Dohner H, Kantarjian H, Martinelli G, Kovacsovics T, et al. Quizartinib, an FLT3 inhibitor, as monotherapy in patients with relapsed or refractory acute myeloid leukemia: An open-label, multicentre, single-arm, phase 2 trial. The Lancet Oncology. 2018;**19**:889-903

[42] Cortes JE, Khaled SK, Martinelli G, Perl AE, Ganguly S, Russell NH, et al. Efficacy and Safety of Single-Agent Quizartinib (Q), a Potent and Selective FLT3 Inhibitor (FLT3i), in Patients (pts) with FLT3-Internal Tandem Duplication (FLT3-ITD)-Mutated

Relapsed/Refractory (R/R) Acute Myeloid Leukemia (AML) Enrolled in the Global, Phase 3, Randomized Controlled Quantum-R Trial. Blood. 2018;**132**:563

[43] Kampa-Schittenhelm KMFJ, Haeusser LA, Illing B, Pavlovsky AA, Blumenstock G, Schittenhelm MM. Crenolanib is a type I tyrosine kinase inhibitor that inhibits mutant KIT D816 isoforms prevalent in systemic mastocytosis and core binding factor leukemia. Oncotarget. 2017;**8**(47):82897-82909

[44] Levis M, Small D. FLT3: ITDoes matter in leukemia. Leukemia. 2003;**17**:1738-1752

[45] Galanis A, Ma H, Rajkhowa T, Ramachandran A, Small D, Cortes J, et al. Crenolanib is a potent inhibitor of FLT3 with activity against resistanceconferring point mutants. Blood. 2014;**123**:94-100

[46] Zimmerman EITD, Buaboonnam J, Hu S, Orwick S, Roberts MS, Janke LJ, et al. Crenolanib is active against models of drug-resistant FLT3-ITD-positive acute myeloid leukemia. Blood. 2013;**122**(22):3607-3615

[47] Cortes JE, Kantarjian HM, Kadia TM, Borthakur G, Konopleva M, Garcia-Manero G, et al. Crenolanib besylate, a type I pan-FLT3 inhibitor, to demonstrateclinical activity in multiply relapsed FLT3-ITD and D835 AML. Journal of Clinical Oncology. 2016;**34**:7008

[48] Wang ES, MST RMS, Walter RB, Karanes C, Jain V, Collins RH. Low relapse rate in younger patients ≤ 60 years old with newly diagnosed FLT3-mutated acute myeloid leukemia (AML) treated with crenolanib and cytarabine/anthracycline chemotherapy. Blood. 2017;**130**:566

[49] Wang ESRMS, Tallman MS, Walter RB, Eckardt JR, Collins R. Crenolanib, a type I FLT3 TKI, can be safely combined with cytarabine and anthracycline induction chemotherapy and results in high response rates in patients with newly diagnosed FLT3 mutant acute myeloid leukemia (AML). Blood. 2016;**128**(22):1071

[50] Iyer SP, Jethava Y, Karanes C, Eckardt JR, Collins R. Safety study of salvage chemotherapy high-dose Ara-C/mitoxantrone (HAM) and type I FLT3-TKI crenolanib in first relapsed/primary refractory AML. Blood. 2016;**128**(22):3983

[51] Maro Ohanian HMK, Borthakur G, Kadia TM, Konopleva M, Garcia-Manero G, Estrov Z, et al. Efficacy of a type I FLT3 inhibitor, crenolanib, with idarubicin and high-dose Ara-C in multiply relapsed/refractory FLT3+ AML. Blood. 2016;**128**:2744

[52] Perl AE, Altman JK, Cortes J, Smith C, Litzow M, Baer MR, et al. Selective inhibition of FLT3 by gilteritinib in relapsed or refractory acute myeloidleukemia: A multicentre, first-in-human, open-label, phase 1-2 study. The Lancet Oncology. 2017;**18**:1061-1075

[53] Usuki KST, Kobayashi Y, Miyamoto T, Iida H, Morita S, Bahceci E, et al. Clinical profile of gilteritinib in Japanese patients with relapsed/refractory AML an open-label phase 1 study. Cancer Science. 2018;**109**(10):3235-3244

[54] Perl AE, Cortes JE, Strickland SA, Ritchie EK, Neubauer A, Martinelli G, et al. An open-label, randomized phase 3 study of gilteritinib versus salvage chemotherapy in relapsed or refractory FLT3 mutation-positive acute myeloid leukemia. Journal of Clinical Oncology. 2017;**35**:TPS7067

[55] Tarabadkar ESTH, Blom A, Parvathaneni U, Olencki T, Nghiem P, Bhatia S. Clinical benefit from tyrosine

kinase inhibitors in metastatic Merkel cell carcinoma: a case series of 5 patients. Am J Case Rep. 2018;**19**:505-511

[56] Osanto S, van der Hulle T. Cabozantinib in the treatment of advanced renal cell carcinoma in adults following prior vascular endothelial growth factor targeted therapy: clinical trial evidence and experience. Therapeutic Advances in Urology. 2018;**10**(3):109-123

[57] Fathi ATBT, Hernandez D, Amrein PC, Ballen KK, McMasters M, Avigan DE, et al. Cabozantinib is well tolerated in acute myeloid leukemia and effectively inhibits the resistance-conferring FLT3/tyrosine kinase domain/F691 mutation. Cancer. 2018;**124**(2):306-314

[58] Mardis ER, Ding L, Dooling DJ, et al. Recurring mutations found by sequencing an acute myeloid leukemia genome. The New England Journal of Medicine. 2009;**361**(11):1058-1066

[59] Buege MJ, DiPippo AJ, DiNardo CD. Evolving treatment strategies for elderly leukemia patients with IDH mutations. Cancers (Basel). 2018;**10**(6):1-20

[60] DiNardo C.D., F. Ravandi, S. Agresta, M. Konopleva, K. Takahashi, T. Kadia, et al., Characteristics, clinical outcome, and prognostic significance of IDH mutations in AML, Am. J. Hematol. 90 (2015) 732-736

[61] Paschka P, Schlenk RF, Gaidzik VI, Habdank M, Krönke J, Bullinger L, et al. IDH1 and IDH2 mutations are frequent genetic alterations in acute myeloid leukemia and confer adverse prognosis in cytogenetically normal acute myeloid leukemia with NPM1 mutation without FLT3 internal tandem duplication. J. Clin. Oncol. 2010;**28**:3636-3643

[62] Stein EM. IDH2 inhibition in AML: finally progress? Best Practice & Research Clinical Haematology. 2015;**28**:112-115

[63] Marcucci G, Maharry K, Wu YZ, Radmacher MD, Mrozek K, Margeson D, et al. IDH1 and IDH2 gene mutations identify novel molecular subsets within de novo cytogenetically normal acute myeloid leukemia: a Cancer and leukemia group B study. Journal of Clinical Oncology. 2010;**28**:2348-2355

[64] Green CL, Evans CM, Zhao L, Hills RK, Burnett AK, Linch DC, et al. The prognostic significance of IDH2 mutations in AML depends on the location of the mutation. Blood. 2011;**118**:409-412

[65] Boissel N, Nibourel O, Renneville A, Gardin C, Reman O, Contentin N, et al. Prognostic impact of isocitrate dehydrogenase enzyme isoforms 1 and 2 mutations in acute myeloid leukemia: a study by the acute leukemia French association group. Journal of Clinical Oncology. 2010;**28**:3717-3723

[66] Amatangelo MD, Quek L, Shih A, Stein EM, Roshal M, David MD, et al. Enasidenib induces acute myeloid leukemia cell diferentiation to promote clinical response. Blood. 2017;**130**:732-741

[67] Stein EM, DiNardo CD, Fathi AT, Pollyea DA, Stone RM, Altman JK, et al. Molecular remission and response patterns in patients with mutant-IDH2 acute myeloid leukemia treated with enasidenib. Blood. 2019;**133**:676-687

[68] Stein EM, DiNardo CD, Fathi AT, Mims AS, Pratz KW, Savona MR, et al. Ivosidenib or Enasidenib Combined with Induction and Consolidation Chemotherapy in Patients with Newly Diagnosed AML with an IDH1 or IDH2 Mutation Is Safe, Effective and Leads to MRD-Negative Complete Remissions. Blood. 2018;**132**:560

[69] DiNardo CD, Stein EM, de Botton S, Roboz GJ, Altman JK, Mims AS, et al. Durable Remissions with Ivosidenib in IDH1-Mutated Relapsed or Refractory AML. The New England Journal of Medicine. 2018;**378**:2386-2398

[70] Tsujimoto Y, Finger LR, Yunis J, Nowell PC, Croce CM. Cloning of the chromosome breakpoint of neoplastic B cells with the t(14;18) chromosome translocation. Science. 1984;**226**(4678):1097-1099

[71] Monaghan P, Robertson D, Amos TAS, et al. Ultrastructural localization of Bcl-2 protein. The Journal of Histochemistry and Cytochemistry. 1992;**40**:1819-1825

[72] Czabotar PE, Lessene G, Strasser A, Adams JM. Control of apoptosis by the BCL-2 protein family: Implications for physiology and therapy. Nat. Rev. Mol. Cell Boil. 2014;**15**:49-63

[73] Testa U, Riccioni R. Deregulation of apoptosis in acute myeloid leukemia. Haematologica. 2007;**92**(1):81-94

[74] Hanahan D, Weinberg RA. Hallmarks of cancer: The next generation. Cell. 2011;**144**:646-674

[75] Souers AJ, Leverson JD, Boghaert ER, et al. ABT-199, a potent and selective BCL-2 inhibitor, achieves antitumor activity while sparing platelets. Nature Medicine. 2013;**19**(2):202-208

[76] Pan R, Ruvolo VR, Wei J, Konopleva M, Reed JC, Pellecchia M, et al. Inhibition of Mcl-1 with the pan-Bcl-2 family inhibitor (–)BI97D6 overcomes ABT-737 resistance in acute myeloid leukemia. Blood. 2015;**126**:363-372

[77] Konopleva M, Pollyea DA, Potluri J, et al. Efficacy and biological correlates of response in a phase ii study of venetoclax monotherapy in patients with acute myelogenous leukemia. Cancer Discovery. 2016;**6**(10):1106-1117

[78] Wei AH, Strickland SA Jr, Hou JZ, Fiedler W, Lin TL, Walter RB, et al. Venetoclax Combined with Low-Dose Cytarabine for Previously Untreated Patients with Acute Myeloid Leukemia: Results from a Phase 1b/2 Study. J. Clin. Oncol. 2019:Jco1801600

[79] Pollyea DADC, Thirman MJ, Letai A, et al. Results of a phase 1b study of venetoclax plus decitabine or azacitidine in untreated acute myeloid leukemia patients $65 years ineligible for standard induction therapy. J Clin Oncol. 2016;**34**(suppl 15)

[80] DiNardo CD, Albitar M, Kadia TM, Naqvi K, Vaughan K, Cavazos A, et al. Venetoclax in Combination with FLAG-IDA Chemotherapy (FLAG-V-I) for Fit, Relapsed/Refractory AML Patients: Interim Results of a Phase 1b/2 Dose Escalation and Expansion Study. Blood. 2018;**132**:4048

[81] Armas-Lopez L, Zuniga J, Arrieta O, Avila-Moreno F. The Hedgehog-GLI pathway in embryonic development and cancer: Implications for pulmonary oncology therapy. Oncotarget. 2017;**8**:60684-60703

[82] Berman DM, Karhadkar SS, Hallahan AR, Pritchard JI, Eberhart CG, Watkins DN, et al. Medulloblastoma growth inhibition by hedgehog pathway blockade. Science. 2002;**297**:1559-1561

[83] Varjosalo M, Taipale J. Hedgehog: functions and mechanisms. Genes & Development. 2008;**22**:2454-2472

[84] Merchant AA, Matsui W. Targeting Hedgehog-a cancer stem cell pathway. Clinical Cancer Research. 2010;**16**:3130-3140

[85] Queiroz KC, Ruela-de-Sousa RR, Fuhler GM, Aberson HL, Ferreira CV,

Peppelenbosch MP, et al. Hedgehog signaling maintains chemoresistance in myeloid leukemic cells. Oncogene. 2010;**29**:6314-6322

[86] Munchhof MJ, Li Q, Shavnya A, Borzillo GV, Boyden TL, Jones CS, et al. Discovery of PF-04449913, a potent and orally bioavailable inhibitor of smoothened. ACS Medicinal Chemistry Letters. 2012;**3**:106-111

[87] Fukushima N, Minami Y, Kakiuchi S, et al. Small-molecule Hedgehog inhibitor attenuates the leukemia-initiation potential of acute myeloid leukemia cells. Cancer Science. 2016;**107**(10):1422-1429. DOI: 10.1111/cas.13019

[88] Martinelli G, Oehler VG, Papayannidis C, Courtney R, Shaik MN, Zhang X, et al. Treatment with PF-04449913, an oral smoothened antagonist, in patients with myeloid malignancies: A phase 1 safety and pharmacokinetics study. Lancet Haematol. 2015;**2**:e339-e346

[89] Cortes JE, Heidel FH, Hellmann A, Fiedler W, Smith BD, Robak T, et al. Randomized comparison of low dose cytarabine with or without glasdegib in patients with newly diagnosed acute myeloid leukemia or high-risk myelodysplastic syndrome. Leukemia. 2019;**33**:379-389

[90] Cortes JE, Douglas Smith B, Wang ES, Merchant A, Oehler VG, Arellano M, et al. Glasdegib in combination with cytarabine and daunorubicin in patients with AML or high-risk MDS: Phase 2 study results. American Journal of Hematology. 2018;**93**:1301-1310

[91] Huang K, Ding B, Zhong Q, Jiang X, Li X, Wang Z, et al. Hh/IGF-1R/PI3K/Akt/MRP1 Pathway Induce Refractory Acute Myeloid Leukemia and Its Targeting Therpy. Blood. 2014;**124**:3612

[92] Tibes R, Kosiorek HE, Dueck A, Palmer J, Slack JL, Knight EA, et al. Phase I/IB study of azacitidine and hedgehog pathway inhibition with Sonidegib (LDE225) in myeloid malignancies. Blood. 2017;**130**:2629

[93] Bixby D, Noppeney R, Lin TL, Cortes J, Krauter J, Yee K, et al. Safety and efficacy of vismodegib in relapsed/refractory acute myeloid leukaemia: Results of a phase Ib trial. British Journal of Haematology. 2018

[94] Schöffski P. Polo-like kinase (PLK) inhibitors in preclinical and early clinical development in oncology. The Oncologist. 2009;**14**(6):559-570

[95] Lens SM, Voest EE, Medema RH. Shared and separate functions of polo-like kinases and aurora kinases in cancer. Nature Reviews. Cancer. 2010;**10**(12):825-841

[96] Renner AG, Dos Santos C, Recher C, et al. Polo-like kinase 1 is overexpressed in acute myeloid leukemia and its inhibition preferentially targets the proliferation of leukemic cells. Blood. 2009;**114**(3):659-662

[97] Rudolph D, Steegmaier M, Hoffmann M, et al. BI 6727, a Polo-like kinase inhibitor with improved pharmacokinetic profile and broad antitumor activity. Clinical Cancer Research. 2009;**15**(9):3094-3102

[98] Döhner H, Lübbert M, Fiedler W, Fouillard L, Haaland A, Brandwein JM, et al. Randomized, phase 2 trial of low-dose cytarabine with or without volasertib in AML patients not suitable for induction therapy. Blood. 2014;**124**:1426-1433

[99] Barbier V, Erbani J, Fiveash C, et al. Endothelial E-selectin inhibition improves acute myeloid leukaemia therapy by disrupting vascular niche-mediated chemoresistance.

Nat Commun. 2020;11(1):2042. Published 2020 Apr 27

[100] Geoffrey L. Uy, Jun Yin, Heidi D. Klepin, Shira Dinner, Anthony J. Jaslowski, Stephen A. Strickland, Jane L. Liesveld, John C. Byrd, Richard M. Stone; Alliance A041701 - a Randomized Phase 2/3 Study of Conventional Chemotherapy +/– Uproleselan (GMI-1271) in Older Adults with Acute Myeloid Leukemia (AML) Receiving Intensive Induction Chemotherapy. Blood 2019; 134 (Supplement_1): 1366

[101] DeAngelo, D.J., Jonas, B.A., Liesveld, J., O'Dwyer, M., Bixby, D., Advani, A.S., Marlton, P., Magnani,J., Thackray, H.M. & Becker, P.S. (2017a) GMI-1271, a novel E-selectin antagonist, in combination with chemotherapy in relapsed/refractory AML. Journal of Clinical Oncology, 35, 2520

[102] Daniel J. DeAngelo, Harry Paul Erba, Brian Andrew Jonas, Michael O'Dwyer, Paula Marlton, Gerwin A Huls, Jane Liesveld, Brenda W. Cooper, Bhavana Bhatnagar, Michael Armstrong, William Fogler, Mary Chen, John Magnani, Helen M. Thackray, Anjali S. Advani, and Pamela Sue Becker Journal of Clinical Oncology 2019 37:15_suppl, TPS7066-TPS7066

[103] Sharma P, Allison JP. The future of immune checkpoint therapy. Science. 2015;**348**:56-61

[104] Topalian SL, Drake CG, Pardoll DM. Immune checkpoint blockade: a common denominator approach to cancer therapy. Cancer Cell. 2015;**27**:450-461

[105] Pardoll DM. The blockade of immune checkpoints in cancer immunotherapy. Nature Reviews. Cancer. 2012;**12**:252-264

[106] Dong H, Strome SE, Salomao DR, Tamura H, Hirano F, Flies DB, et al. Tumor-associated B7-H1 promotes T-cell apoptosis: a potential mechanism of immune evasion. Nature Medicine. 2002;**8**(8):793-800. DOI: 10.1038/nm730

[107] Zhang L, Gajewski TF, Kline J. PD-1/PD-L1 interactions inhibit antitumor immune responses in a murine acute myeloid leukemia model. Blood. 2009;**114**:1545-1552

[108] Gettinger SN, Horn L, Gandhi L, Spigel DR, Antonia SJ, Rizvi NA, et al. Overall Survival and Long-Term Safety of Nivolumab (Anti-Programmed Death 1 Antibody, BMS-936558, ONO-4538) in Patients With Previously Treated Advanced Non-Small-Cell Lung Cancer. Journal of Clinical Oncology. 2015;**33**(18):2004-2012

[109] Topalian SL, Hodi FS, Brahmer JR, Gettinger SN, Smith DC, McDermott DF, et al. Safety, activity, and immune correlates of anti-PD-1 antibody in cancer. The New England Journal of Medicine. 2012;**366**(26):2443-2454

[110] Daver N, Basu S, Garcia-Manero G, Cortes JE, Ravandi F, Jabbour EJ, et al. Phase IB/II study of nivolumab in combination with azacytidine (AZA) in Patients (pts) with relapsed acute myeloid leukemia (AML). Blood. 2016;**128**:763

[111] Assi R, Kantarjian HM, Daver NG, Garcia-Manero G, Benton CB, Thompson PA. Results of a Phase 2, open-label study of idarubicin (I), cytarabine (A) and nivolumab (Nivo) in patients with newly diagnosed acute myeloid leukemia (AML) and high-risk myelodysplastic syndrome (MDS). Blood. 2018;**132**(Suppl 1):905. DOI: 10.1002/cncr.31398

[112] Albring J, Inselmann S, Sauer T, Schliemann C, Altvater B, Kailayangiri S, et al. PD-1 checkpoint blockade in patients with relapsed AML after allogeneic stem cell

transplantation. Bone Marrow Transplantation. 2017;**52**:317-320

[113] Zeidner JF, Vincent BG, Ivanova A, Foster M, Coombs CC, Jamieson K, et al. Genomics reveal potential biomarkers of response to pembrolizumab after high dose cytarabine in an ongoing Phase II Trial in relapsed/refractory AML. In: American Society of Hematology Annual Meeting; 2018 December 6-9 (San Diego: Oral and Poster Abstracts Session 616). 2018

[114] Lindblad KE, Thompson J, Gui G, Valdez J, Worthy T, Tekleab H. Pembrolizumab and decitabine for refractory or relapsed acute myeloid leukemia. In: American Society of Hematology Annual Meeting; 2018 December 6-9 (San Diego: Oral and Poster Abstracts Session 616). 2018

[115] Davids MS, Kim HT, Bachireddy P, Costello C, Liguori R, Savell A, et al. Leukemia and Lymphoma Society Blood Cancer Research Partnership. N Engl J Med. 2016;**375**(2):143-153

[116] Griffin JD, Linch D, Sabbath K, Larcom P, Schlossman SF. A monoclonal antibody reactive with normal and leukemic human myeloid progenitor cells. Leukemia Research. 1984;**8**:521-534

[117] Dinndorf PA, Andrews RG, Benjamin D, Ridgway D, Wolff L, Bernstein ID. Expression of normal myeloid-associated antigens by acute leukemia cells. Blood1986; 67: 1048-1053

[118] Scheinberg DA, Tanimoto M, McKenzie S, Strife A, Old LJ, Clarkson BD. Monoclonal antibody M195: a diagnostic marker for acute myelogenous leukemia. Leukemia. 1989;**3**:440-445

[119] Andrews RG, Torok-Storb B, Bernstein ID. Myeloid-associated differentiation antigens on stem cells and their progeny identified by monoclonal antibodies. Blood. 1983;**62**:124-132

[120] Simmons D, Seed B. Isolation of a cDNA encoding CD33, a differentiation antigen of myeloid progenitor cells. The Journal of Immunology. 1988;**141**:2797-2800

[121] Gao Z, McAlister VC, Williams GM. Repopulation of liver endothelium by bonemarrow- derived cells. The Lancet. 2001;**357**:932-933

[122] Thol F, Schlenk RF. Gemtuzumab ozogamicin in acute myeloid leukemia revisited. Expert Opinion on Biological Therapy. 2014;**14**:1185-1195

[123] Nejadmoghaddam MR, Minai-Tehrani A, Ghahremanzadeh R, Mahmoudi M, Dinarvand R, Zarnani AH. Antibody-drug conjugates: possibilities and challenges. Avicenna J Med Biotechnol. 2019;**11**(1):3-23

[124] Sievers EL, Appelbaum FR, Spielberger RT, Forman SJ, Flowers D, Smith FO, et al. Selective ablation of acute myeloid leukemia using antibody-targeted chemotherapy: a phase I study of an anti-CD33 calicheamicin immunoconjugate. Blood. 1999;**93**(11):3678-3684

[125] Sievers EL, Larson RA, Stadtmauer EA, Estey E, Lowenberg B, Dombret H, et al. Efficacy and safety of gemtuzumab ozogamicin in patients with CD33-positive acute myeloid leukemia in first relapse. Journal of Clinical Oncology. 2001;**19**(13):3244-3254

[126] Petersdorf SH, Kopecky KJ, Slovak M, Willman C, Nevill T, Brandwein J, et al. A phase 3 study of gemtuzumab ozogamicin during induction and postconsolidation therapy in younger patients with acute myeloid leukemia. Blood. 2013;**121**(24):4854-4860

[127] Castaigne S, Pautas C, Terre C, Raoux E, Bordessoule D, Bastie JN, et al. Effect of gemtuzumab ozogamicin on survival of adult patients with de-novoacute myeloid leukemia (ALFA-0701): A randomised, open-label, phase 3 study. Lancet. 2012;**379**:1508-1516

[128] Hills RK, Castaigne S, Appelbaum FR, Delaunay J, Petersdorf S, Othus M, et al. Addition of gemtuzumab ozogamicin to induction chemotherapy in adult patients with acute myeloid leukemia: A meta-analysis of individual patient data from randomised controlled trials. Lancet Oncol. 2014;**15**:986-996

[129] Kung Sutherland MS, Walter RB, Jeffrey SC, Burke PJ, Yu C, Kostner H, et al. SGN-CD33A: a novel CD33-targeting antibody-drug conjugate using a pyrrolobenzodiazepine dimer is active in models of drugresistant AML. Blood. 2013;**122**:1455-1463

[130] Bixby DL, Stein AS, Fathi AT, Kovacsovics TJ, Levy MY, Erba HP, et al. Vadastuximab Talirine monotherapy in older patients with treatment naive CD33-positive acute myeloid leukemia (AML). Blood. 2016;**128**(22)

[131] Stein EM, Walter RB, Erba HP, Fathi AT, Advani AS, Lancet JE, et al. A phase 1 trial of vadastuximab talirine as monotherapy in patients with CD33-positive acute myeloid leukemia. Blood. 2018;**131**(4):387-396

[132] Erba HP, Levy MY, Vasu S, Stein AS, Fathi AT, Maris MB, et al. A phase 1b Study of Vadastuximab Talirine in combination with 7+3 induction therapy for patients with newly diagnosed acute myeloid leukemia (AML). Blood. 2016;**128**(22)

[133] Fathi AT, Erba HP, Lancet JE, Stein EM, Ravandi F, Faderl S, et al. A phase 1 trial of vadastuximab talirine combined with hypomethylating agents in patients with CD33-positive AML. Blood. 2018;**132**(11):1125-1133

Chapter 15

Targeting of Post-Transcriptional Regulation as Treatment Strategy in Acute Leukemia

Paulina Podszywalow-Bartnicka, Magdalena Wolczyk and Katarzyna Piwocka

Abstract

Post-transcriptional regulation is an important step of gene expression that allows to fine-tune the cellular protein profile (so called proteome) according to the current demands. That mechanism has been developed to aid survival under stress conditions, however it occurs to be hijacked by cancer cells. Adjustment of the protein profile remodels signaling in cancer cells to adapt to therapeutic treatment, thereby enabling persistence despite unfavorable environment or accumulating mutations. The proteome is shaped at the post-transcriptional level by numerous mechanisms such as alternative splicing, mRNA modifications and triage by RNA binding proteins, change of ribosome composition or signaling, which altogether regulate the translation process. This chapter is an overview of the translation disturbances found in leukemia and their role in development of the disease, with special focus on the possible therapeutic strategies tested in acute leukemia which target elements of those regulatory mechanisms.

Keywords: leukemia treatment, therapy resistance, mRNA translation, RNA binding proteins, ribosomal proteins

1. Introduction

Translation is one of the regulatory levels that allows cells to adapt the profile of proteins (the proteome) to the current demand of cellular processes like cell division or environmental signals such as hypoxia. Generally, protein synthesis requires activation of the complex mechanisms that are tightly regulated [1]. Since the protein synthesis is related to cell growth and cell cycle, any disturbances of this process can be a mechanism underlying unregulated cell growth, neoplastic transformation and tumor development.

For the great majority of cellular mRNAs, the 5′ cap-dependent translation is the most efficient mechanism of protein synthesis [2]. An alternative mechanism of translation initiation is engaged during cell cycle progression [3], cell differentiation and apoptosis, as well as during cellular stress response [4]. Global regulation of translation is often based on the activation or inhibition of one or more components of the translational machinery (eukaryotic initiation factors, ribosomal proteins, ribosomal RNA), whereas the specific regulation often occurs through the action of two groups of factors: *cis*-acting elements found in mRNA molecule (specific mRNA sequences such as internal ribosome entry sites IRES, mRNA posttranscriptional modifications) and *trans*-acting factors (such as RNA-binding proteins, microRNAs) that bind to mRNA [5]. Furthermore, changes in the cellular signaling can also trigger translational reprogramming. Based on the significant role that all steps of the translation regulation play in development of cancers, including hematological malignancies, and their pro-survival and adaptive function, therapeutic targeting of those mechanisms has been proposed and studied.

2. Modifications of RNA

Posttranscriptional modifications have been found in non-coding RNAs such as ribosomal RNAs (rRNA) and transfer RNAs (tRNA) as well as in messenger RNAs (mRNA). There are about 150 modifications discovered by far. They include pseudouridylation (ψ), methylation or deamination of adenosine to inosine (A-to-I editing). Such modifications have impact on the splicing and translation of mRNA and contribute to epitranscriptional regulation of gene expression. Some modifications exist only in the coding sequence (like A-to-I editing), whilst others are deposited only in a 5′-untranslated regions (5'UTR) such as 5-methylcytosine (m5C) and 7-methylguanosine (m7G). The N6-methyladenosine (m6A) modification is ubiquitously present and deposited in along the mRNA coding sequence and 5′/3′UTRs.

The m6A modification is added to the mRNA in the nucleus by so called 'writers' or removed by 'erasers' and is recognized by proteins which bind to m6A methylated mRNA (so called 'readers'). It has impact on the mRNA stability, export from the nucleus, decay and translation (for recent review on the role of RNA modifications in cancer, including acute myelogenous leukemia (AML) see: [6–8]). The m6A modification has been found to play a critical role in AML development and progression (for review see: [9, 10]).

The m6A writer proteins - methyltransferase-like protein (METTL) 3 and 14 are overexpressed in AML. It was reported that their deletion limits the cancerogenic cellular potential [11, 12]. On the other hand, METTL3 overexpression stimulated the translation of Myc, Bcl-2 and PTEN what contributed to increased proliferation and survival of AML cells [13]. Controversially, increased expression of fat mass and obesity-associated demethylase (FTO), which acts as a m6A eraser, also led to higher level of oncogene expression. Moreover, its inhibition reduced growth of AML cancer cells [14]. Activity of FTO has been found to be directly inhibited by R-2-hydroxyglutarate (R-2HG) leading to loss of stability of Myc mRNA and decreased proliferation rate of leukemic cells [15]. This effect is postulated to result from discrepancy of mRNA triage for translation or decay of pro- and anti-oncogenic proteins in respect to the presence of m6A deposition in mRNA [8].

Though YTHDF2, the m6A reader, appears not to be required for normal hematopoietic stem cells, it occurs to be essential for AML cells similarly to METTL3 and FTO. Its overexpression facilitates AML cells propagation, whereas its silencing disables proliferative and clonogenic potential of leukemia cells. Thus, YTHDF2 seems to be a good therapeutic target in AML, which would enable the selective eradication of cancer cells whilst spearing healthy hematopoietic stem cells [16].

Another m6A reader proteins might also play a key role in the regulation of cancer development. The insulin-like growth factor 2 mRNA-binding protein (IF2BP1–3) stabilizes m6A-modified mRNAs such as *MYC* oncogene, thus enhancing its translation and contributing to oncogenesis [17].

Apart from modification of mRNA, also pseudouridylation of tRNA contributes to AML progression. The tRNAs that contain 5′ terminal oligoguanine (TOG) are the source of 18 nucleotide regulatory sequences (mTOGs), which stimulate differentiation and limit proliferation of hematopoietic stem cells (HSC) by inhibiting translation initiation in HSC. This effect depends on the presence of ψ on the mTOGs. It has been found that development of AML is accompanied by decreased level of pseudouridine synthase 7 (PUS7). Downregulation of PUS7 abolished healthy stem cells differentiation and increased translation demonstrating significance of ψ modification in the development of AML [18]. The oncogenic mTOGs, if attenuated by specific inhibitors, could constitute an effective therapeutic target.

The above examples show that the post-transcriptional regulation of gene expression at the step of RNA modifications constitutes a potent target to disable expression of some oncogenes that should allow to switch the cell fate back towards appropriate hematopoietic differentiation.

3. RNA binding proteins

Activation of RNA binding proteins (RBPs) constitutes an additional layer of posttranscriptional regulation, which has a great impact on the final protein level in the cell. The main function of RNA binding proteins is to recognize the primary transcript (pre-mRNA) and assemble ribonucleoprotein complexes, what governs processes of pre-mRNA maturation i.e. splicing, polyadenylation, attachment of a guanyl cap at the 5′ end of pre-mRNA and RNA modifications. Moreover, RBPs binding to the target mRNA is required for proper mRNA transportation from the nucleus to the cytoplasm and distribution into various cellular compartments. Additionally, *trans*-acting regulatory RNA binding proteins have the ability to affect translation of the specific mRNA, mainly through the interaction with untranslated regions (3′UTR and 5′UTR) and coding region of mature mRNA, what results in changes in ribosome recruitment.

Considering the multifunctional properties of RNA binding proteins, any alterations in those proteins' activity are associated with multiple cancers (reviewed in [19]), including leukemias (reviewed in [20]), and provide a substantial therapeutic opportunity.

The Musashi (MSI) RNA binding proteins (MSI1 and MSI2) contribute to development of various types of cancer. Their elevated expression has been demonstrated in acute myelogenous leukemia (AML), acute lymphoblastic leukemia (ALL) and chronic myelogenous leukemia blastic phase (CML-BP) [21–23]. MSI proteins regulate translation of mRNAs encoding proteins involved in several oncogenic signaling pathways, such as MYC [24], TGFβ/SMAD3 [25] and PTEN/mTOR [26]. Thus, inhibition of MSI RNA-binding activity could demonstrate a novel therapeutic strategy, probably not only in solid tumors but in hematological malignancies as well. A small molecule Ro 08–2750 (Ro) has been shown recently to bind selectively to MSI2 and interfere with its mRNA binding activity, thus triggering increased apoptosis and inhibition of known MSI targets in myeloid leukemia cells [27]. Other agents with presumptive MSI1 inhibitory activity have also been tested and they include (−)-gossypol (natural phenol extracted from cottonseed) [28] and $\omega - 9$ monounsaturated fatty acids (e.g. oleic acid) [29]. Although those agents display inhibitory effects on MSI1 activity, the specificity of both should be further confirmed.

Another RNA binding protein involved in mRNA translation and deregulated in leukemia is DDX3. Mutations in DDX3 gene display oncogenic potential in T-cell lymphoma [30] and lymphocytic leukemia [31]. A small molecule inhibitor (RK-33) targeting DDX3, which has been tested so far, demonstrates the pro-apoptotic activity. Its administration promoted higher sensitivity to radiation in lung cancer

DDX3-overexpressing cells [32, 33], thus providing an argument to develop and improve DDX3 inhibitors, which can target cancer cells, including leukemia.

The activity of HuR RNA binding protein is also deregulated in some types of leukemia [34–37]. Elevated HuR level promotes tumorigenesis, thus targeting HuR could be a promising anti-cancer therapy. A few chemical compounds against HuR activity have been tested so far. MS-444 small molecule inhibitor interfered with HuR binding to target ARE-mRNAs and showed anti-tumor properties in various types of cancers [38–40]. Quercetin and b-40 have been found to inhibit HuR binding to TNFα mRNA, what resulted in TNFα destabilization and decreased TNFα secretion [41]. A coumarin-derived and HuR-targeted small molecule inhibitor CMLD-2, exhibited cytotoxicity towards human lung cancer cells [42], proving that HuR is a good candidate for cancer treatment strategy.

Aberrations of other RNA binding proteins have been linked to the activity of BCR-ABL1, an oncoprotein responsible for chronic myeloid leukemia (CML) development. BCR-ABL1-dependent decrease of CUGBP1 level resulted in repression of the C/EBPβ mRNA translation [43]. As C/EBPβ transcriptional activity controls the maturation of hematopoietic cells in the myeloid lineage, its deficiency contributes to differentiation arrest of CML cells and CML progression to the blast crisis [44]. An increased level and activity of RNA binding proteins: hnRNP K [45], hnRNP A1 [46], hnRNP E2 [46], TLS/FUS [47] and La/SSB [48] have also been observed. These proteins regulate translation of important cancer-related factors: the hnRNP K protein positively regulates c-MYC mRNA translation, protein La/SSB promotes MDM2 mRNA translation, and increased hnRNP E2 activity leads to inhibition of the C/EBP1α protein synthesis.

Activities of RNA binding proteins described above result in the differentiation arrest of CML cell, but also their increased proliferation and survival. Considering the mentioned features, RNA binding proteins provide a significant therapeutic possibility to treat acute leukemia patients.

A single RBP interacts with a number of different mRNAs, and prerequisite for this is a presence of the RBP's binding sequence. The recognition motif for a given protein is often present in mRNAs encoding proteins needed in a certain process. For instance, mRNAs of cell cycle regulating proteins are bound by HuR. Thus, targeting activity of the specific RBP, interfering with its binding ability or masking the targeted sequence would impact the fate of a group of mRNAs. Therefore, this constitutes an opportunity to modulate synthesis of functionally related proteins.

4. Alternative splicing

This post-transcriptional process is one of the key steps of messenger RNA maturation (mRNA) but apart from that, it allows to elevate complexity of the cellular proteome. A core complex called spliceosome is responsible for excision of introns from pre-mRNA in the nucleus. It consists of five small nuclear ribonucleoproteins (snRNPs) – U1, U2, U5, U4/U6 – and small nuclear RNA (snRNA). Splicing is regulated by *cis*-acting elements, which are the nucleotide sequences of primary transcript, *trans*-acting elements, which are the splicing factors or other RNA binding proteins regulating splicing: heterogenous nuclear ribonucleoproteins (hnRNPs) and serine/arginine-rich (SR) proteins. The nucleotide sequence of the transcript promotes or represses splicing at the certain sites. The *trans*-acting elements can antagonize the activity of splicing factors leading to change in splice site selection, known as alternative splicing event. For an overview of the splicing process or interactions of RNA binding proteins with regulators of alternative splicing see: [49–51]. Furthermore, modification of RNA within the *cis*-acting region (like m6A) is one of the major factors that has impact on the binding of *trans*-acting elements (as described above). It has been found that the m6A modification enhances binding by RBPs such as hnRNP A2B1 [52] or SRSF3, whilst respells SRSF10 from transcript [53], exerting the effect on splicing of mRNA. This demonstrates how two distinct post-transcriptional events, RNA methylation and splicing, can cross-talk to tightly control the transcript fate and expression of a particular protein.

Extracellular signals lead to modification of operation of *trans*-acting proteins, affecting or enhancing their action. Therefore, activity of regulatory elements involved in this process is sensitive to environmental signals such as cytokines or hypoxia. Through modulation of alternative splicing, the level of proteins' isoforms can be adjusted according to the circumstances. Additionally to selective intron skipping/excision, alternative splicing can affect length of poly(A) region. As a result, this influence stability of the mRNA, causing its enhanced decay or translation. Apart from that, mutation of the gene sequence modifies binding of RBPs what has impact on the ultimate expression level. Some of the splicing regulators were reported to play an oncogenic role, whilst others act as tumor suppressors.

Apoptosis-stimulating Protein of TP53–2 (ASPP2) is a tumor suppressor enhancing TP53-mediated apoptosis. It has been found that a splice variant ASPP2κ is overexpressed in AML and displays anti-apoptotic function, therefore supporting proliferation of the cells [54].

Analysis of the transcriptome profile revealed that progression of CML from chronic phase (CML-CP) towards acute blastic phase (CML-BP) is accompanied by changes in splicing pattern of genes, thus affecting spliceosome. The exon skipping event in hnRNP A1 led to accumulation of bigger isoform in the CML-BP, though the biological significance of this has not been studied [55].

Altogether, it makes the alternative splicing machinery a powerful tool for cancer cells to support their survival. On the other hand, the necessity to achieve certain modifications through splicing makes cancer cells dependent on this process. Such regulation creates an opportunity for therapeutic targeting.

Activity of SR proteins can be modulated by modifications: phosphorylation of SR proteins can affect activity and switch general splicing repressor to selective activator [56], methylation of SRSF1 by the protein arginine methyltransferase 5 (PRMT5) modulates splicing of many proteins involved in proliferation, therefore supports leukemia development [57]. Its overexpression exerts oncogenic effect increasing aggressiveness of leukemia cells [58]. Specific inhibitors of PRMT5 have been clinically tested for potential treatment of blood and solid cancers [59]. As transcription of PRMT5 it directly stimulated by MYC transcription factor [60], thus leukemia cells overexpressing MYC could be selected for treatment with PRMT5 inhibitors.

A screen of RBPs playing role in AML revealed that RNA binding motif protein 39 (RBM39) plays a significant role in RNA splicing and stimulates proliferation of leukemia cells [61]. A sulfonamid drugs (indisulam, tasisulam, E7820 and CQS,), which are an example of proteolysis-targeting chimeras (PROTACs) compounds, led to polyubiquitination and proteasomal degradation of RBM39, what exerts anticancer activity [62]. The effect depended on the CUL4-DCAF15 E3 ubiquitin ligase, therefore the level of expression of this enzyme could be used as indicative marker in therapy involving sulfonamid drugs [62, 63].

Leukemia development and progression can be triggered by occurrence of point mutations in splicing factors such as SF3B. Activity of spliceosomal complex containing the mutated protein, but not wild type SF3B, can be blocked by a specific small molecule inhibitor H3B-8800 [64]. It has been shown that AML cells with mutated U2 Small Nuclear RNA Auxiliary Factor 1 (U2AF1), a component of spliceosome, display increased sensitivity to sudemycin – a drug targeting SF3BP1, both *in vitro* and *in vivo*. Transcripts altered by sudemycin treatment encoded proteins involved in receptor and signal transduction activities [65]. Noteworthy, SF3B1 has distinct effect on the transcript splicing than SRSF2. Mutation in any of them led to hyperactivation of NF-κB signaling, whilst simultaneous mutation of both SF3B1 and SRSF2 displayed synthetically lethal effect [66].

The splicing regulatory network is complex and full of various cross-talk regulations and interactions. Due to interactive nature of regulatory factors, which influence each other's activity, lowering the level of one factor activates a compensatory mechanism that is mediated by another factor. This refers to both SR [67] as well as hnRNP proteins [68]. Thus, the results should be interpreted cautiously, because the observed effect resulting from a loss of one splicing factor may in fact be the secondary effect of a change in the network. Nevertheless, targeting of the *cis*- or *trans*-regulating elements gives possibility to hit precisely the source of oncogenic transformation.

5. Translation initiation

Previously we described the processes, which regulate translation of the specific RNA in a controlled manner. The initiation of translation is another step on the way of protein synthesis, which is tightly controlled. The process can be remodeled by multiple cellular intrinsic signaling pathways that can be active in malignant cells.

Constitutive activation of the PI3K/Akt/mTOR signaling pathway [69, 70] has been observed in various types of leukemia, including acute lymphoblastic leukemia (ALL), Philadelphia (Ph) chromosome positive and Ph-like acute lymphoblastic leukemia (BCR-ABL1-like ALL) or AML. Continuous activity of the PI3K/Akt/mTOR pathway contributes to unregulated proliferation and leads to resistance to therapy with tyrosine kinase inhibitors (TKI) [71]. Activation of mTOR results in phosphorylation of S6K kinase and eukaryotic translation initiation factor 4E binding protein (4E-BP1), promoting cap-dependent mRNA initiation of translation and increased protein synthesis in leukemia cells [72]. On the other hand, mTOR pathway stimulates cap-independent translation mediated by internal ribosome entry sites IRES, mainly by activation of eIF4A helicase [73]. Another signaling pathway that regulates initiation of translation is the Ras/MAPK/ERK pathway. Its activity has also been found in leukemia cells [71, 74]. Activation of that pathway resulted in phosphorylation of the translation initiation factor eIF4E by MNK1/2 kinases. This contributed to increased β-catenin mRNA translation efficiency and activation of the Wnt/β-catenin signaling pathway, which plays an important role in differentiation and proliferation of leukemia cells [71, 75]. Microenvironmental signals, such as acute hypoxia or nutrient deprivation, trigger so called Integrated Stress Response (ISR) pathway, which shapes the mRNA translation. There are four protein kinases activated dependently on the stressor type: GCN – amino acid deprivation, PKR – appearance of viral RNA, PERK – accumulation of unfolded/misfolded proteins in the ER and HRI – oxidative stress, heme deficiency, osmotic shock and heat shock. Activation of these kinases in response to stress leads to phosphorylation of eukaryotic initiation factor 2 subunit alpha (eIF2α) and 4E-BP, which orchestrate number of downstream events regulating translation. ISR has been shown to be active in leukemia cells and displayed pro-survival properties of those cells [76].

Changes in cellular signaling provide a great opportunity for the anti-leukemia treatment strategy. One is based on the inhibition of PI3K/Akt/mTOR [77] and Ras/MAPK/ERK [78] signaling pathways. Rapamycin, an inhibitor of the mTOR signaling pathway, has been tested in the context of leukemia treatment [79].

Moreover, PP242 and hippuristanol, inhibitors of mTOR-eIF4A pathways, also have the potential to overcome TKI resistance [73]. Recent reports have shown that ribavirin, which is used as an antiviral drug, inhibits the mTOR/eIF4E and ERK/Mnk1/eIF4E pathways in leukemia cells expressing BCR-ABL1 oncogene and ultimately leads to reduction of anti-apoptotic proteins, inhibition of proliferation and consequently apoptosis of leukemia cells [80]. Salubrinal, guanabenz and Sephin1 are known agents inhibiting activity of phosphatase, which dephosphorylates eIF2α. Their effectiveness has been studied mainly in the context of neurological disorders, but leukemia should also be included into this research. Inactivation of ISR pathway can constitute a significant treatment strategy. The best described group of molecules targeting ISR are inhibitors of the kinases phosphorylating eIF2α, i.e. PERK kinase. The compounds GSK2606414 and GSK2656157 were designed to bind selectively to the ATP binding pocket of the PERK kinase and to inhibit PERK activity. Their potency has been studied in a vast number of cancers. Unfortunately, the use of those inhibitors caused serious side effects [81] and recently not specific effects have been reported [82]. Alternatively, a small molecule ISRIB (ISR inhibitor) is another example of the drug that inhibits general translation. It acts downstream of the eIF2α factor in the ISR signaling pathway and through direct interaction with eIF2B abolishes the phosphorylation effect of eIF2α [83].

Initiation of the translation process can be altered by aberrant cell signaling leading to enhanced expression of proteins, which play a pro-survival role and support cell proliferation. Therefore, interference with elements enabling the stimulated translation, could be one of the strategies that, by targeting general protein synthesis, restrict propagation potential of acute leukemia cells. The broad spectrum of proteins which synthesis might be disturbed by such treatment, has both advantages and disadvantages. On one hand such treatment will affect most of actively translating cells in the body. On the other hand however, this attitude represents a powerful tool to block highly proliferative acute leukemia cells by limiting their ability to propagate. Moreover, taking into account the heterogeneity of cancer, it might be effective towards broader spectrum of leukemia cell clones and push the clonal selection towards less proliferative, so less aggressive form of cancer. This in turn enables other drugs, which can be then used in combinatory treatment to exert the beneficial effect.

6. Ribosomal proteins

Machinery that physically executes the protein synthesis on the matrices of mRNA is based on ribosomes. This complex entities are formulated of rRNA core and ribosomal proteins (RPs) of small (RPS) or large (RPL) subunit. Recent evidence demonstrated that ribosomes can contain different RPL/RPS, thus indicating a heterogeneity among ribosomes. Additionally, different expression of some RPL and RPS in the tissues has been observed. There are RPs, such as RPL38, which regulate translation of the Homeobox genes during embryo development [84], showing involvement of RPs in directing tissue organization. This heterogeneity of the translational machinery is further amplified by proteins associating/interacting with ribosomes [85, 86] (reviewed in more detail here [87]).

Existence of ribosomopathies demonstrates that RPs can play significant role in determining the cell fate. The first ribosomopathy which has been recognized was the Diamond-Blackfan anemia (DBA) caused by defect in RPS19 gene, what leads to the bone marrow failure [88]. Since then, more similar aberrations related to pathological state have been discovered. It has been observed that ribosomopathies are often related to cancers including leukemia, bone marrow failure and anemia.

Difference in expression of ribosomal proteins between normal and malignant tissues has been found [89] (for review see [90]). It has also been proposed that aberrant expression of ribosomal proteins might support cancer progression. Overexpression of RPL23 in CD34-positive myelodysplastic cells (MDS) had impact on therapy effectiveness and was associated with poor prognosis [91]. Moreover, CD34-positive cells refractory to azacitidine treatment, displayed upregulation of RPL15, RPL28, RPL31 and RPL32 ribosomal proteins [92]. Recent study of MDS revealed that progression to AML is accompanied by elevated expression of some ribosomal proteins in CD123-positive cells [93]. Contrary to this, some ribosomal proteins play a tumor suppressor role in development of leukemia. Loss of RPL11 promoted lymphomagenesis [94], deletion in RPL5 gene has been found in multiple myeloma [95] and mutations in RPL5 and RPL10 contribute to development of T-cell acute lymphoblastic leukemia [96]. Additionally, mutation in RPL10 caused upregulation of phosphoserine phosphatase, which stimulated proliferation of cancer cells [97], deletion of a fragment of chromosome 5 led to myelodysplastic syndrome, which may progress to AML caused by RPS14 haploinsufficiency [98], deletion of RPL22 led to T-cell ALL by inducing a stemness factor [99] and mutation of RPS15 has been discovered to drive chronic lymphoblastic leukemia (CLL) development [100] and to cause cancer relapse [101]. Altogether, these examples clearly show that abnormally expressed ribosomal proteins are strong candidates for leukemia drivers.

It has been shown that ribosomal proteins associated with the ribosome define pool of mRNA transcripts that are selectively translated by this ribosome [102]. There are RPs that facilitate translation upon stress by interacting with IRES or allowing for translation with the use of alternative upstream open reading frames [uORFs]. For instance, RPS5 regulates binding of transcripts with IRES-2 [103] and RPS25 regulates binding of IRES-1 in 40S subunit [104].

Phosphorylation or other modifications of ribosomal proteins might also have impact on the spectrum of translated proteins. However, even if the phosphorylation of RPS6 is well documented, its physiological role remains not clear (for review see [105]). More recently, a phosphorylation of RPL12 has been identified to facilitate translation of AU-rich mRNAs during mitosis [86].

Selectivity for mRNA binding by the particular RPs shows that besides being a part of the translational machinery, they might actually play an important regulatory role of this process. Furthermore, identification of numerous proteins that interact with ribosome, so called ribosome associated proteins, has revealed that its activity is shaped by the microenvironment [85]. Changes of mRNA translation upon RPL12 phosphorylation during cell cycle progression [86] represent an example of how cells could use the translational machinery itself, to adapt the proteome to the current demands. This creates possibility for cellular signals to have impact on the translation machinery, allowing adjustment of the profile of synthesized proteins and by that way contributing to leukemia progression.

Targeting of ribosome activity could be a strategy of leukemia treatment. Based on cryo-EM structure, an antibiotic called cycloheximide (CHX) has been designed, that stalls ribosomes on mRNA [106]. However, due to high toxicity level, CHX is mainly used in molecular biology assays nowadays. Homoharringtonine (omacetaxine, HHT) is now the only FDA approved drug to treat CML patients refractory to TKIs [107]. Its mechanism of action is based on prevention of binding of tRNA to the ribosome [108], while at the cellular level this compound reduces the level of anti-apoptotic proteins Bcl2 and MCL-1, thus guiding leukemic cells into the apoptotic pathway [109]. Targeting of monosome translation by HHT has been recently intensively tested. This drug is also examined in terms of AML treatment. Omacetaxine occurred to be highly potent in subpopulation of myelodysplastic cells progressing towards AML [93]. Apart from that, usage of HHT has shown the synergistic effect in combinatory therapy (as reviewed in [110]).

Additionally, there are strategies to target ribosomal proteins biosynthesis at the step of transcription by using DNA intercalating agents such as: oxaliplatin, cisplatin or carboplatin [111] or by specific inhibition of ribosomal genes transcription by Polimerase I inhibitor CX-5461 [112]. This inhibitor showed the clinical potential in Myc expressing multiple myeloma [113, 114]. The Phase I clinical study in hematological malignancies has reported the increased patients survival/enhanced elimination of cancer cells [115].

The fact that the presence of ribosomal protein or its modification might be different in cancer versus healthy cells creates opportunity to target cancer cells in more precise way, limiting the damage of healthy tissue. Design of specific small molecule inhibitors or other drugs targeting precisely the deregulated ribosomes would allow effective elimination of leukemia cells 'hiding' quiescently in the niche.

7. Conclusions

Translation regulation is a key process, which enables cancer cells to adapt the proteome according to the cellular demands and therefore survive the therapeutic treatment. Moreover, it can contribute to oncogenic transformation, because deranged translation can be a source of enhanced expression of such oncogenes as Myc. This includes modification of activity of certain RNA binding proteins or stimulation of signaling, what leads to increase of global protein synthesis rate. Thus, targeting the translation regulatory mechanisms can be an effective way to eliminate the oncogene-driven malignant cells or just limit cancer cells potential for survival. In other words, therapeutic targeting of post-transcriptional regulation of gene expression gives possibility for both, precise medicine approach as well as blockade of cancer cells proliferation, irrespective of the evolving cancer clones or oncogene expression.

Acknowledgements

This work was supported by research grants from the National Science Centre UMO-2018/30/M/NZ3/00274 (PP-B) and UMO-2016/23/N/NZ3/02232 (MW).

Conflict of interest

The authors declare no competing interests.

Author details

Paulina Podszywalow-Bartnicka*, Magdalena Wolczyk and Katarzyna Piwocka
Nencki Institute of Experimental Biology, Polish Academy of Sciences, Warsaw, Poland

*Address all correspondence to: p.podszywalow@nencki.edu.pl

References

[1] Holcik M, Sonenberg N. Translational control in stress and apoptosis. Nature Reviews. Molecular Cell Biology. 2005 Apr;**6**(4):318-327. DOI: 10.1038/nrm1618

[2] Sonenberg N, Dever TE. Eukaryotic translation initiation factors and regulators. Current Opinion in Structural Biology. 2003 Feb;**13**(1):56-63. DOI: 10.1016/s0959-440x(03)00009-5

[3] Pyronnet S, Sonenberg N. Cell-cycle-dependent translational control. Current Opinion in Genetics & Development. 2001 Feb;**11**(1):13-18. DOI: 10.1016/s0959-437x(00)00150-7

[4] Clemens MJ. Translational regulation in cell stress and apoptosis. Roles of the eIF4E binding proteins. Journal of Cellular and Molecular Medicine. 2001 Sep;**5**(3):221-239. DOI: 10.1111/j.1582-4934.2001.tb00157.x

[5] Gebauer F, Preiss T, Hentze MW. From cis-regulatory elements to complex RNPs and back. Cold Spring Harbor Perspectives in Biology. 2012 Jul 1;**4**(7):a012245. DOI: 10.1101/cshperspect.a012245

[6] Frye M, Harada BT, Behm M, He C. RNA modifications modulate gene expression during development. Science. 2018;**361**(6409):1346-1349. DOI: 10.1126/science.aau1646

[7] Delaunay S, Frye M. RNA modifications regulating cell fate in cancer. Nature Cell Biology. 2019;**21**(5):552-559. DOI: 10.1038/s41556-019-0319-0

[8] Barbieri I, Kouzarides T. Role of RNA modifications in cancer. Nature Reviews. Cancer. 2020 Jun;**20**(6):303-322. DOI: 10.1038/s41568-020-0253-2

[9] Ianniello Z, Fatica A. N6-Methyladenosine Role in Acute Myeloid Leukaemia. International Journal of Molecular Sciences. 2018 Aug 9;**19**(8). DOI: 10.3390/ijms19082345

[10] Rosselló-Tortella M, Ferrer G, Esteller M. Epitranscriptomics in Hematopoiesis and Hematologic Malignancies. Blood Cancer Discov [Internet]. 2020 Jul 1 [cited 2020 Aug 18];1(1):26-31. Available from: https://bloodcancerdiscov.aacrjournals.org/content/1/1/26. DOI: 10.1158/2643-3249.BCD-20-0032.

[11] Barbieri I, Tzelepis K, Pandolfini L, Shi J, Millán-Zambrano G, Robson SC, et al. Promoter-bound METTL3 maintains myeloid leukaemia by m6A-dependent translation control. Nature. 2017 07;552(7683):126-31. DOI: 10.1038/nature24678

[12] Weng H, Huang H, Wu H, Qin X, Zhao BS, Dong L, et al. METTL14 Inhibits Hematopoietic Stem/Progenitor Differentiation and Promotes Leukemogenesis via mRNA m6A Modification. Cell Stem Cell. 2018;22(2):191-205.e9. DOI: 10.1016/j.stem.2017.11.016

[13] Vu LP, Pickering BF, Cheng Y, Zaccara S, Nguyen D, Minuesa G, et al. The N6-methyladenosine (m6A)-forming enzyme METTL3 controls myeloid differentiation of normal hematopoietic and leukemia cells. Nature Medicine. 2017 Nov;**23**(11):1369-1376. DOI: 10.1038/nm.4416

[14] Li Z, Weng H, Su R, Weng X, Zuo Z, Li C, et al. FTO Plays an Oncogenic Role in Acute Myeloid Leukemia as a N6-Methyladenosine RNA Demethylase. Cancer Cell. 2017;31(1):127-41. DOI: 10.1016/j.ccell.2016.11.017

[15] Su R, Dong L, Li C, Nachtergaele S, Wunderlich M, Qing Y, et al. R-2HG Exhibits Anti-tumor Activity by Targeting FTO/m6A/MYC/CEBPA

Signaling. Cell. 2018 11;172(1-2):90-105.e23. DOI: 10.1016/j.cell.2017.11.031

[16] Paris J, Morgan M, Campos J, Spencer GJ, Shmakova A, Ivanova I, et al. Targeting the RNA m6A Reader YTHDF2 Selectively Compromises Cancer Stem Cells in Acute Myeloid Leukemia. Cell Stem Cell. 2019 03;25(1):137-148.e6. DOI: 10.1016/j.stem.2019.03.021

[17] Huang H, Weng H, Sun W, Qin X, Shi H, Wu H, et al. Recognition of RNA N6-methyladenosine by IGF2BP proteins enhances mRNA stability and translation. Nature Cell Biology. 2018;**20**(3):285-295. DOI: 10.1038/s41556-018-0045-z

[18] Guzzi N, Cieśla M, Ngoc PCT, Lang S, Arora S, Dimitriou M, et al. Pseudouridylation of tRNA-Derived Fragments Steers Translational Control in Stem Cells. Cell. 2018 17;173(5):1204-1216.e26. DOI: 10.1016/j.cell.2018.03.008

[19] Pereira B, Billaud M, Almeida R. RNA-Binding Proteins in Cancer: Old Players and New Actors. Trends Cancer. 2017;**3**(7):506-528. DOI: 10.1016/j.trecan.2017.05.003

[20] Hodson DJ, Screen M, Turner M. RNA-binding proteins in hematopoiesis and hematological malignancy. Blood. 2019;**133**(22):2365-2373. DOI: 10.1182/blood-2018-10-839985

[21] Griner LN, Reuther GW. Aggressive myeloid leukemia formation is directed by the Musashi 2/Numb pathway. Cancer Biology & Therapy. 2010 Nov 15;**10**(10):979-982. DOI: 10.4161/cbt.10.10.14010

[22] Ito T, Kwon HY, Zimdahl B, Congdon KL, Blum J, Lento WE, et al. Regulation of myeloid leukaemia by the cell-fate determinant Musashi. Nature. 2010 Aug 5;**466**(7307):765-768. DOI: 10.1038/nature09171

[23] Kharas MG, Lengner CJ, Al-Shahrour F, Bullinger L, Ball B, Zaidi S, et al. Musashi-2 regulates normal hematopoiesis and promotes aggressive myeloid leukemia. Nature Medicine. 2010 Aug;**16**(8):903-908. DOI: 10.1038/nm.2187

[24] Park S-M, Gönen M, Vu L, Minuesa G, Tivnan P, Barlowe TS, et al. Musashi2 sustains the mixed-lineage leukemia-driven stem cell regulatory program. The Journal of Clinical Investigation. 2015 Mar 2;**125**(3):1286-1298. DOI: 10.1172/JCI78440

[25] Park S-M, Deering RP, Lu Y, Tivnan P, Lianoglou S, Al-Shahrour F, et al. Musashi-2 controls cell fate, lineage bias, and TGF-β signaling in HSCs. The Journal of Experimental Medicine. 2014 Jan 13;**211**(1):71-87. DOI: 10.1084/jem.20130736

[26] Wang S, Li N, Yousefi M, Nakauka-Ddamba A, Li F, Parada K, et al. Transformation of the intestinal epithelium by the MSI2 RNA-binding protein. Nature Communications. 2015 Mar 16;**6**:6517. DOI: 10.1038/ncomms7517

[27] Minuesa G, Albanese SK, Xie W, Kazansky Y, Worroll D, Chow A, et al. Small-molecule targeting of MUSASHI RNA-binding activity in acute myeloid leukemia. Nature Communications. 2019;**10**(1):2691. DOI: 10.1038/s41467-019-10523-3

[28] Lan L, Appelman C, Smith AR, Yu J, Larsen S, Marquez RT, et al. Natural product (−)-gossypol inhibits colon cancer cell growth by targeting RNA-binding protein Musashi-1. Molecular Oncology. 2015 Aug;**9**(7):1406-1420. DOI: 10.1016/j.molonc.2015.03.014

[29] Clingman CC, Deveau LM, Hay SA, Genga RM, Shandilya SM, Massi F, et al. Allosteric inhibition of a stem cell RNA-binding protein by an intermediary metabolite. Black DL, editor. eLife

[Internet]. 2014 Jun 16;3:e02848. DOI: 10.7554/eLife.02848

[30] Jiang L, Gu Z-H, Yan Z-X, Zhao X, Xie Y-Y, Zhang Z-G, et al. Exome sequencing identifies somatic mutations of DDX3X in natural killer/T-cell lymphoma. Nature Genetics. 2015 Sep;**47**(9):1061-1066. DOI: 10.1038/ng.3358

[31] Wang L, Lawrence MS, Wan Y, Stojanov P, Sougnez C, Stevenson K, et al. SF3B1 and other novel cancer genes in chronic lymphocytic leukemia. The New England Journal of Medicine. 2011 Dec 29;**365**(26):2497-2506. DOI: 10.1056/NEJMoa1109016

[32] Bol GM, Vesuna F, Xie M, Zeng J, Aziz K, Gandhi N, et al. Targeting DDX3 with a small molecule inhibitor for lung cancer therapy. EMBO Molecular Medicine. 2015 May;**7**(5):648-669. DOI: 10.15252/emmm.201404368

[33] Heerma van Voss MR, Vesuna F, Bol GM, Afzal J, Tantravedi S, Bergman Y, et al. Targeting mitochondrial translation by inhibiting DDX3: a novel radiosensitization strategy for cancer treatment. Oncogene. 2018;**37**(1):63-74. DOI: 10.1038/onc.2017.308

[34] Annabi B, Currie J-C, Moghrabi A, Béliveau R. Inhibition of HuR and MMP-9 expression in macrophage-differentiated HL-60 myeloid leukemia cells by green tea polyphenol EGCg. Leukemia Research. 2007 Sep;**31**(9):1277-1284. DOI: 10.1016/j.leukres.2006.10.001

[35] Ishimaru D, Ramalingam S, Sengupta TK, Bandyopadhyay S, Dellis S, Tholanikunnel BG, et al. Regulation of Bcl-2 expression by HuR in HL60 leukemia cells and A431 carcinoma cells. Molecular Cancer Research. 2009 Aug;**7**(8):1354-1366. DOI: 10.1158/1541-7786.MCR-08-0476

[36] Ko C-Y, Wang W-L, Li C-F, Jeng Y-M, Chu Y-Y, Wang H-Y, et al. IL-18-induced interaction between IMP3 and HuR contributes to COX-2 mRNA stabilization in acute myeloid leukemia. Journal of Leukocyte Biology. 2016 Jan;**99**(1):131-141. DOI: 10.1189/jlb.2A0414-228RR

[37] Blackinton JG, Keene JD. Functional coordination and HuR-mediated regulation of mRNA stability during T cell activation. Nucleic Acids Research. 2016 Jan 8;**44**(1):426-436. DOI: 10.1093/nar/gkv1066

[38] Meisner N-C, Hintersteiner M, Mueller K, Bauer R, Seifert J-M, Naegeli H-U, et al. Identification and mechanistic characterization of low-molecular-weight inhibitors for HuR. Nature Chemical Biology. 2007 Aug;**3**(8):508-515. DOI: 10.1038/nchembio.2007.14

[39] Blanco FF, Preet R, Aguado A, Vishwakarma V, Stevens LE, Vyas A, et al. Impact of HuR inhibition by the small molecule MS-444 on colorectal cancer cell tumorigenesis. Oncotarget. 2016 Nov 8;**7**(45):74043-74058. DOI: 10.18632/oncotarget.12189

[40] Filippova N, Yang X, Ananthan S, Sorochinsky A, Hackney JR, Gentry Z, et al. Hu antigen R (HuR) multimerization contributes to glioma disease progression. The Journal of Biological Chemistry. 2017;**292**(41):16999-17010. DOI: 10.1074/jbc.M117.797878

[41] Chae M-J, Sung HY, Kim E-H, Lee M, Kwak H, Chae CH, et al. Chemical inhibitors destabilize HuR binding to the AU-rich element of TNF-alpha mRNA. Experimental & Molecular Medicine. 2009 Nov 30;**41**(11):824-831. DOI: 10.3858/emm.2009.41.11.088

[42] Muralidharan R, Mehta M, Ahmed R, Roy S, Xu L, Aubé J, et al.

HuR-targeted small molecule inhibitor exhibits cytotoxicity towards human lung cancer cells. Scientific Reports. 2017;**7**(1):9694. DOI: 10.1038/s41598-017-07787-4

[43] Timchenko NA, Welm AL, Lu X, Timchenko LT. CUG repeat binding protein (CUGBP1) interacts with the 5′ region of C/EBPbeta mRNA and regulates translation of C/EBPbeta isoforms. Nucleic Acids Research. 1999 Nov 15;**27**(22):4517-4525. DOI: 10.1093/nar/27.22.4517

[44] Guerzoni C, Bardini M, Mariani SA, Ferrari-Amorotti G, Neviani P, Panno ML, et al. Inducible activation of CEBPB, a gene negatively regulated by BCR/ABL, inhibits proliferation and promotes differentiation of BCR/ABL-expressing cells. Blood. 2006 May 15;**107**(10):4080-4089. DOI: 10.1182/blood-2005-08-3181

[45] Notari M, Neviani P, Santhanam R, Blaser BW, Chang J-S, Galietta A, et al. A MAPK/HNRPK pathway controls BCR/ABL oncogenic potential by regulating MYC mRNA translation. Blood. 2006 Mar 15;**107**(6):2507-2516. DOI: 10.1182/blood-2005-09-3732

[46] Iervolino A, Santilli G, Trotta R, Guerzoni C, Cesi V, Bergamaschi A, et al. hnRNP A1 nucleocytoplasmic shuttling activity is required for normal myelopoiesis and BCR/ABL leukemogenesis. Molecular and Cellular Biology. 2002 Apr;**22**(7):2255-2266. DOI: 10.1128/mcb.22.7.2255-2266.2002

[47] Perrotti D, Bonatti S, Trotta R, Martinez R, Skorski T, Salomoni P, et al. TLS/FUS, a pro-oncogene involved in multiple chromosomal translocations, is a novel regulator of BCR/ABL-mediated leukemogenesis. The EMBO Journal. 1998 Aug 3;**17**(15):4442-4455. DOI: 10.1093/emboj/17.15.4442

[48] Trotta R, Vignudelli T, Candini O, Intine RV, Pecorari L, Guerzoni C, et al. BCR/ABL activates mdm2 mRNA translation via the La antigen. Cancer Cell. 2003 Feb;**3**(2):145-160. DOI: 10.1016/s1535-6108(03)00020-5

[49] Fu X-D, Ares M. Context-dependent control of alternative splicing by RNA-binding proteins. Nature Reviews. Genetics. 2014 Oct;**15**(10):689-701. DOI: 10.1038/nrg3778

[50] da Silva MR, Moreira GA, Gonçalves da Silva RA, de Almeida Alves Barbosa É, Pais Siqueira R, Teixera RR, et al. Splicing Regulators and Their Roles in Cancer Biology and Therapy. BioMed Research International. 2015;2015:150514. DOI: 10.1155/2015/150514

[51] Wang E, Aifantis I. RNA Splicing and Cancer. Trends Cancer. 2020 Aug;**6**(8):631-644. DOI: 10.1016/j.trecan.2020.04.011

[52] Alarcón CR, Goodarzi H, Lee H, Liu X, Tavazoie S, Tavazoie SF. HNRNPA2B1 Is a Mediator of m(6)A-Dependent Nuclear RNA Processing Events. Cell. 2015 Sep 10;**162**(6):1299-1308. DOI: 10.1016/j.cell.2015.08.011

[53] Xiao W, Adhikari S, Dahal U, Chen Y-S, Hao Y-J, Sun B-F, et al. Nuclear m(6)A Reader YTHDC1 Regulates mRNA Splicing. Molecular Cell. 2016 Feb 18;**61**(4):507-519. DOI: 10.1016/j.molcel.2016.01.012

[54] Schittenhelm MM, Walter B, Tsintari V, Federmann B, Bajrami Saipi M, Akmut F, et al. Alternative splicing of the tumor suppressor ASPP2 results in a stress-inducible, oncogenic isoform prevalent in acute leukemia. eBioMedicine. 2019 Apr;**42**:340-351. DOI: 10.1016/j.ebiom.2019.03.028

[55] Li S-Q, Liu J, Zhang J, Wang X-L, Chen D, Wang Y, et al. Transcriptome profiling reveals the high incidence of hnRNPA1 exon 8 inclusion in chronic myeloid leukemia. Journal of Advanced

Research. 2020 Jul;**24**:301-310. DOI: 10.1016/j.jare.2020.04.016

[56] Feng Y, Chen M, Manley JL. Phosphorylation switches the general splicing repressor SRp38 to a sequence-specific activator. Nature Structural & Molecular Biology. 2008 Oct;**15**(10):1040-1048. DOI: 10.1038/nsmb.1485

[57] Radzisheuskaya A, Shliaha PV, Grinev V, Lorenzini E, Kovalchuk S, Shlyueva D, et al. PRMT5 methylome profiling uncovers a direct link to splicing regulation in acute myeloid leukemia. Nature Structural & Molecular Biology. 2019;**26**(11):999-1012. DOI: 10.1038/s41594-019-0313-z

[58] Shailesh H, Zakaria ZZ, Baiocchi R, Sif S. Protein arginine methyltransferase 5 (PRMT5) dysregulation in cancer. Oncotarget. 2018 Nov 30;**9**(94):36705-36718. DOI: 10.18632/oncotarget.26404

[59] Li X, Wang C, Jiang H, Luo C. A patent review of arginine methyltransferase inhibitors (2010-2018). Expert Opinion on Therapeutic Patents. 2019;**29**(2):97-114. DOI: 10.1080/13543776.2019.1567711

[60] Koh CM, Bezzi M, Low DHP, Ang WX, Teo SX, Gay FPH, et al. MYC regulates the core pre-mRNA splicing machinery as an essential step in lymphomagenesis. Nature. 2015 Jul 2;**523**(7558):96-100. DOI: 10.1038/nature14351

[61] Wang E, Lu SX, Pastore A, Chen X, Imig J, Chun-Wei Lee S, et al. Targeting an RNA-Binding Protein Network in Acute Myeloid Leukemia. Cancer Cell. 2019;**35**(3):369-384.e7. DOI: 10.1016/j.ccell.2019.01.010

[62] Han T, Goralski M, Gaskill N, Capota E, Kim J, Ting TC, et al. Anticancer sulfonamides target splicing by inducing RBM39 degradation via recruitment to DCAF15. Science. 2017;**356**(6336). DOI: 10.1126/science.aal3755

[63] Faust TB, Yoon H, Nowak RP, Donovan KA, Li Z, Cai Q, et al. Structural complementarity facilitates E7820-mediated degradation of RBM39 by DCAF15. Nature Chemical Biology. 2020;**16**(1):7-14. DOI: 10.1038/s41589-019-0378-3

[64] Seiler M, Yoshimi A, Darman R, Chan B, Keaney G, Thomas M, et al. H3B-8800, an orally available small-molecule splicing modulator, induces lethality in spliceosome-mutant cancers. Nature Medicine. 2018;**24**(4):497-504. DOI: 10.1038/nm.4493

[65] Shirai CL, White BS, Tripathi M, Tapia R, Ley JN, Ndonwi M, et al. Mutant U2AF1-expressing cells are sensitive to pharmacological modulation of the spliceosome. Nature Communications. 2017;8:14060. DOI: 10.1038/ncomms14060

[66] Lee SC-W, North K, Kim E, Jang E, Obeng E, Lu SX, et al. Synthetic Lethal and Convergent Biological Effects of Cancer-Associated Spliceosomal Gene Mutations. Cancer Cell. 2018 13;34(2):225-241.e8. DOI: 10.1016/j.ccell.2018.07.003

[67] Pandit S, Zhou Y, Shiue L, Coutinho-Mansfield G, Li H, Qiu J, et al. Genome-wide analysis reveals SR protein cooperation and competition in regulated splicing. Molecular Cell. 2013 Apr 25;**50**(2):223-235. DOI: 10.1016/j.molcel.2013.03.001

[68] Huelga SC, Vu AQ, Arnold JD, Liang TY, Liu PP, Yan BY, et al. Integrative genome-wide analysis reveals cooperative regulation of alternative splicing by hnRNP proteins. Cell Reports. 2012 Feb 23;**1**(2):167-178. DOI: 10.1016/j.celrep.2012.02.001

[69] Ly C, Arechiga AF, Melo JV, Walsh CM, Ong ST. Bcr-Abl kinase

modulates the translation regulators ribosomal protein S6 and 4E-BP1 in chronic myelogenous leukemia cells via the mammalian target of rapamycin. Cancer Research. 2003 Sep 15;**63**(18):5716-5722

[70] Mirabilii S, Ricciardi MR, Piedimonte M, Gianfelici V, Bianchi MP, Tafuri A. Biological Aspects of mTOR in Leukemia. International Journal of Molecular Sciences. 2018 Aug 14;**19**(8). DOI: 10.3390/ijms19082396

[71] Redig AJ, Vakana E, Platanias LC. Regulation of mammalian target of rapamycin and mitogen activated protein kinase pathways by BCR-ABL. Leukemia & Lymphoma. 2011 Feb;**52**(Suppl 1):45-53. DOI: 10.3109/10428194.2010.546919

[72] Hirao A, Hoshii T. Mechanistic / mammalian target protein of rapamycin signaling in hematopoietic stem cells and leukemia. Cancer Science. 2013 Aug;**104**(8):977-982. DOI: 10.1111/cas.12189

[73] Tsai BP, Jimenez J, Lim S, Fitzgerald KD, Zhang M, Chuah CTH, et al. A novel Bcr-Abl-mTOR-eIF4A axis regulates IRES-mediated translation of LEF-1. Open Biology. 2014 Nov;**4**(11):140180. DOI: 10.1098/rsob.140180

[74] Xian J, Shao H, Chen X, Zhang S, Quan J, Zou Q, et al. Nucleophosmin Mutants Promote Adhesion, Migration and Invasion of Human Leukemia THP-1 Cells through MMPs Up-regulation via Ras/ERK MAPK Signaling. International Journal of Biological Sciences. 2016;**12**(2):144-155. DOI: 10.7150/ijbs.13382

[75] Wang X, Pesakhov S, Weng A, Kafka M, Gocek E, Nguyen M, et al. ERK 5/MAPK pathway has a major role in 1α,25-(OH)2 vitamin D3-induced terminal differentiation of myeloid leukemia cells. J Steroid Biochem Mol Biol. 2014 Oct;144 Pt A:223-227. DOI: 10.1016/j.jsbmb.2013.10.002

[76] Kusio-Kobialka M, Podszywalow-Bartnicka P, Peidis P, Glodkowska-Mrowka E, Wolanin K, Leszak G, et al. The PERK-eIF2α phosphorylation arm is a pro-survival pathway of BCR-ABL signaling and confers resistance to imatinib treatment in chronic myeloid leukemia cells. Cell Cycle. 2012 Nov 1;**11**(21):4069-4078. DOI: 10.4161/cc.22387

[77] Dinner S, Platanias LC. Targeting the mTOR Pathway in Leukemia. Journal of Cellular Biochemistry. 2016;**117**(8):1745-1752. DOI: 10.1002/jcb.25559

[78] Dreas A, Mikulski M, Milik M, Fabritius C-H, Brzózka K, Rzymski T. Mitogen-activated Protein Kinase (MAPK) Interacting Kinases 1 and 2 (MNK1 and MNK2) as Targets for Cancer Therapy: Recent Progress in the Development of MNK Inhibitors. Current Medicinal Chemistry. 2017;**24**(28):3025-3053. DOI: 10.2174/0929867324666170203123427

[79] Truitt ML, Ruggero D. New frontiers in translational control of the cancer genome. Nature Reviews. Cancer. 2016;**16**(5):288-304. DOI: 10.1038/nrc.2016.27

[80] Shi F, Len Y, Gong Y, Shi R, Yang X, Naren D, et al. Ribavirin Inhibits the Activity of mTOR/eIF4E, ERK/Mnk1/eIF4E Signaling Pathway and Synergizes with Tyrosine Kinase Inhibitor Imatinib to Impair Bcr-Abl Mediated Proliferation and Apoptosis in Ph+ Leukemia. PLoS One. 2015;**10**(8):e0136746. DOI: 10.1371/journal.pone.0136746

[81] Axten JM, Romeril SP, Shu A, Ralph J, Medina JR, Feng Y, et al. Discovery of GSK2656157: An Optimized PERK Inhibitor Selected

for Preclinical Development. ACS Medicinal Chemistry Letters. 2013 Oct 10;**4**(10):964-968. DOI: 10.1021/ml400228e

[82] Rojas-Rivera D, Delvaeye T, Roelandt R, Nerinckx W, Augustyns K, Vandenabeele P, et al. When PERK inhibitors turn out to be new potent RIPK1 inhibitors: critical issues on the specificity and use of GSK2606414 and GSK2656157. Cell Death Differ. 2017;24(6):1100-10. DOI: 10.1038/cdd.2017.58

[83] Sidrauski C, McGeachy AM, Ingolia NT, Walter P. The small molecule ISRIB reverses the effects of eIF2α phosphorylation on translation and stress granule assembly. eLife. 2015 Feb 26;**4**. DOI: 10.7554/eLife.05033

[84] Kondrashov N, Pusic A, Stumpf CR, Shimizu K, Hsieh AC, Ishijima J, et al. Ribosome-mediated specificity in Hox mRNA translation and vertebrate tissue patterning. Cell. 2011 Apr 29;**145**(3):383-397. DOI: 10.1016/j.cell.2011.03.028

[85] Simsek D, Tiu GC, Flynn RA, Byeon GW, Leppek K, Xu AF, et al. The Mammalian Ribo-interactome Reveals Ribosome Functional Diversity and Heterogeneity. Cell. 2017 Jun 1;**169**(6):1051-1065.e18. DOI: 10.1016/j.cell.2017.05.022

[86] Imami K, Milek M, Bogdanow B, Yasuda T, Kastelic N, Zauber H, et al. Phosphorylation of the Ribosomal Protein RPL12/uL11 Affects Translation during Mitosis. Mol Cell. 2018 04;72(1):84-98.e9. DOI: 10.1016/j.molcel.2018.08.019

[87] Genuth NR, Barna M. The Discovery of Ribosome Heterogeneity and Its Implications for Gene Regulation and Organismal Life. Mol Cell. 2018 02;71(3):364-74. DOI: 10.1016/j.molcel.2018.07.018

[88] Gustavsson P, Willing TN, van Haeringen A, Tchernia G, Dianzani I, Donnér M, et al. Diamond-Blackfan anaemia: genetic homogeneity for a gene on chromosome 19q13 restricted to 1.8 Mb. Nature Genetics. 1997 Aug;**16**(4):368-371. DOI: 10.1038/ng0897-368

[89] Guimaraes JC, Zavolan M. Patterns of ribosomal protein expression specify normal and malignant human cells. Genome Biol. 2016 24;17(1):236. DOI: 10.1186/s13059-016-1104-z

[90] Bastide A, David A. The ribosome, (slow) beating heart of cancer (stem) cell. Oncogene. 2018 Apr 20;7(4):34. DOI: 10.1038/s41389-018-0044-8

[91] Wu L, Li X, Xu F, Chang C, He Q, Zhang Z, et al. Over-expression of RPL23 in myelodysplastic syndromes is associated with apoptosis resistance of CD34+ cells and predicts poor prognosis and distinct response to CHG chemotherapy or decitabine. Annals of Hematology. 2012 Oct;**91**(10):1547-1554. DOI: 10.1007/s00277-012-1486-2

[92] Monika Belickova M, Merkerova MD, Votavova H, Valka J, Vesela J, Pejsova B, et al. Up-regulation of ribosomal genes is associated with a poor response to azacitidine in myelodysplasia and related neoplasms. International Journal of Hematology. 2016 Nov;**104**(5):566-573. DOI: 10.1007/s12185-016-2058-3

[93] Stevens BM, Khan N, D'Alessandro A, Nemkov T, Winters A, Jones CL, et al. Characterization and targeting of malignant stem cells in patients with advanced myelodysplastic syndromes. Nat Commun. 2018 12;9(1):3694. DOI: 10.1038/s41467-018-05984-x

[94] Morgado-Palacin L, Varetti G, Llanos S, Gómez-López G, Martinez D, Serrano M. Partial Loss of Rpl11 in Adult Mice Recapitulates

Diamond-Blackfan Anemia and Promotes Lymphomagenesis. Cell Reports. 2015 Oct 27;**13**(4):712-722. DOI: 10.1016/j.celrep.2015.09.038

[95] Hofman IJF, van Duin M, De Bruyne E, Fancello L, Mulligan G, Geerdens E, et al. RPL5 on 1p22.1 is recurrently deleted in multiple myeloma and its expression is linked to bortezomib response. Leukemia. 2017;**31**(8):1706-1714. DOI: 10.1038/leu.2016.370

[96] De Keersmaecker K, Atak ZK, Li N, Vicente C, Patchett S, Girardi T, et al. Exome sequencing identifies mutation in CNOT3 and ribosomal genes RPL5 and RPL10 in T-cell acute lymphoblastic leukemia. Nature Genetics. 2013 Feb;**45**(2):186-190. DOI: 10.1038/ng.2508

[97] Kampen KR, Fancello L, Girardi T, Rinaldi G, Planque M, Sulima SO, et al. Translatome analysis reveals altered serine and glycine metabolism in T-cell acute lymphoblastic leukemia cells. Nat Commun. 2019, 2542;**10**(1). DOI: 10.1038/s41467-019-10508-2

[98] Ebert BL, Pretz J, Bosco J, Chang CY, Tamayo P, Galili N, et al. Identification of RPS14 as a 5q- syndrome gene by RNA interference screen. Nature. 2008 Jan 17;**451**(7176):335-339. DOI: 10.1038/nature06494

[99] Rao S, Lee S-Y, Gutierrez A, Perrigoue J, Thapa RJ, Tu Z, et al. Inactivation of ribosomal protein L22 promotes transformation by induction of the stemness factor, Lin28B. Blood. 2012 Nov 1;**120**(18):3764-3773. DOI: 10.1182/blood-2012-03-415349

[100] Landau DA, Tausch E, Taylor-Weiner AN, Stewart C, Reiter JG, Bahlo J, et al. Mutations driving CLL and their evolution in progression and relapse. Nature. 2015 Oct 22;**526**(7574):525-530. DOI: 10.1038/nature15395

[101] Ljungström V, Cortese D, Young E, Pandzic T, Mansouri L, Plevova K, et al. Whole-exome sequencing in relapsing chronic lymphocytic leukemia: clinical impact of recurrent RPS15 mutations. Blood. 2016 Feb 25;**127**(8):1007-1016. DOI: 10.1182/blood-2015-10-674572

[102] Shi Z, Fujii K, Kovary KM, Genuth NR, Röst HL, Teruel MN, et al. Heterogeneous Ribosomes Preferentially Translate Distinct Subpools of mRNAs Genome-wide. Molecular Cell. 2017 Jul 6;**67**(1):71-83.e7. DOI: 10.1016/j.molcel.2017.05.021

[103] Bhat P, Shwetha S, Sharma DK, Joseph AP, Srinivasan N, Das S. The beta hairpin structure within ribosomal protein S5 mediates interplay between domains II and IV and regulates HCV IRES function. Nucleic Acids Research. 2015 Mar 11;**43**(5):2888-2901. DOI: 10.1093/nar/gkv110

[104] Hertz MI, Landry DM, Willis AE, Luo G, Thompson SR. Ribosomal protein S25 dependency reveals a common mechanism for diverse internal ribosome entry sites and ribosome shunting. Molecular and Cellular Biology. 2013 Mar;**33**(5):1016-1026. DOI: 10.1128/MCB.00879-12

[105] Meyuhas O. Ribosomal Protein S6 Phosphorylation. Four Decades of Research. Int Rev Cell Mol Biol. 2015;**320**:41-73. DOI: 10.1016/bs.ircmb.2015.07.006

[106] Myasnikov AG, Kundhavai Natchiar S, Nebout M, Hazemann I, Imbert V, Khatter H, et al. Structure-function insights reveal the human ribosome as a cancer target for antibiotics. Nature Communications. 2016 Sep 26;7:12856. DOI: 10.1038/ncomms12856

[107] Huang B-T, Zeng Q-C, Zhao W-H, Tan Y. Homoharringtonine

contributes to imatinib sensitivity by blocking the EphB4/RhoA pathway in chronic myeloid leukemia cell lines. Med Oncol Northwood Lond Engl. 2014 Feb;**31**(2):836. DOI: 10.1007/s12032-013-0836-9

[108] Tujebajeva RM, Graifer DM, Karpova GG, Ajtkhozhina NA. Alkaloid homoharringtonine inhibits polypeptide chain elongation on human ribosomes on the step of peptide bond formation. FEBS Letters. 1989 Nov 6;**257**(2):254-256. DOI: 10.1016/0014-5793(89)81546-7

[109] Lü S, Wang J. Homoharringtonine and omacetaxine for myeloid hematological malignancies. Journal of Hematology & Oncology. 2014 Jan 3;**7**(2). DOI: 10.1186/1756-8722-7-2

[110] Gilles A, Frechin L, Natchiar K, Biondani G, Loeffelholz O von, Holvec S, et al. Targeting the Human 80S Ribosome in Cancer: From Structure to Function and Drug Design for Innovative Adjuvant Therapeutic Strategies. Cell 2020 Mar 5;9(3). DOI: 10.3390/cells9030629

[111] nBruno PM, Liu Y, Park GY, Murai J, Koch CE, Eisen TJ, et al. A subset of platinum-containing chemotherapeutic agents kills cells by inducing ribosome biogenesis stress. Nature Medicine. 2017 Apr;**23**(4):461-471. DOI: 10.1038/nm.4291

[112] Bywater MJ, Poortinga G, Sanij E, Hein N, Peck A, Cullinane C, et al. Inhibition of RNA polymerase I as a therapeutic strategy to promote cancer-specific activation of p53. Cancer Cell. 2012 Jul 10;**22**(1):51-65. DOI: 10.1016/j.ccr.2012.05.019

[113] Devlin JR, Hannan KM, Hein N, Cullinane C, Kusnadi E, Ng PY, et al. Combination Therapy Targeting Ribosome Biogenesis and mRNA Translation Synergistically Extends Survival in MYC-Driven Lymphoma. Cancer Discovery. 2016 Jan;**6**(1):59-70. DOI: 10.1158/2159-8290.CD-14-0673

[114] Lee HC, Wang H, Baladandayuthapani V, Lin H, He J, Jones RJ, et al. RNA Polymerase I Inhibition with CX-5461 as a Novel Therapeutic Strategy to Target MYC in Multiple Myeloma. British Journal of Haematology. 2017;**177**(1):80-94. DOI: 10.1111/bjh.14525

[115] Khot A, Brajanovski N, Cameron DP, Hein N, Maclachlan KH, Sanij E, et al. First-in-Human RNA Polymerase I Transcription Inhibitor CX-5461 in Patients with Advanced Hematologic Cancers: Results of a Phase I Dose-Escalation Study. Cancer Discovery. 2019;**9**(8):1036-1049. DOI: 10.1158/2159-8290.CD-18-1455

Chapter 16

Mechanisms of Resistence of New Target Drugs in Acute Myeloid Leukemia

Debora Capelli, Francesco Saraceni, Diego Menotti, Alessandro Fiorentini and Attilio Olivieri

Abstract

New drugs targeting single mutations have been recently approved for Acute Myeloid Leukemia (AML) treatment, but allogeneic transplant still remains the only curative option in intermediate and unfavorable risk settings, because of the high incidence of relapse. Molecular analysis repertoire permits the identification of the target mutations and drives the choice of target drugs, but the etherogeneity of the disease reduces the curative potential of these agents. Primary and secondary AML resistance to new target agents is actually an intriguing issue and some of these mechanisms have already been explored and identified. Changes in mutations, release of microenvironment factors competing for the same therapeutic target or promoting the survival of blasts or of the leukemic stem cell, the upregulation of the target-downstream pathways and of proteins inhibiting the apoptosis, the inhibition of the cytochrome drug metabolism by other concomitant treatments are some of the recognized patterns of tumor escape. The knowledge of these topics might implement the model of the 'AML umbrella trial' study through the combinations or sequences of new target drugs, preemptively targeting known mechanisms of resistance, with the aim to improve the potential curative rates, expecially in elderly patients not eligible to transplant.

Keywords: acute myeloid Leukemia, FLT3 inhibitors, IDH inhibitors, BCL2 inhibitors, mechanisms of resistance, immunotherapy, target therapy

1. Introduction

The better knowledge of leukemogenesis has led in the last few years to approval of new target drugs for AML treatment. The availability of these drugs has dramatically changed the AML treatment guidelines, supported by the evidence of their efficacy on a molecular driven basis approach. Neverthless primary resistance and clonal evolution leading to adaptive resistance is a recurring theme even in this setting.

Actually acute myeloid leukemia (AML) is the result of a multi-step sequence of events resulting in impairment of lineage differentiation, hematopoiesis and enhanced self-renewal. Somatic mutations contribute to AML pathogenesis in different manner. Analysis of healthy population exomic and genomic sequencing [1] showed a correlation between pre-leukemic somatic mutations (IDH1/2, SRSF2, U2AF1, TP53, RUNX1, PPM1D) and subsequent development of AML, as first step

 IntechOpen

process towards leukemogenesis. The subsequent acquisition of mutations appeared to be related with different AML phenotypes. The Cancer genome atlas research network [2] identified eight different genetic pathways responsable of leukemogenesis in 200 adult patients, shown in **Table 1** (trancriptor factor genes fusion and hyper-expression; nucleophosmin 1 delocalization; tumor suppressor genes inhibition; mutations of: DNA-methylation related genes, activated signaling genes, chromatin-modifying genes, cohesin-complex genes, spliceosoma-complex genes). Afterwards Papaemmanuil et al. [3] identified three other molecular subgroups including: IDH2R172 mutation in 1% of AML, mutually exclusive with NPM1, associated with more severe alterations of metabolic activity in comparison to other IDH2 mutations; CCAAT/enhancer binding protein alpha (CEBPA) biallelic mutated AML and inv3 or t(3;3) AML with MECOM (EVI1) and GATA2 mutations. Furthermore Ibanez et al. [4] analyzed 100 patients with normal karyotype AML, lacking NPM1, FLT3, and CEBPA mutations, identifying thirteen seed-genes involved in leukemogenesis with a mean of 4.89 mutations per sample. The network analysis showed a high heterogeneity of gene mutations in this setting and suggested that a specific alteration could not be essential for leukemogenesis, as the interaction between several deregulated pathways.

Mechanisms of action	Class of mutations	Mutations/translocations (prevalence)
Transcription deregulation and impaired hematopoietic differentation.	Class 1 Transcription factor fusions*	t(8;21), t(16;16), t(15;17), MLL fusions (18%)
Aberrant localizationn of NPM1 and MPM1-interacting protein.	Class 2 NUCLEOPHOSMIN 1	NPM1 mutations (27%)
transcriptional deregulation and impaired degradation through the mouse double minute 2 homolog (MDM2) and the phosphatase and tensin homolog (PTEM).	Class 3 Tumor suppressor genes	TP53, WT1, PHF6 (16%)
Epigenetic modification and accumulation of 2-hydroxyglutarate (2HG) which deregulates DNA methylation	Class 4 DNA-methylation-related genes: DNA hydroxymethylation	TET2, IDH1, IDH2, DNA methyltransferases DNMT3A (44%)
Proliferative advantage through the RAS– RAF, JAK–STAT, and PI3K–AKT signaling pathways.	Class 5 Activated signaling genes	FLT3, KIT, RAS mutations (59%)
Deregulation of chromatin modification through methylation of histone or impairment of DOT1L (DOT1-like histone H3K79 methyltransferase).	Class 6 Chromatin-modifying genes	ASXL1, EZH2 mutations, MLL fusions, MLL partial tandem duplications (30%)
Transcription deregulation	Class 7 Myeloid transcription factor genes*	CEBPA, RUNX1 mutations (22%)
Chromosome segregation and transcriptional regulation.	Class 8 Cohesin-complex genes	STAG2, RAD21, SMC1, SMC2 (13%)
Deregulation of RNA processing.	Class 9 Spliceosoma-complex genes	SRSF2, U2AF3S, ZRSR2 (14%)

**Class 1 and 7 mutations are both included in the category of mutations of transcription factors genes.*

Table 1.
Cathegories of AML mutations and their role in leukemogenesis.

The perspective of the comprehension of the eterogeneity of the disese inspired recent studies exploring genetic and transcriptomic single leukemic cell analysis with the following aims:

- find the correlation with mutations and subclonal architecture;
- define a hierarchies of leukemic clones, compared to normal hemapotoiesis;
- identify new markers and leukemic stem cell (LSC) specific gene repertoire.

The aknowledgement of these data will promote the finding of future targets for the eradication of the disease even in the biologically chemoresistant setting of LSC.

Uptoday the understanding of leukemogenesis mechanisms have led to the recent approval of FLT3, BCL2 and IDH inhibitors (FLT3i, BCL2i, IDHi).

We briefly resume the mechanisms of leukemogenesis addressed by these drugs. FLT3 tirosin kinase receptor mutations determines the constitutive activation and dimerization status of the receptor itself, indipendently from FLT3 ligand binding, and the downstream activation of leukemic cells prolipheration and pro-survival pathways (RAS-NFKB, JAK–STAT, PI3K, BCL2) as showed in **Figure 1** [5]. BCL2 is an antiapoptotic protein of BCL2 family which compete with

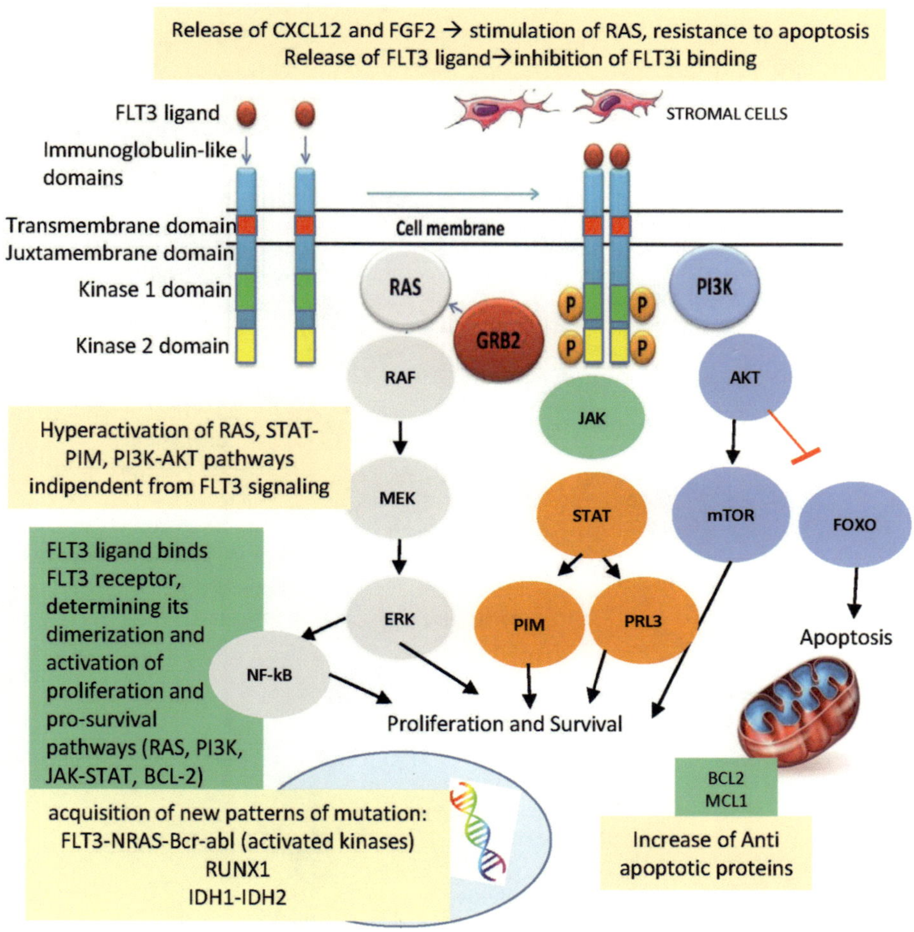

Figure 1.
FLT3 pathway (green label) and mechanisms of resistance to FLT3i (light yellow labels).

BH3 for the binding with the pro-apoptotic proteins BAK/BAX [6]. It inhibits the BH3-BAK/BAX domain and its interaction with the mitochondrial membrane, blocking the p53 dependent mitochondrial apoptosis pathway of the leukemic cell (**Figure 2**). Isocitrate dehydrogenases are cytoplasmic (IDH1) and mitochondrial (IDH2) enzymes cathalyse the reduction of a-ketoglutarate (a-KG) to citrate in krebs cycle in a NADPH-dependent way. NADPH is important for the reduction of glutathione, which in the reduced state is a major antioxidant and protects the cell against reactive-oxygen species (ROS) and other free radicals. IDH mutations have a loss of function effect, producing the accumulation of the oncometabolite R2-hydroxyglutarate (2-HG) which competitively inhibits multiple α-ketoglutarate dependent dioxygenases such as lysine (K)-specific demethylase (KDM) and ten eleven translocation methylcytosine dioxygenase 2 (TET2), causing widespread epigenetic changes with global dysregulation of gene expression and abnormal differentiation and proliferation of leukemic cells (**Figure 3**) [7]. Furthermore 2-HG activates the EglN family of prolyl 4-hydroxylases (EglN), with consequent ubiquitination and degradation of HIF1a, impairing p53 dependent apoptosis. IDH1

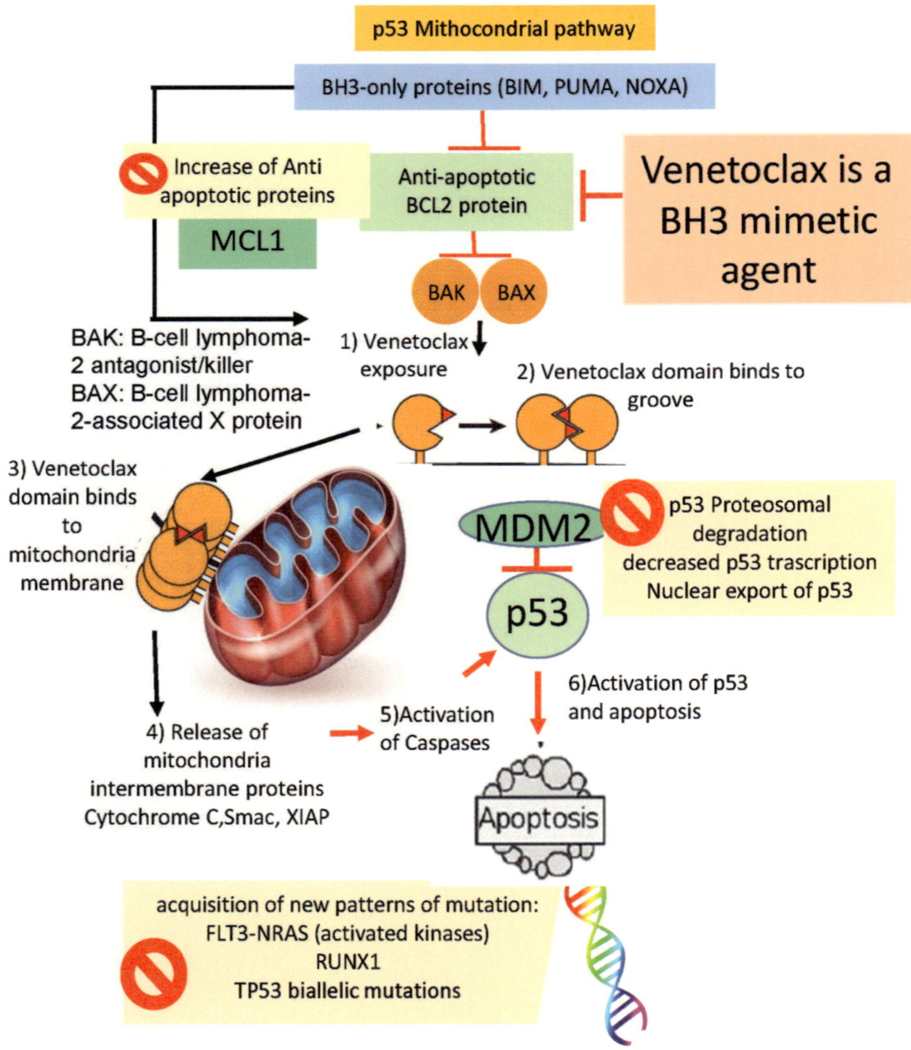

Figure 2.
p53 mitochondrial pathway and mechanisms of resistance to Venetoclax (light yellow labels).

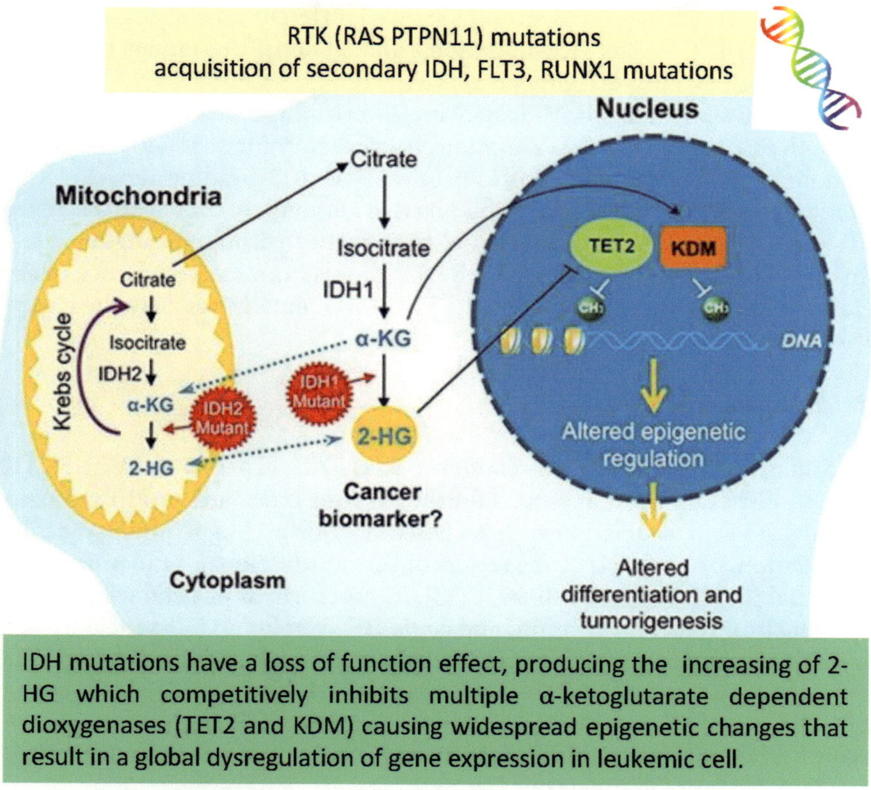

2-HG, 2-hydroxyglutarate; α-KG, α-ketoglutarate; IDH, isocitrate dehydrogenase; KDM, lysine (K)-specific demethylase; TET2, ten eleven translocation methylcytosine dioxygenase 2.

Figure 3.
Mechanism of leukemogenesis of IDH mutations (green label) and mechanisms of resistance to IDHi (light yellow label).

mutations also result in a lack of crucial metabolites including a decrease in the NADPH pool and inhibition of krebs cycle with metabolic changes conferring chemotherapy resistance of leukemic cell. At last 2-HG determines a leukemic status highly BCL-2 dependent, preventing the hypoxia mediated apoptosis, determined by cytochrome c oxidase inhibiton.

Recent studies utilizing NGS and single-cell technologies have also illustrated the complex and polyclonal nature of resistance to targeted therapeutics including FLT3, BCL2 and IDH inhibitors (FLT3i, BCL2i, IDHi) [8, 9]. Here we report the results of the principle studies aiming to analyze mechanism of primary and secondary leukemic resistance to new approved target therapies.

2. New target therapies in AML

2.1 FLT3 inhibitors (FLT3i)

FLT3 is a Tirosin Kinase receptor expressed by hematopoietic progenitors and mutated in 25-30% AML. The mutations involve two different domains: the iuxtamembrane domain (FLT3 ITD) in 20-25% AML and the tirosin kinase domain (TKD) in 5-10% AML, expecially at codon D835. They both determine the constitutive activation of the FLT3 receptor tyrosine kinase, inducing cellular proliferation and survival and inhibiting differentiation, through the activation of PI3K/AKT/mTOR pathway, with a critical role in leukemogenesis [10] (**Figure 1**).

Target drugs inhibiting FLT3 receptor showed different potency of inhibition, activity on FLT3-ITD versus TKD mutations, and on non-FLT3 targets (i.e., kinome specificity), with variable off-target toxicities [11].

Type I FLT3i (Lestaurtinib, Midostaurin, Gilteritinib, Crenolanib) are active against both FLT3-ITD and TKD mutations because they interact with the gate-keeper domain near to the activation loop or with the ATP binding site, expleting their activity on both active dimeric and inactive monomeric tirosin kinase receptor. Type II FLT3i (Quizartinib and Sorafenib) bind to the hydrophobic region adjacent to the ATP binding site only when the receptor is in an inactive form and are therefore ineffective in the forms with the FLT3TKD mutations where the receptor is always in the dimeric active form.

2.1.1 Midostaurin

Midostaurin, a type I FLT3i, also targets c-KIT, PKC, PDGFR, and VEGFR [12] and is FDA, EMA and AIFA approved for the first line treatment of FLT3 mutated (FLT3-mut) AML in association with 7 + 3 in induction and high dose Cytarabine in consolidation, on the basis of the results of the multinational, randomized phase III trial RATIFY (CALBG 10603) [13]. Midostaurin or placebo were given during induction and consolidation, and could be given for up to one year as post-consolidation maintenance, allogeneic transplant was admitted after the stop of the experimental treatment. Midostaurin was associated with a significant improvement in OS (4-year OS rate: 51.4% versus 44.3%; median OS: 74.7 months versus 25.6 months, HR = 0.78; P = 0.009) regardless of the type of *FLT3* mutation (e.g., ITD or D835 TKD) or ITD allele burden, ($<0.7/\geq 0.7$).

2.1.2 Quizartinib

Quizartinib is a type II FLT3i, but also a potent inhibitor of c-KIT, PDGFR, and RET achieving 45-50% marrow remission rates as single-agent in relapsed/refractory (R/R) *FLT3*-mut AML with an OS advantage over investigator choice salvage chemotherapy in the Quantum R-trial, a phase III randomized study of 367 patients with relapsed or refractory *FLT3*-ITD mutated AML (CRc rate 48% vs. 27%; median OS 6.2 months vs. 4.7 months, P = 0.0177) [14]. Neverthless Quizartinib failed FDA approval for this indication, due in part to concerns over treatment equipoise and robustness of OS improvement, while obtained approval in Japan in June 2019 and is being considered for approval in other countries.

2.1.3 Gilteritinib

Gilteritinib is another potent second-generation type I inhibitor with activity against AXL, a receptor tyrosine kinase that may play a role in mediating resistance to earlier generation FLT3 inhibitors [15]. Gilteritinib was found to be well tolerated as single-agent in a randomized phase III study enrolling R/R FLT3-mut AML, with marrow remission rates of 54% superior to the 22% CRc rate observed after investigator choice salvage chemotherapy (both high- and low-dose chemotherapy), with also a longer median OS (9.3 months vs. 5.6 months, HR = 0.79; P = 0.007) [16]. More patients (26% vs. 15%) were able to proceed to HSCT with gilteritinib compared with salvage chemotherapy. These results led to Gilteritinib FDA approval for the treatment of R/R FLT3-mut AML (both ITD and TKD) in November 2018.

2.1.4 Considerations on phase III trials in R/R FLT3-mut AML

Some concerns on these last two trials have been recently raised by a french retrospective analysis of 160 patients with R/R (114 relapsed and 46 refractory) FLT3-mut AML after a first-line TKI-free treatment, 92 of whom fulfilling the main criteria of the QUANTUM-R study, with CR1 durations <6 months, who received an intensive salvage regimen in 48.9% of cases achieving a 52.8% CRc rate and a bridge to transplant rate of 39.6%, superior to 27% of CR and 11% of bridge to transplant rates observed in the same setting in QUANTUM-R. The Median OS of 7 months observed in the French study was also superior to the Quantum-R OS of 4.7 months. The authors argue that the possible bias, caused by the inclusion in the control arm of patients receiving low-intensity regimens, such as low-dose cytarabine or hypomethylating agents, might compromise the results of similar phase 3 trials [17].

2.1.5 Mechanisms of resistance to FLT3i

Neverthless hematopoietic stem cell transplant (HSCT) is still necessary and recommended for the cure of the disease, since retrospective studies [18, 19] showed that HSCT improves RFS and OS and reduces incidence of relapse. The favorable predictive role of FLT3 allelic ratio in NPM1 mutated AML is still controversial due to lack of standardization of techniques and thresholds of this factor [20, 21]. Novel FLT3i might increase outcomes in this setting, but researchers have already identified multiple mechanisms of resistance as hereby reported [11].

- The acquisition of secondary mutations of single amino acids of the activation loop of the FLT3 receptor (D835, I836, D839, Y842) or of the gate-keeper residue (F691) called 'TKD' mutations are reported in 22% of FLT3 AML [22] and are responsible for the resistance specially to type II FLT3i (Quizartinib and Sorafenib) ineffective in targeting TKD mutations [23, 24].

- The activity of fibroblast growth factor 2 (FGF2) and CXCL12/CXCR4 pathways in FLT3 mutated leukemic cells can induce their chemoresistance. The increase in FGF2 is an autocrine response mechanism of stromal cells to all phenomena of hematopoietic stress, including that induced by Quizartinib. Paracrine production of FL (FLT3 ligand) by stromal cells also inhibits the action of FLT3 inhibitors with competitive mechanism, but removal of FL from stromal and leukemic cell cultures does not stop the chemoresistance process due to activation of RAS-MAPK mediated by the FGF2-FGFR1 interaction. The increase in FGF2 secreted by stromal cells has been reported to precede the relapse of mutated FLT3ITD mut AML treated with Quizartinib, through activation of the RAS–MEK/MAPK signal [25]. The combination of FGFR and FLT3 inhibitors is being studied, the rationale is represented by the inhibition of the autocrine and paracrine stimulus favoring the survival of the stromal and leukemic cells, respectively.

- Furthermore FLT3ITD mutated leukemic cells express CXCR4 and are CXCL12 dependent for growth and survival, which makes them resistant to the action of chemotherapy [26]. Activation of Nutlin-3a reduces mRNA levels and CXCL12 secretion through activation of p53 and consequent down-regulation of HIF-1 alpha. Nutlin-3a also binds MDM2 in the p53 binding domain, inhibiting its interaction with p53 which, remaining free, recovers its function.

MDM2 inhibitors such as Nutlin-3a are under study (NCT00623870) and there is a rationale for their association with FLT3 inhibitors [27].

- The activation of RAS/RAF/MEK/ERK is independent of the activation of FLT3 as it is constantly present during therapy with FLT3 inhibitors and can represent a mechanism of resistance to inhibitors in some subclones. Inhibitors of these signals could play a role in counteracting resistance to FLT3 inhibitors [28].

- The PI3K/AKT/mTOR pathway is activated and upregulated in FLT3 mut AML resistant to FLT3i, suggesting the efficacy of AKT and mTOR inhibitors in this setting. In vitro studies have shown that Sorafenib is able to inhibit FLT3 in leukemia cells of resistant patients without blocking colony formation and survival, due to a replication mechanism independent of FLT3. The GEP analysis of these cells and cell lines resistant to FLT3 inhibitors has shown downstream activation of PI3K/mTOR and in vitro and in vivo studies have shown that Gedatolisib is able, by inhibiting this pathway, to block the formation of colonies and to improve the survival of mice transplanted with Sorafenib-resistant cells [29].

- The activation of the FLT3 receptor also promotes leukemogenesis through the trigger of STAT5 and Pim-1 (serine–threonine oncogenic kinase). The FLT3ITD receptor is partially reteined in the endoplasmic reticulum as a 130 kDa protein that interacts with calnexin and heat shock protein 90 (HSP90), resulting in the upregulation of STAT5 and the consequent Pim-1 increase. Pim-1 promotes the phosphorylation at the level of serine and tyrosine 591 of the 130 kDa isoform of FLT3ITD, blocking its glycosylation and degradation, with consequent hyperactivation of calnexin, HSP90 and STAT5 by establishing a FLT3-STAT5-Pim-1 hyperactivation loop that determines the proliferation of mutated FLT3ITD cells and their resistance to FLT3i. STAT5 and Pim-1 inhibitors might therefore have a rationale in resistant FLT3 mut AML [30].

- CDK4 and CDK6 regulate the transcription of FLT3 and Pim-1 therefore CDK4 and CDK6 inhibitors, such as Palbociclib, are also useful in this setting [31].

- The upregulation of anti-apoptotic proteins Bcl-2, Bcl-xl, Mcl-1 proteins has been described in AML resistant to second generation FLT3 inhibitors. In particular, the FLT3-ITD627E mutation, located in the beta-2 sheet of the first kinase domain, induces a dramatic increase in anti-apoptotic protein MCL-1 suggesting a possible role of MCL-1 inhibitor drugs in blocking resistance to FLT3 inhibitors [32].

- The concentration in the marrow at suboptimal doses represents an additional mechanism of resistance, specially of inhibitors that have interactions with drugs metabolized by cytochrome P450 [33].

- Recently NGS and single cell analysis were performed in 41 patients with FLT3mut AML relapsing after Gilteritinib monotherapy, permitting the identification of mechanisms of resistance in 22 cases. RAS and FLT3 F691L mutations were found in 15 and 5 patients respectively and acquisition of Bcr Abl fusion protein was found in 2 samples. The FLT3 F691L mutation was more frequent in patients receiving Gilteritinib at dose lower than 200 mg, suggesting a dose dependent resistance and the importance of using higher doses to prevent this mechanism of failure [8]. FLT3 pathway and mechanisms of resistance to FLT3i are illustrated in **Figure 1**.

2.1.6 Novel FLT3i and future perspectives

Crenolanib is a potent novel type I pan-FLT3 inhibitor, effective against both ITD and TKD, but the response in monotherapy is unfortunately transient. Zhang et al. performed WES of samples from R/R FLT3 pos AML patients before and after Crenolanib, administered in a phase II study (NCT 01522469, NCT 01657682). They interestingly observed that patients previously treated with FLT3i expressed RAS mutations at baseline more frequently than naive patients and were less likely to respond to Crenolanib. They identified mutations of NRAS and IDH2 arising in FLT3-independent subclones and of TET2 and IDH1 in FLT3-subclones as possible

Combination regimen	Mechanism of action of combination agent	Mechanism rationale for combination	Clinicaltrials.gov identifier
LGH447 + midostaurin	Pim kinasi inhibitor	Pim kinasi activity mediates FLT3 inhibitor resistance; combination increases apoptosis	NCT02078609
Milademetan (DS-3032b) + quizartinib	MDM2 inhibitor	MDM2 inhibitor restore p53 tumor suppression function	NCT03552029
Omacetaxine mepesuccinate + sorafenib Omacetaxine mepesuccinate + quizartinib	Protein synthesis inhibitor	Synergistic with FLT3 inhibitors to suppress leukemic proliferation	NCT03170895 NCT03135054
Palbociclib + sorafenib	CDK4/6 inhibitor	CDK4/6 regulate transcription of FLT3 and Pim kinases (mechanism of FLT3 inhibitor resistance)	NCT03132454
SEL24 (dual pan Pim/FLT3 inhibitor)	Pim kinase inhibitor	Pim kinase activity mediates FLT3 inhibitor resistance; combination increases apoptosis	NCT03008187
Venetoclax + gilteritinb	Bcl-2 inhibitor	Upregolation of anti-apoptotic proteins (e.g. Bcl-2, BCL-xL and Mcl-1) mediates FLT3 inhibitor resistance	NCT03625505
Azacitidine + venetoclax + gilteritinib	Hypomethylating agent Bcl-2 inhibitor	Hypomethylation of target genes	NCT04140487
Vorinostat + bortezomib + sorafenib	Hystone deacetylase inhibitor (vorinostat) Proteasome inhibitor (bortezomib)	Histone deacetylase inhibitors synergistically induce apoptosis with FLT3 inhibitors; Proteasome inhibitors induce FLT3 ITD degradation through autophagy	NCT101534260

Table 2.
Trials with combinations of FLT3i and target drugs.

mechanisms of resistance. Post-crenolanib expansion of mutations associated with epigenetic regulators, transcription factors, and cohesion factors was also detected suggesting diverse genetic/epigenetic mechanisms of crenolanib resistance. Drug combinations in experimental models restore crenolanib sensitivity [34].

FLT3 F691L mutation was shown to be resistant to the majority of FLT3 TKIs including crenolanib, but not ponatinib and pexidartinib (PLX3397) [35]. In addition, a novel FLT3 extracellular mutation at K429E was detected in one patient with high VAF, which showed increased crenolanib IC50. The structural basis for the drug resistance of FLT3 K429E requires further investigations.

Given the expanding spectrum of FLT3 inhibitors FDA-approved, randomized phase III studies of conventional chemotherapy in combination with midostaurin versus gilteritinib (NCT03836209) and with midostaurin versus crenolanib (NCT03258931) are ongoing to establish wich FLT3i should be used in first line. Phase III study of gilteritinib versus placebo and phase II Crenolanib trial as maintenance after HSCT in FLT3-mutated AML are ongoing and may help to more definitively address the benefit of FLT3 inhibition in this setting (BMT CTN 1506; ClinicalTrials.gov identifier: NCT02997202, NCT02400255). Last but not least, the recent findings of intra- and extracellular mechanisms of FLT3i resistance, provided the background of ongoing trials, rationally including combinations with agents targeting specific resistance pathways. Current approaches include adding FLT3i to antiapoptotic drugs such as Venetoclax or milademetan or with drugs inhibiting other target such as PIM kinasi or CDK4/6. The addition of chemotherapy or hypomethylating agents (HMA) to this backbone could be the following step in patients eligible and not to intensive chemotherapy. **Table 2** reports the ongoing studies exploring association of FLT3i with other drugs.

2.2 Venetoclax

One of the possible mechanisms of leukemogenesis is represented by the functional loss of p53 or by an altered balance of antiapoptotic and proapoptotic protein expression [36]. Apoptosis is controlled by two parallel pathways, intrinsic and extrinsic, leading to activation of intracellular caspases, ending with cell death. The intrinsic pathway is under the control of the BCL2 family proteins, including antiapoptotic proteins (e.g., BCL2, BCL-XL, and MCL1), proapoptotic BH3-only proteins (e.g., BIM, BAD, PUMA, and NOXA), and proapoptotic effector proteins (e.g., BAK and BAX) (**Figure 2**). Leukemic cells showed to overexpress BCL2 making of Venetoclax, an oral inhibitor of BCL2, an ideal target therapy. Venetoclax acts as BH3 mimetic protein and restors apoptosis without interacting with other antiapoptotic proteins such as BCL-XL or MCL-1. Based on phase II study outstanding results [37] venetoclax has been approved by FDA, EMA and AIFA for first line treatment of elderly AML over 75 years or unfit for intensive chemotherapy. The trial associated venetoclax at the doses of 400 or 800 mg daily in combination with either decitabine (20 mg/m^2, days 1-5, intravenously [IV]) or azacitidine (75 mg/m^2, days 1-7, IV or subcutaneously) in 145 AML patients, not eligible to intensive chemotherapy, in first line. CRc (CR and CRi) rate was 73% with a median duration of 11.3 months and a median overall survival of 17.5 months.

2.2.1 Mechanism of resistance to Venetoclax

Avoidance of apoptosis and the acquisition of BCL-2 mutations such as BCL2 Gly101Val are among the mechanisms currently identified for resistance in chronic lymphocitic leukemia. MCL-1 inhibitors appear to bypass this mutation in preclinical studies and preliminary clinical studies with these agents are ongoing [38].

Mechanisms of resistance to Venetoclax, have been further investigated in AML. A recent study of DiNardo [39] performed NGS at baseline and relapse and follow-up and single cell analysis at baseline and relapse in 81 AML patients receiving HMA (N: 58) or low dose cytarabine (LDAC) (N: 23) with Venetoclax in frontline (NCT02287233 and NCT02203773) at the MD Anderson Cancer Center (Houston) or at the Alfred Hospital (Melbourne). The median age of this elderly cohort was 74 years (range, 62-87 years). The HMA group excluded prior HMA therapy. In contrast, the LDAC group included patients with prior HMA exposure. The target dose of venetoclax was also different in the 2 studies (HMA study: 400 mg/day; LDAC study: 600 mg/day).

Twenty-five cases had adaptive resistance, representing 31% of the total cohort of 81 patients. The median time to relapse was 6.4 months (95% confidence interval, 4.5-10.6 months); 5 patients relapsed after 12 months. To identify dynamic molecular changes indicative of adaptive resistance, the VAFs of individual mutations were compared at diagnosis, in remission, and at relapse to identify clones expanded at relapse. Two important findings emerged: progressive expansion of clones with activated kinases, particularly FLT3-ITD, and in other cases, selection of clones with likely biallelic perturbation of TP53. The single cell analysis of the relapsed clones also showed the selective impact of the expansion of FLT3-ITD or other kinase (CBL, NRAS) in mediating resistance with FLT3-ITD loss of heterozygosity (LOH) at relapse.

In contrast, NPM1mut and IDH2mut were associated with high rates of response and durable remissions. In NPM1mut AML, measurable residual disease (MRD) was eliminated in most cases. Median OS for patients with either NPM1mut or IDH2mut was not reached, with 2-year OS of 71.8% and 79.5%, respectively. In the durable remission group, DNMT3A mut was present in 44% of cases (8/18), and 6 out of 8 of these cases were among patients with concurrent NPM1 or IDH2mut. The association between IDH1mut and prognosis was less clear. There were 2 IDH1mut cases in the durable remission subgroup, and both had a co-occurring NPM1mut. Among the 7 IDH1mut cases occurring in patients with relapsing or primary refractory disease, 5 cases had a concurrent TP53, FLT3-ITD, or RAS mutation. The median OS for patients with IDH1mut was not significantly different from patients with IDH1 wild-type (WT) AML (18.3 vs. 12.7 months; P = 0.79).

Primary refractory AML had 3 patterns of resistance: TP53 abnormality, RUNX1 and activating kinase mutations (FLT3-ITD, N/KRAS, CBL, or KIT). The VAF of TP53 mutation was higher in refractory patients, while RUNX1 mutations were also found in responder patients, in association with IDH1 and SRSF2 mutations, suggesting that larger studies are needed to refine their role in resistance to Venetoclax. **Figure 2** shows the mithocondrial pathway of p53 and the mechanisms of resistance to venetoclax.

2.2.2 Future perspectives

On the basis of the results of the analysis performed by DiNardo et al. [39], a baseline molecular characterization may allow patients to be risk stratified into a favorable risk NPM1mut subgroup, where molecular MRD monitoring, and even consideration of treatment cessation, could be employed within a future clinical trial. Patients with IDHmut could be considered for postremission IDH inhibitor maintenance-based approaches, aimed at eradicating residual molecular disease, and patients with FLT3-ITD mutations could also benefit from the addition of targeted FLT3 inhibitors to prevent failures. Relapsed and refractory patients with TP53 mutations actually still represent an unmet medical need. Clinical trials incorporating new agents targeting TP53mut/del(17p) drug resistant clones should be pursued. APR 246 showed encouraging results in a phase I/IIa clinical trial of patients with hematological malignancies or prostate cancer [40] due to the reactivation of the disrupted TP53 through the conversion to methylene quinuclidinone (MQ), a Michael acceptor that reacts with cysteines in the p53 core domain restoring its activity [41]. However, the mechanism by which APR-246/MQ reactivates mutant p53 is not fully understood. In early results from an ongoing phase Ib/II study in patients with high-risk *TP53*-mutated MDS or oligoblastic AML (20–30% blasts), the combination of APR-246 and azacitidine resulted in a composite CR, CRi, and morphologic leukemia-free state (MLFS) rate of 100% (11 of 11 evaluable patients), with 82% CR and 72% of responders having undetectable *TP53* mutation by nextgeneration sequencing [42].

Transcriptomic analysis after run-in of single-agent APR-246 confirmed on-target effects, including transcriptional activation of p53 targets. A phase III randomized study of azacitidine with or without APR-246 in MDS and AML with 20–30% blasts is ongoing (NCT03745716).

Preclinical studies showed sinergy between MCL1 inhibition and venetoclax [43] and therefore MCL1 inhibitors are now being explored in early clinical trials, both as single agents and in combination with venetoclax. Interestingly BH3 profiling might predict sensitivity to specific BH3 agents helping the choice between BCL2 or MCL1 inhibition or a combination of both [44].

In vitro studies also showed a synergistic effect of MDM2 inhibitors in combination with BCL2i due to the downregulation of MCL1 through the inhibition of RAS–RAF–MEK–ERK pathway. In an ongoing international phase Ib study of venetoclax and idasanutlin, in patients aged >60 years with relapsed or refractory AML, the marrow remission rate was 37% (11 of 30 evaluable patients) in the entire population, and 50% (9 of 18 evaluable patients) at the recommended phase II dose of venetoclax. As with other venetoclax-based regimens, higher ratios of BCL2/BCL-XL and BCL2/MCL1 were predictive of response [45].

2.3 IDHi

IDH1 and 2 are targetable mutations occurring in approximately 20% of Acute Myeloid Leukemia (AML) patients [IDH1 (8%) and IDH2 (12%)] and are more common in the elderly (25-28%). They are usually associated with intermediate-risk cytogenetics, FLT3 and NPM1 mutations [46, 47] and mutually exclusive with the TET2 mutation [48].

Hotspot IDH1 mutations, affecting the catalytic domains, commonly involve a cysteine (R132C) or histidine (R132H) substitution for arginine. In IDH2 mutations, arginine is most often replaced by glutamine at residue 140 (R140Q) or by lysine at residue 172 (R172K) [49]. Further, IDH2 R172 and NPM1 mutations were not detected in the same patient samples [50]. The incidences of IDH1 and IDH2 mutations are equivalent and mutually exclusive [51]; however, the incidence rate of IDH2 R140Q was found to be higher than that of IDH2 R172K (9.2% vs. 2.9%) [52]. Somatic mutations in catalytically active arginine residues decrease their enzymatic activity as well as confer a gain of function activity leading to the production of the oncometabolite 2 hydroxyglutate (2-HG) instead of alpha-ketoglutarate (α-KG). 2-HG competitively inhibits the function of αKG-dependent oxygenases involved in DNA or histone demethylation, increases the production of ROS (reactive oxygen species) through the oxydation of Glutathione and determines metabolic changes interfering with NF-Kb and BCL-2 proteins, such as ten-eleven translocation (TET2) DNA methylases, and Jumonji C (JmjC) domain containing histone demethylases, resulting in global DNA hypermethylation of regulatory genes and arrested myeloid differentiation [53] (**Figure 3**). Mutant IDH has therefore become a viable target in AML treatment.

The prognostic value of the different mutation isoforms remain controversial [54]. Some AML patients with IDH mutation, especially IDH2 R172 mutation, have a poor response to traditional chemotherapy and have a higher relapse rate [55]. Therefore, individualized treatment, specially targeted therapy for IDH mutations, may be an important option for such patients. In recent years, IDH inhibitors have shown good clinical response in AML patients. Based on phase 1/2 clinical trials, enasidenib and ivosidenib have been approved by the FDA on 1 August 2017 and 20 July 2018 for the treatment of adult R/R AML with IDH2 and IDH1 mutations, respectively [56, 57]. Ivosidenib 500 mg/day in combination with subcutaneous azacitidine was associated with an ORR of 78% (18/23) and 30% of CRs with a median OS of 12.6 months, while in patients with IDH2 mutation, enasidenib (100 mg once daily) plus azacitidine was associated with an ORR of 67% with 20.6% of CRs and median OS of 9.3 months. No patient in the ivosidenib group and one patient in the enasidenib group had progressive disease.

2.3.1 Mechanisms of resistance to IDHi

To fully characterize the mechanisms of response and relapse to ivosidenib monotherapy, Choe et al. [58] conducted a comprehensive genomic analysis of samples from a cohort of 179 patients with m*IDH1* (IDH1 mutated) R/R AML, treated in a phase 1 study with ivosidenib at the starting approved dose of 500 mg once daily (QD), confirming that RTK pathway mutations (NRAS, PTPN11) are associated with primary and secondary resistance to ivosidenib. Emergence or outgrowth of AML-related mutations, such as RTK pathway genes, and *IDH*-related mutations (comprising second-site mutations in *IDH1* and mutations in *IDH2)*, which were associated with increased 2-HG, contribute to relapse after ivosidenib therapy. These various mechanisms of resistance occurred in isolation or in combination, underscoring the complex biology of treatment resistance.

Single-cell DNA sequencing analyses also found co-occurring mutations at single-cell resolution, including genes of the RTK pathway (eg, *NRAS*, *KRAS*, *PTPN11*, *FLT3*), transcription factors (*RUNX1*), chromatin/epigenetic regulators (*DNMT3A*, *ASXL1*), and splicing factors (*U2AF*, *SF3B1*). These co-occurring mutations indicate functional interplay between these genes and m*IDH1*, and reflect a more complex role of m*IDH1* during leukemogenesis or maintenance of m*IDH1*AML, such as cooperation with the constitutively activated RTK pathway to promote cell proliferation, and/or cooperation with chromatin/epigenetic regulators and transcription regulators to block cell differentiation.

The analysis of baseline mutational profiles of 101 mIDH1 AML patients [59] showed similar results with the following comutations: DNMT3A (35%), NPM1 (26%), SRSF2 (24%), ASXL1 (18%), RUNX1 (18%), NRAS (14%), and TP53 (13%); FLT3TKD (9%), FLT3ITD (2%), TET2 (14%). The achievement of CR was analogously related to lower genomic complexity with lower number of comutations in responders compared to non responders (2.8 vs. 3.7), with $P < .001$. RTK pathway mutations, along with an increased number of mutations, are conversely associated with primary treatment resistance.

Actually, although 2-HG–restoring mutations are a major pathway of resistance, other 2-HG-independent pathways, such as RAS and FLT3 mutations, are important and may be dominant over 2-HG restoration.

This finding is consistent with a similar work showing an association between NRAS mutations and a lower likelihood of response to enasidenib in patients with mIDH2 R/R AML [60].

Amatangelo et al. showed emergence of AML-related mutations, such as *RUNX1*, FLT3, and IDH-related mutations in patients relapsing after enasidenib in mIDH2 R/R AML. Outgrowth of mIDH1 in patients who initially had mIDH2 (isoform switching) [61, 62] and the emergence of second-site IDH2 mutations [63] were confirmed in other series. However, these reports were based on a limited number of patients, and the frequency and breadth of resistance mechanisms have not been comprehensively characterized.

Some reports have shown that FLT3 inhibitors induce granulocytic differentiation and differentiation syndrome symptoms in some patients with *FLT3*-mutated AML [64, 65]. Thus, the combination of mIDH inhibitors with RTK pathway inhibitors, including FLT3 inhibitors, may present a rational treatment strategy. Choe et al. [58] also showed that *JAK2* mutations were associated with a high CR/CRh rate (64%), with the caveat of the limited number of patients (n = 11). Although *JAK2* mutations are often classed together with other mutations affecting MAPK pathway signaling, their different pattern of response to ivosidenib treatment depends on the distinct biology of *JAK2* mutations, such as STAT pathway activation, frequent ancestral status during clonal evolution, and association with prior myeloproliferative neoplasm. The number of patients in Choe analysis is insufficient to determine whether de novo or secondary disease has a prognostic role in the context of *JAK2* mutation. Data on additional patients with *JAK2* mutations are needed to gain a more robust picture of this patient subset. **Figure 3** summerizes the IDH pathway and the main mechanisms of resistance of IDHi.

2.3.2 Future perspectives

These findings highlight the interplay among baseline mutation profiles, response, and clonal evolution during ivosidenib therapy. The complex and polyclonal mechanism of resistance to ivosidenib has implications for mIDH1/2 inhibitor treatment strategies, and supports the use of combination therapies or sequential treatment modifications at early relapse before overt clinical progression, rather than monotherapy with mIDH1/2 inhibitors. It will also be important to understand whether or not these patterns of resistance are replicated with combination therapies. Because individual patients often show multiple resistance mechanisms at relapse, combination of ivosidenib with nontargeted agents, such as intensive chemotherapy/cytotoxic therapies, hypomethylating agents, and venetoclax (BCL-2 inhibitor), may improve responses and decrease the likelihood of relapse.

2-HG accumulation lead to cytochrome c oxidase activity, mimicking an oxygen-deprived state and decreasing the mitochondrial threshold for induction of apoptosis.

The association of IDHi to BCL2i might represents the exciting possibility of a chemotherapy free oral combination for IDH mut AML and a phase Ib/II clinical trial (NCT03471260) confirmed a surprisingly high 75% CRc rate in a cohort of 12 patients [66, 67].

2.4 Fighting policlonal resistance

As we have seen that RAS mutation are often involved in resistance to all new approved target therapies, RAS pathway–targeting agents may be useful, either concomitantly with FLT3i or IDHi to avoid primary resistance in patients with RAS mutations at baseline, or sequentially in patients who have a newly detectable RAS mutation while on therapy with a FLT3, IDH, or BCL2 inhibitor. MEK1/MEK2 inhibitors selumetinib and trametinib unfortunately did not confirm this potential efficacy since modest response rates of 17–20% were seen in relapsed or refractory RAS-mutated AML [68]. An established mechanism of resistance to MEK inhibition is the compensatory activation of PI3K–AKT–mTOR pathway.

The targeted downmodulation of pERK and pS6 was shown in a study of 23 RAS-mutated AML patients treated with trametinib plus an AKT inhibitor (GSK2141795), without producing any clinical response [69].

At last but not least immune evasion represents one of the main mechanism of resistance common to all target drugs. Actually the exhaustion of the host's own immune system contribute to cancer growth. Murine and human studies have shown association between AML and increased infiltration of T-regulatory cell and expression of immune checkpoint proteins on CD8 positive T cells, including PD-1, TIM3, and LAG3 [70] which might induce immune exhaustion and early relapse [71]. The immunotherapies with antibody targeting leukemic antigens, such as CD123 might be an effective strategy to target measurable residual disease (MRD) in maintenance therapy in high-risk AML. The IL3 receptor alpha chain, CD123, is notably expressed on leukemic stem cells (LSC) and is expressed at lower levels on normal hematopoietic stem cells (HSC) than CD33 [72].

Antibody-drug-conjugate (ADCs) and bispecific antibodies targeting CD123 have shown promising clinical activity in phase I studies and are rapidly moving to multicenter studies as single-agent expansions and in combination approaches [73, 74]. Pre therapy low levels of bone marrow CD3+ or CD8+ and overexpression of CTLA4 predict resistance to check point inhibitors [75]. These may be potential biomarkers to prospectively select patients most likely to respond. Inhibitors of "macrophage checkpoints" could be another interesting chance for immunomodulation. In particular CD47, highly expressed on LSCs, is associated with unfavorable outcomes [76]. Upregulation of CD47 on AML cells allows the binding to the signal-regulatory protein-α (SIRPα) receptor on macrophages, providing a "don't eat me" signal [77].

Hu5F9-G4 is an anti-CD47 antibody that inhibits the binding of LSC with SIRPα, promoting macrophage-mediated phagocytosis of leukemic cells [78].

The combination of Hu5F9-G4 with azacitidine in unfit newly diagnosed AML produced 64% of CR/CRi/MLFS (9/14) [79]. The study is ongoing at multiple centers (NCT03248479). Unfortunately the lack of an AML specific antigen restricted to the leukemic cell is the main reason of unsatisfactory results of vaccines and chimeric antigen receptor (CAR) T-cell therapies in this setting [80]. CD33, CD123, CLEC12A are expressed on normal cells leading to potential "on-target, off-tumor" toxicity.

3. Conclusions

In conclusion the knowledge of the mechanism of resistance might help the design of future studies with sequences (**Figure 4**) or combinations (**Figure 5**) of new target drugs. Furthermore the policlonal nature of leukemia resistance might

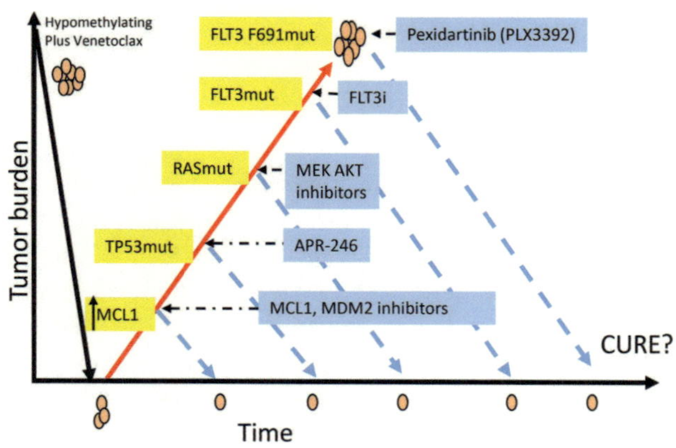

Figure 4.
Model of kinetics of chemoresistant leukemic clones after treatment with hypomethylating agents plus Venetoclax when target drugs are administered sequentially at the onset of chemoresistant clones.

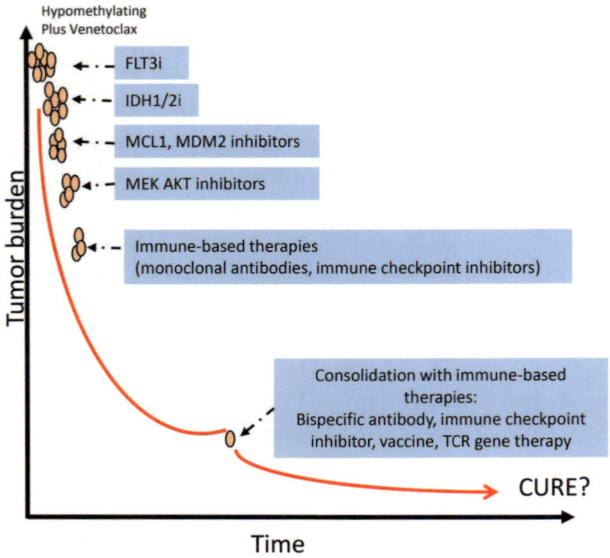

Figure 5.
Model of kinetics of chemoresistant leukemic clones after a total therapy approach including treatment with hypomethylating agents plus Venetoclax, plus combination of target drugs and immune therapies, preventively administerd to avoid emergence of chemoresistant leukemic clones. Consolidation with immune based therapies might be administered in order to reduce MRD and possibly cure AML.

reduce the efficacy of target therapies leaving a role to immune therapies such as checkpoint inhibitors, vaccines, and adoptive T-cell therapies, in decreasing the burden of residual disease. Several studies of consolidative or maintenance immune modulation in this context are ongoing [81].

These approaches may be particularly appealing in patients not eligible to allogeneic transplant. The polyclonal mechanisms of resistence to new drugs, hereby illustrated, underline an urgent need for future trials in this setting, based on total therapy approach, including initial chemotherapy or HMA with targeted or apoptosis-inducing drugs, sequentially adjusted, on the basis of emerging early clones, with immune or target-based therapies, to eradicate reservoirs of residual disease (**Figure 5**).

Author details

Debora Capelli*, Francesco Saraceni, Diego Menotti, Alessandro Fiorentini and Attilio Olivieri
Departement of Haematology, Azienda Universitaria Ospedali Riuniti di Ancona, Italy

*Address all correspondence to: debora.capelli@ospedaliriuniti.marche.it

References

[1] Jaiswal S, Fontanillas P, Flannick J, Manning A, Grauman PV, et al. Age related clonal hematopoiesis associated with adverse outcome. N Engl J Med 2013; 371: 2488-2498. doi: 10.1056/ NEJMoa1408617.

[2] Cancer Genome Atlas Research Network. Genomic and epigenomic landscapes of adult de novo acute myeloid leukemia. N Engl J Med. 2013 May 30; 368(22):2059±74. doi. org/10.1056/ NEJMoa1301689.

[3] Papaemmanuil E, Gerstung M, Bullinger L, Gaidzik VI, Paschka P, et al. Genomic Classification and Prognosis in Acute Myeloid Leukemia. N Engl J Med. 2016; 374(23):2209-2221. doi: 10.1056/ NEJMoa1516192.

[4] Ibañez M, Carbonell-Caballero JA, Such E, Garcõa-Alonso L, Liquori A, et al. The modular network structure of the mutational landscape of Acute Myeloid Leukemia PLoS ONE 13: 1-16. doi.org/10.1371/journal.pone. 0202926.

[5] Kazi JU, Rönnstrand L. FMS-like Tyrosine Kinase 3/FLT3: From Basic Science to Clinical Implications. Physiol Rev. 2019;99:1433-1466. doi: 10.1152/ physrev.00029.2018.

[6] Casas S, Ollila J, Aventín A, Vihinen M, Sierra J, Knuutila S. Changes in apoptosis-related pathways in acute myelocytic leukemia. Cancer Genet Cytogenet. 2003;146: 89-101. doi: 10.1016/s0165-4608(03)00102-x.

[7] Nassereddine S, Lap CJ, Haroun F, Tabbara I.The role of mutant IDH1 and IDH2 inhibitors in the treatment of acute myeloid leukemia. Ann Hematol. 2017; 96:1983-1991. doi: 10.1007/ s00277-017-3161-0.

[8] McMahon CM, Ferng T, Canaani J, Wang ES, Morrissette JJD et al. Clonal selection with RAS pathway activation mediates secondary clinical resistance to selective FLT3 inhibition in acute myeloid leukemia. Cancer Discov. 2019; 9:1050-1063. DOI: 10.1182/ bloodadvances.2018029496.

[9] Quek L, David MD, Kennedy A, Metzner M, Amatangelo M, et al. Clonal heterogeneity of acute myeloid leukemia treated with the IDH2 inhibitor enasidenib. Nat Med. 2018;24(8):1167-1177. DOI: 10.1038/s41591-018-0115-6.

[10] Brandts CH, Sargin B, Rode M, Biermann C, Lindtner B, et al. Constitutive activation of Akt by Flt3 internal tandem duplications is necessary for increased survival, proliferation, and myeloid transformation. Cancer Res 2005; 65:9643-50. doi: 10.1158/0008-5472. CAN-05-0422.

[11] Short NJ, Kantarjian H, Ravandi F, Daver N. Emerging treatment paradigms with FLT3 inhibitors in acute myeloid leukemia. Ther Adv Hematol 2019; 10:1-18. doi: 10.1177/2040620719827310.

[12] Weisberg E, Boulton C, Kelly LM, Manley P, Fabbro D, Meyer T, et al. Inhibition of mutant FLT3 receptors in leukemia cells by the small molecule tyrosine kinase inhibitor PKC412. Cancer Cell 2002;1: 433-43. DOI: 10.1016/s1535-6108(02)00069-7.

[13] Stone RM, Mandrekar SJ, Sanford BL, Laumann K, Geyer S, Bloomfield CD, et al. Midostaurin plus chemotherapy for acute myeloid leukemia with a FLT3 mutation. N Engl J Med 2017; 377:454-64. DOI: 10.1056/ NEJMoa1614359.

[14] Cortes JE, Khaled S, Martinelli G, Perl AE, Ganguly S, Russell N, Krämer A, Dombret H, Hogge D, Jonas BA, Leung AY, Mehta P, Montesinos P, Radsak M, Sica S, Arunachalam M, Holmes M,

Kobayashi K, Namuyinga R, Ge N, Yver A, Zhang Y, Levis MJ. Quizartinib versus salvage chemotherapy in relapsed or refractory FLT3-ITD acute myeloid leukaemia (QuANTUM-R): a multicentre, randomised, controlled, open-label, phase 3 trial. Lancet Oncol. 2019; 20: 984-997. DOI: 10.1016/S1470-2045(19)30150-0.

[15] Park IK, Mundy-Bosse B, Whitman SP, Zhang X, Warner SL, Bearss DJ, et al. Receptor tyrosine kinase Axl is required for resistance of leukemic cells to FLT3-targeted therapy in acute myeloid leukemia. Leukemia 2015; 29:2382-9. DOI: 10.1038/leu.2015.147.

[16] Perl AE, Martinelli G, Cortes JE, Neubauer A, Berman E, Paolini S, Montesinos P, Baer MR, Larson RA, Ustun C, Fabbiano F, Erba HP, Di Stasi A, Stuart R, Olin R, Kasner M, Ciceri F, Chou WC, Podoltsev N, Recher C, Yokoyama H, Hosono N, Yoon SS, Lee JH, Pardee T, Fathi AT, Liu C, Hasabou N, Liu X, Bahceci E, Levis MJ. Gilteritinib or Chemotherapy for Relapsed or Refractory FLT3-Mutated AML. N Engl J Med. 2019; 381(18):1728-1740. doi: 10.1056/NEJMoa1902688.

[17] Dumas PY, Bertoli S, Bérard E, Largeaud L, Bidet A, Delabesse E, Leguay T, Leroy H, Gadaud N, Rieu JB, Vial JP, Vergez F, Lechevalier N, Luquet I, Klein E, Sarry A, de Grande AC, Pigneux A, Récher. Real-World Outcomes of Patients with Refractory or Relapsed FLT3-ITD Acute Myeloid Leukemia: A Toulouse-Bordeaux DATAML Registry Study. Cancers (Basel). 2020; 12: E2044. DOI: 10.3390/cancers12082044.

[18] Taylor E, Morris K, Ellis M, Marlton P, Baveshi K, Clarey J, Irving I, Cochrane T, Kennedy G. FLT3-ITD positive acute myeloid leukemia: A retrospective analysis of the role of allogeneic transplant and allelic ratio in patient management. Asia Pac J Clin Oncol. 2018; 14:426-430. DOI: 10.1111/ajco.12827.

[19] Sakaguchi M, Yamaguchi H, Najima Y, Usuki K, Ueki T et al. Prognostic impact of low allelic ratio FLT3-ITD and NPM1 mutation in acute myeloid leukemia. Blood Adv. 2018;2: 2744-2754. DOI:10.1182/bloodadvances.2018020305.

[20] Alvarado Y, Kantarjian HM, Luthra R, et al. Treatment with FLT3 inhibitor in patients with FLT3-mutated acute myeloid leukemia is associated with development of secondary FLT3-tyrosine kinase domain mutations. Cancer 2014; 120: 2142-2149. DOI: 10.1002/cncr.28705.

[21] Daver N, Cortes J, Ravandi F, Patel KP, Burger JA et al. Secondary mutations as mediators of resistance to targeted therapy in leukemia. Blood 2015; 125: 3236– 3245. DOI: 10.1182/blood-2014-10-605808.

[22] Cools J, Mentens N, Furet P, et al. Prediction of resistance to small molecule FLT3 inhibitors: implications for molecularly targeted therapy of acute leukemia. Cancer Res 2004; 64: 6385– 6389.

[23] Traer E, Martinez J, Javidi-Sharifi N, Agarwal A, Dunlap J et al. FGF2 from marrow microenvironment promotes resistance to FLT3 inhibitors in acute myeloid leukemia. Cancer Res 2016; 76: 6471-6482. DOI: 10.1158/0008-5472.CAN-15-3569.

[24] Onishi C, Mori-Kimachi S, Hirade T, Abe M, Taketani T et al. Internal tandem duplication mutations in FLT3 gene augment chemotaxis to Cxcl12 protein by blocking the down-regulation of the Rho associated kinase via the Cxcl12/Cxcr4 signaling axis. Journal Biol Chem 2014; 289: 31053– 31065. DOI: 10.1074/jbc.M114.568287.

[25] Kojima K, McQueen T, Chen Y, Konopleva M, Shinojima N, et al. p53 activation of mesenchymal stromal cells partially abrogates microenvironment-mediated resistance to FLT3 inhibition in AML through HIF1alpha-mediated down-regulation of CXCL12. Blood 2011; 118: 4431-4439. DOI: 10.1182/blood-2011-02-334136.

[26] Zhang W, Borthakur G, Gao C, , Chen Y, Mu H, et al The dual MEK/FLT3 inhibitor E6201 exerts cytotoxic activity against Acute Myeloid Leukemia cells harboring resistance-conferring FLT3 mutations. Cancer Research 2016; 76: 1528-1536. DOI: 10.1158/0008-5472.CAN-15-1580.

[27] Lindblad O, Cordero E, Puissant A, Macaulay L, Ramos A et al. Aberrant activation of the PI3K/mTOR pathway promotes resistance to sorafenib in AML. Oncogene. 2016; 35:5119-31. DOI: 10.1038/onc.2016.41

[28] Natarajan K, Xie Y,Burcu M, Linn DE, Qiu Y, Baer MR. Pim-1 kinase phosphorylates and stabilizes 130 kDa FLT3 and promotes aberrant STAT5 signaling in acute myeloid leukemia with FLT3 internal tandem duplication. PLoS One. 2013;8: 746-753. doi: 10.1371/journal.pone.0074653.

[29] Uras I, Walter G, Scheicher R, Bellutti F, Prchal-Murphy M et al. Palbociclib treatment of FLT3- ITD + AML cells uncovers a kinase-dependent transcriptional regulation of FLT3 and PIM1 by CDK6. Blood 2016; 127: 2890-2902. DOI: 10.1182/blood-2015-11-683581.

[30] Breitenbuecher F, Markova B, Kasper S, Carius B, Stauder T et al. A novel molecular mechanism of primary resistance to FLT3-kinase inhibitors in AML. Blood 2009; 113: 4063-73. DOI: 10.1182/blood-2007-11-126664.

[31] Alonso S, Su M, Jones J, Ganguly S, Kane MA et al. Human bone marrow niche chemoprotection mediated by cytochrome P450 enzymes. Oncotarget 2015; 6: 14905-14912. doi: 10.18632/oncotarget.3614.

[32] Zhang H, Savage S, Schultz AR, Bottomly D, White L et al. Clinical resistance to crenolanib in acute myeloid leukemia due to diverse molecular mechanisms. Nat Commun. 2019 Jan 16;10(1):244. DOI: 10.1038/s41467-018-08263-x.

[33] Smith CC, Lin K, Stecula A, Sali A, Shah NP. FLT3D835 mutations confer differential resistance to type II FLT3 inhibitors. Leukemia. 2015; 29:2390-2. DOI: 10.1038/leu.2015.165

[34] Letai AG. Diagnosing and exploiting cancer's addiction to blocks in apoptosis. Nat Rev Cancer 2008; 8:121-32.

[35] DiNardo CD, Pratz K, Pullarkat V, et al. Venetoclax combined with decitabine or azacitidine in treatment-naive, elderly patients with acute myeloid leukemia. Blood. 2019; 133:7-17. DOI: 10.1038/nrc2297.

[36] Blombery P, Anderson MA, Gong JN, Thijssen R, Birkinshaw RW et al. Acquisition of the recurrent Gly101Val mutation in BCL2 confers resistance to Venetoclax in patients with progressive chronic lymphocytic leukemia. Cancer discovery 2019; 9: 342-353. DOI: 10.1158/2159-8290.CD-18-1119.

[37] DiNardo C, Tiong I, Quaglieri A, MacRaild S, Loghavi S et al. Molecular Patterns of Response and Treatment Failure After Frontline Venetoclax Combinations in Older Patients With AML. Blood, 2020; 135: 791-803. DOI: 10.1158/2159-8290.CD-18-0387.

[38] Lehmann S, Bykov VJ, Ali D, Andrén O, Cherif H, et al. Targeting p53 in vivo: a first-in-human study with p53-targeting compound APR-246 in

refractory hematologic malignancies and prostate cancer. J. Clin. Oncol. 2012; 30: 3633-3639. DOI: 10.1200/JCO.2011.40.7783.

[39] Lambert JM, Gorzov P, Veprintsev DB, Söderqvist M, Segerbäck D et al. PRIMA-1 reactivates mutant p53 by covalent binding to the core domain. Cancer Cell. 2009; 15:376-388. DOI: 10.1016/j.ccr.2009.03.003.

[40] Sallman DA, DeZern AE, Steensma D, Sweet KL, Cluzeau T, Sekkeres M, et al. Phase 1b/2 combination study of APR-246 and azacitidine (AZA) in patients with *TP53* mutant myelodysplastic syndromes (MDS) and acute myeloid leukemia (AML). Blood 2018;132(Suppl 1):3091.

[41] Moujalled DM, Pomilio G, Ghiurau C, Ivey A, Salmon J, Rijal S, et al. Combining BH3-mimetics to target both BCL-2 and MCL1 has potent activity in pre-clinical models of acute myeloid leukemia. Leukemia 2019; 33:905-17. doi: 10.1038/s41375-018-0261-3.

[42] Kadia TM, Kantarjian HM, Konopleva M. Myeloid cell leukemia-1 dependence in acute myeloid leukemia: a novel approach to patient therapy. Oncotarget 2019; 10:1250-65. DOI: 10.18632/oncotarget.26579

[43] Daver NG, Pollyea DA, Garcia JS, Jonas BA, Yee KWL, Fenaux P, et al. Safety, efficacy, pharmacokinetic (PK) and biomarker analyses of BCL2 inhibitor venetoclax (Ven) plus MDM2 inhibitor idasanutlin (idasa) in patients (pts) with relapsed or refractory (R/R) AML: a phase Ib, non-randomized, open-label study. Blood 2018;132(Suppl 1): 767.

[44] Chou WC, Lei WC, Ko BS, Hou HA, Chen CY, Tang JL, et al. The prognostic impact and stability of Isocitrate dehydrogenase 2 mutation in adult patients with acute myeloid leukemia. Leukemia. 2011;25(2): 246-53. doi: 10.1038/leu.2010.267

[45] Chou WC, Hou HA, Chen CY, Tang JL, Yao M, Tsay W, et al. Distinct clinical and biologic characteristics in adult acute myeloid leukemia bearing the isocitrate dehydrogenase 1 mutation. Blood. 2010;115(14):2749-54. doi: 10.1182/blood-2009-11-253070.

[46] Gaidzik VI, Paschka P, Spath D, Habdank M, Kohne CH, Germing U, et al. TET2 mutations in acute myeloid leukemia (AML): results from a comprehensive genetic and clinical analysis of the AML study group. J Clin Oncol. 2012; 30:1 350-1357. doi: 10.1200/JCO.2011.39.2886.

[47] Ward PS, Patel J, Wise DR, Abdel-Wahab O, Bennett BD, Coller HA, et al. The common feature of leukemia-associated IDH1 and IDH2 mutations is a neomorphic enzyme activity converting alpha-ketoglutarate to 2-hydroxyglutarate. Cancer Cell. 2010; 17:225-234. doi: 10.1016/j.ccr.2010.01.020.

[48] Stein EM, DiNardo D, Fathi AT, Pollyea DA, Stone RM, Altman JK, et al. Molecular remission and response patterns in patients with mutant-IDH2 acute myeloid leukemia treated with enasidenib. Blood. 2019; 133:676-687. doi: 10.1182/blood-2018-08-869008.

[49] Abbas S, Lugthart S, Kavelaars FG, Schelen A, Koenders JE, Zeilemaker A, et al. Acquired mutations in the genes encoding IDH1 and IDH2 both are recurrent aberrations in acute myeloid leukemia: prevalence and prognostic value. Blood. 2010; 116:2122-2126. doi: 10.1182/blood-2009-11-250878.

[50] Sharma H. Development of novel therapeutics targeting Isocitrate dehydrogenase mutations in Cancer. Curr Top Med Chem. 2018; 18:505-524. doi: 10.2174/1568026618666180518091144.

[51] Figueroa ME, Abdel-Wahab O, Lu C, Ward PS, Patel J, Shih A, et al. Leukemic IDH1 and IDH2 mutations result in a hypermethylation phenotype, disrupt TET2 function, and impair hematopoietic differentiation. Cancer Cell. 2010; 18: 553-67. doi: 10.1016/j.ccr.2010.11.015.

[52] Bertoli S, Tavitian S, Delabesse E, Sarry A, Huguet F, Recher C. Outcome of AML patients with IDH1 or IDH2 mutations from diagnosis and refractory/relapse phase of the disease in routine practice. Blood. 2016;128(22):1718.

[53] Green CL, Evans CM, Zhao L, Hills RK, Burnett AK, Linch DC, et al. The prognostic significance of IDH2 mutations in AML depends on the location of the mutation. Blood. 2011;118(2):409-412. doi: 10.1182/blood-2010-12-322479.

[54] Kim ES. Enasidenib: First Global Approval. Drugs. 2017;77(15):1705-11. doi: 10.1007/s40265-017-0813-2

[55] Dhillon S. Ivosidenib: First Global Approval. Drugs. 2018;78(14):1509-16. doi: 10.1007/s40265-018-0978-3.

[56] Choe S, Wang H, DiNardo CD, Stein EM, de Botton S, Roboz GJ et al. Molecular mechanisms mediating relapse following ivosidenib monotherapy in *IDH1*-mutant relapsed or refractory AML. Blood Adv. 2020; 4: 1894-1905.Blood Adv. 2020 May 12;4(9):1894-1905. doi: 10.1182/bloodadvances.2020001503

[57] DiNardo CD, Stein EM, de Botton S, Roboz GJ, Altman JK, Mims AS, Swords R et al. Durable remissions with ivosidenib in *IDH1*-mutated relapsed or refractory AML. N Engl J Med. 2018;378(25):2386-2398. doi: 10.1056/NEJMoa1716984.

[58] Amatangelo MD, Quek L, Shih A, Stein EM, Roshal M, David MD, Marteyn B et al. Enasidenib induces acute myeloid leukemia cell differentiation to promote clinical response. Blood. 2017;130(6):732-741. doi: 10.1182/blood-2017-04-779447.

[59] Quek L, David MD, Kennedy A, Metzner M, Amatangelo MD, Shih A, Stoilova B, Quivoron C et al. Clonal heterogeneity of acute myeloid leukemia treated with the IDH2 inhibitor enasidenib. Nat Med. 2018;24(8):1167-1177. doi: 10.1038/s41591-018-0115-6.

[60] Harding JJ, Lowery MA, Shih AH, Schvartzman JM, Hou S, Famulare C, Patel M et al. Isoform switching as a mechanism of acquired resistance to mutant isocitrate dehydrogenase inhibition. Cancer Discov. 2018;8(12): 1540-1547. doi: 10.1158/2159-8290. CD-18-0877.

[61] Intlekofer AM, Shih AH, Wang B, Nazir A, Rustenburg AS, Albanese SK, Patel M, et al. Acquired resistance to IDH inhibition through trans or cisdimer-interface mutations. Nature. 2018;559(7712):125-129. doi: 10.1038/s41586-018-0251-7

[62] Sexauer A, Perl A, Yang X, Borowitz M, Gocke C, Rajkhowa T, Thiede C, Frattini M et al. Terminal myeloid differentiation in vivo is induced by FLT3 inhibition in FLT3/ITD AML. Blood. 2012;120(20):4205-4214. doi: 10.1182/blood-2012-01-402545

[63] McMahon CM, Canaani J, Rea B, Sargent RL, Qualtieri JN, Watt CD, Morrissette JJD et al. Gilteritinib induces differentiation in relapsed and refractory FLT3-mutated acute myeloid leukemia. Blood Adv. 2019;3(10):1581-1585. doi: 10.1182/bloodadvances.2018029496.

[64] Chan SM, Thomas D, Corces-Zimmerman MR, Xavy S, Rastogi S, Hong WJ, et al. Isocitrate dehydrogenase 1 and 2 mutations induce BCL-2 dependence in acute myeloid leukemia. Nat Med 2015;21: 178-84. DOI: 10.1038/nm.3788.

[65] Dinardo C, Takahashi K, Kadia T, Loghavi S, Naqvi K, Bose P, et al. A phase 1b/2 clinical study of targeted IDH1 inhibition with ivosidenib, in combination with the BCL-2 inhibitor venetoclax, for patients with IDH1-mutated (MIDH1) myeloid malignancies. HemaSphere 2019; 3:97.

[66] Jain N, Curran E, Iyengar NM, Diaz-Flores E, Kunnavakkam R, Popplewell L, et al. Phase II study of the oral MEK inhibitor selumetinib in advanced acute myelogenous leukemia: a University of Chicago phase II consortium trial. Clin Cancer Res 2014; 20:490-8. doi: 10.1158/1078-0432.CCR-13-1311.

[67] Ragon BK, Odenike O, Baer MR, Stock W, Borthakur G, Patel K, et al. Oral MEK 1/2 inhibitor trametinib in combination with AKT inhibitor GSK2141795 in patients with acute myeloid leukemia with RAS mutations: a phase II study. Clin Lymphoma Myeloma Leuk 2019;19: 431-40. doi: 10.1016/j.clml.2019.03.015.

[68] Williams P, Basu S, Garcia-Manero G, Hourigan CS, Oetjen KA, Cortes JE, et al. The distribution of T-cell subsets and the expression of immune checkpoint receptors and ligands in patients with newly diagnosed and relapsed acute myeloid leukemia. Cancer 2019;125: 1470-81. doi: 10.1002/cncr.31896.

[69] Zhou Q, Munger ME, Veenstra RG, Weigel BJ, Hirashima M, Munn DH, et al. Coexpression of Tim-3 and PD-1 identifies a CD8+ T-cell exhaustion phenotype in mice with disseminated acute myelogenous leukemia. Blood 2011; 117:4501-10. doi: 10.1182/blood-2010-10-310425.

[70] Testa U, Pelosi E, Frankel A. CD 123 is a membrane biomarker and a therapeutic target in hematologic malignancies. Biomark Res 2014; 2:4. doi: 10.1186/2050-7771-2-4.

[71] Uy GL, Rettig MP, Vey N, Godwin J, Foster MC, Rizzieri D, et al. Phase 1 cohort expansion of flotetuzumab, a CD123-CD3 bispecific Dart® protein in patients with relapsed/refractory acute myeloid leukemia (AML). Blood 2018;132(Suppl 1):764.

[72] Kovtun Y, Jones GE, Adams S, Harvey L, Audette CA, Wilhelm A, et al. A CD123-targeting antibody-drug conjugate, IMGN632, designed to eradicate AML while sparing normal bone marrow cells. Blood Adv 2018; 2:848-58. doi: 10.1182/bloodadvances.2018017517.

[73] Daver N, Garcia-Manero G, Basu S, Boddu PC, Alfayez M, Cortes JE, et al. Efficacy, safety, and biomarkers of response to azacitidine and nivolumab in relapsed/refractory acute myeloid leukemia: a nonrandomized, open-label, phase II study. Cancer Discov 2019; 9: 370-83. doi: 10.1158/2159-8290.CD-18-0774.

[74] Majeti R, Chao MP, Alizadeh AA, Pang WW, Jaiswal S, Gibbs KD Jr, et al. CD47 is an adverse prognostic factor and therapeutic antibody target on human acute myeloid leukemia stem cells. Cell 2009; 138:286-99. DOI: 10.1016/j.cell.2009.05.045.

[75] Willingham SB, Volkmer JP, Gentles AJ, Sahoo D, Dalerba P, Mitra SS, et al. The CD47-signal regulatory protein alpha (SIRPα) interaction is a therapeutic target for human solid tumors. Proc Natl Acad Sci U S A 2012; 109: 6662-7. doi: 10.1073/pnas.1121623109.

[76] Pietsch EC, Dong J, Cardoso R, Zhang X, Chin D, Hawkins R, et al. Anti-leukemic activity and tolerability of anti-human CD47 monoclonal antibodies. Blood Cancer J 2017;7: e536. doi: 10.1038/bcj.2017.7.

[77] Sallman D, Donnellan W, Asch A, Lee D, Al Malki M, Pollyea D, et al.

The first-in-class anti-CD47 antibody HU5F9-G4 is active and well tolerated alone or in combination with azacitidine in AML and MDS patients: initial phase 1b results: S878. HemaSphere 2019; 3: 394.

[78] Fan M, Li M, Gao L, Geng S, Wang J, Wang Y, et al. Chimeric antigen receptors for adoptive T cell therapy in acute myeloid leukemia. J Hematol Oncol 2017; 10: 151. doi: 10.1186/s13045-017-0519-7.

[79] Short NJ, Ravandi F. How close are we to incorporating measurable residual disease into clinical practice for acute myeloid leukemia? Haematologica 2019; 104:1532-41. doi: 10.3324/haematol.2018.208454.